# Microsurgery: Global Perspectives

*Editors*

JIN BO TANG
MICHEL SAINT-CYR

# CLINICS IN
# PLASTIC SURGERY

www.plasticsurgery.theclinics.com

April 2017 • Volume 44 • Number 2

**ELSEVIER**

1600 John F. Kennedy Boulevard • Suite 1800 • Philadelphia, Pennsylvania, 19103-2899

http://www.theclinics.com

**CLINICS IN PLASTIC SURGERY Volume 44, Number 2**
**April 2017 ISSN 0094-1298, ISBN-13: 978-0-323-52427-8**

*Editor:* Jessica McCool
*Developmental Editor:* Donald Mumford

*Clinics in Plastic Surgery* (ISSN 0094-1298) is published quarterly by Elsevier Inc., 360 Park Avenue South, New York, NY 10010-1710. Months of issue are January, April, July, and October. Business and Editorial Offices: 1600 John F. Kennedy Blvd., Suite 1800, Philadelphia, PA 19103-2899. Periodicals postage paid at New York, NY and additional mailing offices. Subscription prices are $495.00 per year for US individuals, $825.00 per year for US institutions, $100.00 per year for US students and residents, $561.00 per year for Canadian individuals, $982.00 per year for Canadian institutions, $636.00 per year for international individuals, $982.00 per year for international institutions, and $305.00 per year for Canadian and foreign students/residents. To receive student/resident rate, orders must be accompanied by name of affiliated institution, date of term, and the *signature* of program/residency coordinator on institution letterhead. Orders will be billed at individual rate until proof of status is received. Foreign air speed delivery is included in all *Clinics* subscription prices. All prices are subject to change without notice. **POSTMASTER:** Send address changes to *Clinics in Plastic Surgery*, Elsevier Health Sciences Division, Subscription Customer Service, 3251 Riverport Lane, Maryland Heights, MO 63043. **Customer Service: 1-800-654-2452 (US and Canada). From outside of the United States and Canada, call 314-447-8871. Fax: 314-447-8029. E-mail: JournalsCustomerService-usa@elsevier.com (for print support); JournalsOnlineSupport-usa@ elsevier.com (for online support).**

*Reprints.* For copies of 100 or more of articles in this publication, please contact the Commercial Reprints Department, Elsevier Inc., 360 Park Avenue South, New York, New York 10010-1710. Tel.: +1-212-633-3874; Fax: +1-212-633-3820; E-mail: reprints@elsevier.com.

*Clinics in Plastic Surgery* is covered in *Current Contents, EMBASE/Excerpta Medica, Science Citation Index, MEDLINE/ PubMed (Index Medicus), ASCA, and ISI/BIOMED.*

# Contributors

## EDITORS

**JIN BO TANG, MD**
Professor and Chair, Department of Hand Surgery, Affiliated Hospital of Nantong University, Chair, The Hand Surgery Research Center, Nantong University, Nantong, Jiangsu, China; Professor of Surgery (Adjunct), The Alpert Medical School of Brown University, Providence, Rhode Island

**MICHEL SAINT-CYR, MD, FRCS(C)**
Director, Division of Plastic Surgery, Wigley Professor in Plastic Surgery, Baylor Scott & White Health, Scott & White Memorial Hospital, Temple, Texas

## AUTHORS

**JASSON T. ABRAHAM, MD**
Division of Plastic Surgery, Baylor Scott & White Health, Temple, Texas

**ROHIT ARORA, MD**
Professor of Trauma Surgery, Department of Trauma Surgery and Sports Medicine, Medical University Innsbruck, Innsbruck, Austria

**KARIM BAKRI, MBBS**
Assistant Professor of Surgery, Division of Plastic and Reconstructive Surgery, Mayo Clinic, Rochester, Minnesota

**BRUNO BATTISTON, MD**
Consultant, U.O.C. Traumatology, Hand Surgery, Microsurgery, A.S.O. Città della Salute e della Scienza, Torino, Italy

**HEINZ K. BÜRGER, MD**
Privat Hospital Maria Hilf, Klagenfurt, Austria

**BRIAN T. CARLSEN, MD**
Consultant and Associate Professor of Plastic, Reconstructive, and Orthopedic Surgery, Division of Plastic and Reconstructive Surgery, Mayo Clinic, Rochester, Minnesota

**PEDRO C. CAVADAS, MD, PhD**
Chief, Reconstructive Surgery Unit, Clinica Cavadas, Valencia, Spain

**CURTIS L. CETRULO Jr, MD, FACS, FAAP**
Assistant Professor of Surgery, Division of Plastic and Reconstructive Surgery; Vascularized Composite Allotransplantation Laboratory, Center for Transplantation Sciences, Massachusetts General Hospital, Boston, Massachusetts

**CHAO CHEN, MD**
Attending Surgeon, Department of Hand and Foot Surgery, Shandong Provincial Hospital, Shandong University, Jinan, Shandong, China

**JING CHEN, MD**
Attending Surgeon, Department of Hand Surgery, Affiliated Hospital of Nantong University, Nantong, Jiangsu, China

**DAVIDE CICLAMINI, MD**
Consultant, U.O.C. Traumatology, Hand Surgery, Microsurgery, A.S.O. Città della Salute e della Scienza, Torino, Italy

**FRANCISCO DEL PIÑAL, MD, PhD**
Instituto de Cirugía Plástica y de la Mano, Private Practice, Hospital La Luz and Hospital Mutua Montañesa, Madrid/Santander, Spain

**AI DONG DENG, MD**
Lecturer and Attending Surgeon, Department of Hand Surgery, Affiliated Hospital of Nantong University, Nantong, Jiangsu, China

**KYLE R. EBERLIN, MD**
Assistant Professor of Surgery, Division of Plastic and Reconstructive Surgery, Massachusetts General Hospital, Harvard Medical School, Boston, Massachusetts

**MARKUS GABL, MD**
Professor of Trauma Surgery, Department of Trauma Surgery and Sports Medicine, Medical University Innsbruck, Innsbruck, Austria

**WALEED GIBREEL, MD**
Division of Plastic and Reconstructive Surgery, Mayo Clinic, Rochester, Minnesota

**LI WEN HAO, MD**
Attending Surgeon, Department of Hand and Foot Surgery, Shandong Provincial Hospital, Shandong University, Jinan, Shandong, China

**JAMES P. HIGGINS, MD**
Chief, Curtis National Hand Center, MedStar Union Memorial Hospital, Baltimore, Maryland

**OMAR N. HUSSAIN, MD**
Division of Plastic and Reconstructive Surgery, Mayo Clinic, Rochester, Minnesota

**AMIR E. IBRAHIM, MD**
Division of Plastic Surgery, Department of Surgery, American University of Beirut Medical Center, Beirut, Lebanon

**MARCO INNOCENTI, MD**
Director, Plastic and Reconstructive Microsurgery; Associate Professor, Plastic Surgery, University of Florence Careggi University Hospital, Florence, Italy

**ALI IZADPANAH, MD**
Hand Fellow, Department of Orthopedic Surgery, Mayo Clinic, Rochester, Minnesota

**MACIEJ KLICH, MD**
Instituto de Cirugía Plástica y de la Mano, Private Practice, Hospital La Luz and Hospital Mutua Montañesa, Madrid/Santander, Spain; Department of Traumatology and Orthopedics, Clinical Hospital, Warsaw, Otwock, Poland

**LUIS LANDÍN, MD, PhD**
Consultant, Plastic and Reconstructive Surgery, Hospital Universitario La Paz, Madrid, Spain

**LIN FENG LIU, MD**
Attending Surgeon, Department of Hand Surgery, Weinan Hand and Foot Surgery Hospital, Weinan, Shanxi, China

**SAMIR MARDINI, MD**
Professor, Division of Plastic and Reconstructive Surgery, Mayo Clinic, Rochester, Minnesota

**JAUME MASIÀ, MD, PhD**
Department of Plastic Surgery, Hospital de la Santa Creu I Sant Pau, Universitat Autònoma de Barcelona, Barcelona, Spain

**ANITA MOHAN, MBBS**
Division of Plastic and Reconstructive Surgery, Mayo Clinic, Rochester, Minnesota

**STEVEN L. MORAN, MD**
Professor and Chair of Plastic Surgery, Professor of Plastic, Reconstructive, and Orthopedic Surgery, Division of Plastic and Reconstructive Surgery, Department of Surgery, Mayo Clinic, Rochester, Minnesota

**ZHI YANG NG, MD**
Research Fellow, Division of Plastic and Reconstructive Surgery; Vascularized Composite Allotransplantation Laboratory, Center for Transplantation Sciences, Massachusetts General Hospital, Boston, Massachusetts

**NAKUL GAMANLAL PATEL, BSc (Hons), MBBS (Lond), FRCS (Plastic Surgery)**
Consultant Plastic Surgeon, Department of Plastic Surgery and Burns, The Royal Infirmary Hospital, University Hospital of Leicester, Leicester, United Kingdom

**GEMMA PONS, MD, PhD**
Consultant, Department of Plastic Surgery, Hospital de la Santa Creu I Sant Pau, Universitat Autònoma de Barcelona, Barcelona, Spain

**VENKAT RAMAKRISHNAN, MS, FRCS, FRACS (Plastic Surgery)**
Consultant Plastic Surgeon, St. Andrew's Centre for Plastic Surgery and Burns, Broomfield Hospital, Chelmsford, Essex, United Kingdom

**M. DIYA SABBAGH, MD**
Division of Plastic and Reconstructive Surgery, Mayo Clinic, Rochester, Minnesota

**MICHEL SAINT-CYR, MD, FRCS(C)**
Director, Division of Plastic Surgery, Wigley Professor in Plastic Surgery, Baylor Scott & White Health, Scott & White Memorial Hospital, Temple, Texas

**KARIM A. SARHANE, MD, MSc**
Department of Surgery, University of Toledo Medical Center, Toledo, Ohio

**JESSE C. SELBER, MD, MPH, FACS**
Department of Plastic Surgery, University of Texas MD Anderson Cancer Center, Houston, Texas

**BASEL SHARAF, MD, DDS**
Assistant Professor of Surgery, Division of Plastic and Reconstructive Surgery, Mayo Clinic, Rochester, Minnesota

**MARISSA SUCHYTA, BA**
Division of Plastic and Reconstructive Surgery, Mayo Clinic, Rochester, Minnesota

**CHENG HUA TANG, MD**
Former Chief, Replantation Research Laboratory, Extremity Microsurgery Institute, Shanghai, China

**JIN BO TANG, MD**
Professor and Chair, Department of Hand Surgery, Affiliated Hospital of Nantong University, Chair, The Hand Surgery Research Center, Nantong University, Nantong, Jiangsu, China; Professor of Surgery (Adjunct), The Alpert Medical School of Brown University, Providence, Rhode Island

**ALESSANDRO THIONE, MD, PhD**
Senior Consultant, Reconstructive Surgery Unit, Clinica Cavadas, Valencia, Spain

**ESTEBAN URRUTIA, MD**
Instituto de Cirugía Plástica y de la Mano, Private Practice, Hospital La Luz and Hospital Mutua Montañesa, Madrid/Santander, Spain; Department of Orthopaedic Surgery, School of Medicine, Pontificia Universidad Catolica de Chile, Santiago, Chile

**APARNA VIJAYASEKARAN, MBBS, MS**
Division of Plastic and Reconstructive Surgery, Mayo Clinic, Rochester, Minnesota

**ZENG TAO WANG, MD**
Professor and Chair, Department of Hand and Foot Surgery, Shandong Provincial Hospital, Shandong University, Jinan, Shandong, China

**JONATHAN M. WINOGRAD, MD**
Assistant Professor of Surgery, Division of Plastic and Reconstructive Surgery, Massachusetts General Hospital, Harvard Medical School, Boston, Massachusetts

**JASON WONG, MBChB, PhD**
Honorary Senior Lecturer, Department of Plastic and Reconstructive Surgery, The University of Manchester, Manchester, United Kingdom

**LI FENG XIA, MD**
Attending Surgeon, Department of Hand and Foot Surgery, The Fourth People's Hospital of Shanxi Province, Xian, Shanxi, China

**YA BIN ZHANG, MD**
Chief, Department of Hand and Foot Surgery, The Fourth People's Hospital of Shanxi Province, Xian, Shanxi, China

**YOU MAO ZHENG, MD**
Chief, Department of Hand and Foot Surgery, Enze Hospital of Taizhou Enze Medical Center (Group), Taizhou, Zhejiang, China

**LEI ZHU, MD**
Chief, Department of Hand and Foot Surgery, Qilu Hospital of Shandong University, Jinan, Shandong, China

**LIN ZHU, MD**
Attending Surgeon, Department of Plastic Surgery, Peking Union Medical College Hospital, Beijing, China

# Contents

Survival rates of digital replantation vary in different regions and countries, and Asian surgeons see more challenging cases and have developed some unique methods. Replantation of multiple digits in one or both hands can follow a structure-by-structure method or a digit-by-digit method. For replanting all 10 digits, 3 or 4 teams should be organized. Flow-through flaps, often venous flaps, can be taken from the distal forearm or lower extremity to repair defects of soft tissues and arteries. A pedicled digital artery flap from the adjacent digit can also repair tissue defects and supply blood to the replanted digit.

This article presents the authors' understanding and experience concerning anatomic studies and clinical methods in microsurgical hand reconstruction. The 4 parts of this article include anatomic study of the hand for developing new flaps; application of mini-flaps from the hand, including clinical experience with 8 unique flaps in the hand; anatomic and clinical considerations concerning several flaps from other parts of the human body; and our experience with vascularized free toe joint transfer.

The main goals of treating severe crush injuries are debriding away devitalized tissue and filling any resultant dead space with vascularized tissue. In the authors' experience, the most ideal methods for soft tissue coverage in treating crush injuries are the iliac flap, the adipofascial lateral arm flap, and the gracilis flap. Accompanying bone defects respond very well to free corticoperiosteal flaps. Digital defects often require the use of complete or subtotal toe transfer to avoid amputation and restore function to the hand.

Vascularized osteochondral flaps are a new technique described for the reconstruction of challenging articular defects of the carpus. The medial femoral trochlea osteochondral flap is supplied by the descending geniculate artery. This osteochondral flap has shown promise in the treatment of recalcitrant scaphoid proximal pole nonunions and advanced avascular necrosis of the lunate. The anatomy, surgical technique, and results are discussed, with clinical cases provided.

Vascularized small-bone grafting is an efficient and often necessary surgical approach for nonunion or necrosis of several bones in particular sites of the body, including scaphoid, lunate, distal ulna, and clavicle. The medial femoral condyle is an excellent graft source that can be used in treating scaphoid, ulna, clavicle, or lower-extremity bone defects, including nonunion. Vascularized bone grafting to the small bones, particularly involving reconstruction of damaged cartilage surfaces, should enhance subchondral vascular supply and help prevent cartilage regeneration. Vascularized osteoperiosteal and corticoperiosteal flaps are useful for treating nonunion of long bones.

Novel and combined tissue transfers from the lower extremity provide new tools to combat soft tissue defects of the hand, foot, and ankle, or fracture nonunion. Flaps can be designed for special purposes, such as providing a gliding bed for a grafted or repaired tendon or for thumb or finger reconstruction. Propeller flaps can cover soft tissue defects of the leg and foot. In repairing severe bone and soft tissue defects of the lower extremity, combined approaches, including external fixators, one-stage vascularized bone grafting, and skin or muscle flap coverage of the traumatized leg and foot, have become popular.

Reconstruction of soft tissue defects following tumor ablation procedures in the trunk and extremities can challenge the microsurgeon. The goal is not just to provide adequate soft tissue coverage but also to restore form and function and minimize donor site morbidity. Although the principles of the reconstructive ladder still apply in the trunk and extremities, free tissue transfer is used in many cases to optimally restore form and function. Microsurgery has changed the practice in soft tissue tumors and amputation is less frequently necessary.

As microsurgical expertise has improved, allowing for the safe transfer of smaller and more refined flaps, free tissue transfer has continued to gain popularity for the management of pediatric soft tissue and bony defects. For the past 2 decades pediatric microsurgery has been shown to be technically feasible and reliable. The major advantage of free tissue transfer in children is the ability to reconstruct defects in a single stage, avoiding the historic treatments of skin grafting, tissue expansion, and pedicled flaps. This article reviews the present state-of-the-art in pediatric microsurgery.

Head and neck reconstructive microsurgery is constantly innovating because of a combination of multidisciplinary advances. This article examines recent innovations that have affected the field as well as presenting research leading to future advancement. Innovations include the use of virtual surgical planning and three-dimensional printing in craniofacial reconstruction, advances in intraoperative navigation and imaging, as well as postoperative monitoring, development of minimally invasive reconstructive microsurgery techniques, integration of regenerative medicine and stem cell biology with reconstruction, and the dramatic advancement of face transplant.

Autologous breast reconstructions have grown in popularity because of their durability, aesthetic outcomes, symmetry, increase in external beam radiotherapy use, and potential aesthetic enhancement at the donor site. Increasing patient expectations for predictable high aesthetic outcomes with minimal complications or need for further procedures has been met by refinement in the use of flaps. The authors' microsurgical breast reconstruction center aims to provide this while delivering efficient service. The deep inferior epigastric flaps form 85% and transverse upper gracilis and profunda artery perforator flaps account for 10%; lumbar artery perforator flaps are a new addition to the authors' armamentarium.

Use of the retrograde limb of the internal mammary vein has been described previously as a lifeboat for venous congestion but not prophylactically. Maximizing the length of the deep inferior artery perforator (DIEP) flap pedicle, identifying and dissecting the superficial inferior epigastric vein proximally in every patient, and taking advantage of the retrograde internal mammary vein are all technical details that facilitate the additional venous anastomosis and flap inset. Performing a second venous anastomosis routinely using the superficial inferior epigastric vein to the retrograde internal mammary vein helps with flap inset.

The pedicled anterolateral thigh (PALT) flap is an underutilized flap for locoregional reconstruction largely because methods to maximize its reach are neither universally implemented nor fully understood. In addition, most of the available literature has focused on the utility of the free anterolateral thigh flap with less emphasis on the PALT flap. Moreover, flap design concepts to maximize its utility and reach and optimize outcomes have not been comprehensively described. In an effort to address this knowledge gap, the authors sought to review their institution's experience with the PALT flap for locoregional reconstruction.

Pedicle perforator flaps and keystone perforator island flaps are additional tools for reconstructive surgeons. Advances in understanding of vascular anatomy, the dynamic nature of perforator perfusion, inter-perforator flow and the hot-spot principle have led to reconstructive techniques that allow innovative autologous tissue transfer while limiting donor site morbidity. Further modifications of the pedicle perforator flap have led to a multitude of freestyle pedicle perforator flap options, as well as freestyle free flaps for soft tissue reconstruction. Modifications in the keystone perforator island flap have increased the degrees of freedom for soft tissue coverage of large defects, with reliable and aesthetically pleasing results.

 Video content accompanies this article at http://www.plasticsurgery.theclinics.com.

Several methods can be used for identifying tissues for transfer in donor-site–depleted patients. A fillet flap can be temporarily stored in other parts of the body and transferred back to the site of tissue defect, including covering the amputated stump of the lower extremity. Human arm transplant is rare and has some unique concerns for the surgery and postsurgical treatment. Cosmetics of the narrow neck of transferred second toes can be improved with insertion of a flap. Lymphedema of the breast after cancer treatment can be diagnosed with several currently available imaging techniques and treated surgically with lymphaticovenous anastomosis.

Robotic surgery has revolutionized minimally invasive surgery. Owing to its unique features and key advantages, robotic surgery is being used for complex cases across surgical specialties. It has been introduced into reconstructive surgery, and is being applied in microsurgery. Robotic surgery combines properties of conventional microsurgery, endoscopic surgery, and telesurgery. It holds great promise in expanding the boundaries of reconstructive microsurgery. However, there are constraints that limit its widespread use. We present the different clinical applications of robotic microsurgery, highlighting its advantages over conventional microsurgery, and outlining the main limitations that might prevent its widespread use.

Modern microsurgical techniques have made possible a broad spectrum of novel means for the reconstruction of complex bone and soft tissue defects. These techniques, in combination with developments in transplant immunology, have led to successful hand and facial allotransplantation and achievement of the highest rung in the reconstructive ladder – truly replacing like with like. The utilization of contemporary microsurgical technique in the context of vascularized composite allotransplantation (VCA) (1) permits successful technical execution and feasibility of VCA, (2) facilitates the study of immunologic tolerance in VCA preclinical models, and (3) optimizes functional VCA outcomes.

# CLINICS IN PLASTIC SURGERY

**THE CLINICS ARE AVAILABLE ONLINE!**
Access your subscription at:
www.theclinics.com

# Preface

# Microsurgery Half a Century After Establishment: Global Perspectives

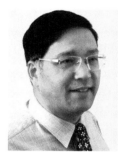

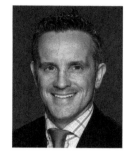

Jin Bo Tang, MD    Michel Saint-Cyr, MD, FRCS(C)

*Editors*

We are proud to assemble and edit this issue offering global perspectives on microsurgery for the jubilee commemoration of the technical establishment and advent of many clinical techniques of microsurgery in the middle of the twentieth century. We are especially grateful to the authors of the review articles presented here; they are world experts in individual topics and have devoted enormous effort to summarizing their innovations and cutting-edge techniques in microsurgery. Of particular note are accounts of work at the very frontier of our field, such as approaches to difficult replantation; transfer of mini-flaps; comprehensive treatment of crush injuries of the hand and forearm; novel vascularized bone grafting; up-to-date techniques for breast, hand, and neck reconstruction; pediatric microsurgery; microlymphatic surgery; and complex reconstruction after tumor excision in the trunk, neck, or extremities.

For this *Clinics in Plastic Surgery* issue on microsurgery half a century after its technical establishment, we include an editorial on the development of fundamental techniques currently in routine use and about the early days of microsurgery. At the end of the issue, we included two articles on future perspectives, about evolving work on use of robots in microsurgical repair and investigations into composite tissue

allografts. We hope to offer readers some perspective on the dramatic changes in microsurgery since the discipline was established, summarize the current state of the field, and provide a glimpse of what may be expected and what challenges remain to be conquered.

Microsurgery has deep roots in plastic surgery, where several of our core techniques originated. Because technical innovations vary widely, with some being very advanced, and new procedures emerging constantly, we feel obliged to remind readers that microsurgery is most powerful when used out of clinical necessity. There are many instances in which simpler and more traditional options achieve similar outcomes, and surgeons should always consider the least complex and technically less demanding options when deciding on treatment. The contents of this issue reflect cutting-edge techniques in microsurgery, which you can use for your own patients when necessary or may inspire you to advance the field in years to come.

We thank all the authors for expert contributions and the publisher for the inspiration to dedicate this issue to commemorating the first half-century of thriving and widespread clinical use of microsurgery. We acknowledge editorial contribution from Drs Daniel Kwan, Jonathan Bass, and Bella Avanessian for their insightful

Clin Plastic Surg 44 (2017) xiii–xiv
http://dx.doi.org/10.1016/j.cps.2017.01.001
0094-1298/17/© 2017 Published by Elsevier Inc.

comments and review for some of the articles in this issue. Special thanks are given to Dr Luis Landin for coordinating the article on unique techniques and clinical approaches, and Drs Marco Innocenti and Rohit Arora for thoroughly reviewing their cases and techniques for an article on vascularized bone grafting in this issue. Planning this issue and collecting the articles began in the summer of 2015 and ended in early 2017. Considerable editorial effort was devoted to each of those articles by authors from multiple countries or clinical units, with which we aim to offer comprehensive international views. This effort has been warmly supported by experts from different countries in Europe, America, and Asia. They kindly contributed their wisdom, case materials, and technical points to comprehensive reviews on individual subjects. We humbly acknowledge that the experience of many eminent microsurgeons has not been included, simply because their work was either reflected in recent issues of *Clinics in Plastic Surgery* or has been well known to our readers, and the work being presented here is fresher.

Development of microsurgery started in the first half of the twentieth century; its foundation for clinical techniques was established about half a century ago. In the mid-1960s and later years, digital replantation and free vascularized tissue transfers came into clinical use; today we enjoy the fruits of the early work. It was an honor to edit this issue. We dedicate it to the many pioneers who established the foundation of the special surgical field we now call *microsurgery*.

Jin Bo Tang, MD
Department of Hand Surgery
Affiliated Hospital of Nantong University
The Hand Surgery Research Center
Nantong University
20 West Temple Road
Nantong 226001, Jiangsu, China

Michel Saint-Cyr, MD, FRCS(C)
Division of Plastic Surgery
Baylor Scott & White Health
Scott & White Memorial Hospital
MS-01-E443, 2401 South 31st Street
Temple, TX 76508, USA

E-mail addresses:
jinbotang@yahoo.com (J.B. Tang)
michel.saintcyr@bswhealth.org (M. Saint-Cyr)

# Erratum

Please note that the name of the 2nd author of the article "Transconjunctival lower lid blepharoplasty with and without fat repositioning", appearing in Volume 42, Issue 1 (January 2015) of *Clinics in Plastic Surgery*, was misspelled. The correct spelling is Matthew L. Iorio.

Clin Plastic Surg 44 (2017) xv
http://dx.doi.org/10.1016/j.cps.2017.03.001
0094-1298/17/© 2014 Elsevier Inc. All rights reserved.

# Editorial
# Microsurgical Technical Training: Differences Between China and the United States

I have been fortunate to work in two different countries in treating hand-related trauma and disorders, in which microvascular anastomosis is sometimes necessary. Though surgeons in both China and United States are considered to have advanced microsurgical techniques—and might themselves assume their practices are quite similar—in fact, I have noticed differences in their training, judgment, and practice in these two quite dissimilar cultures.

## TRAINING

Training in microvascular anastomosis is commonly included at the very beginning of the training of hand surgeons, mostly during orthopedic surgery residency in China, because orthopedic surgeons commonly perform soft tissue reconstructions and any on-call resident is likely to need to connect vessels during his or her third or fourth year of residency. Rat tails are usually used for practice, because the vessels are long and can be repaired at each segment under an operating microscope. Clinically digital replantation is usually performed by rather young surgeons, from fourth-year residents to junior attendings. However, there is no requirement that an attending be present for replantation; if the attending surgeon considers a senior resident sufficiently proficient, the attending may not scrub. If trauma is extensive or more than one digit are severed, replantation is usually performed by a team of two or three attending surgeons with assistants. Replantation is also done very frequently in non–teaching hospitals: one attending surgeon usually works with two assistants (hand or non–hand surgeons). Thus, training of microsurgical anastomosis is routine during very early hand surgery training. Consequently, one may also find some young surgeons who are very proficient at vascular anastomosis, yet still just beginning to learn classic hand surgery. In the United States, orthopedic or plastic surgery residents are often more exposed to classical hand surgery, but practice and training in microvascular anastomosis are usually delayed compared with those in the Chinese system; such training is also less mandatory in the United States than it is in China. When I compare residents at year four or five, I feel that those in the United States have much greater knowledge of disease classification and the mechanics of deformities in the hand, but some have had few opportunities to use microscopes and are virtually unable to dissect under a microscope. In contrast, after 4 or 5 years, it is common for a Chinese surgeon in a hand surgery center to perform a skillful replantation and to be very comfortable with microscopic dissection. These differences reflect variations in the requirements set by the department or training program in either country.

Proficiency of microsurgical skills at expert levels likely is very similar in the two countries and in top microsurgical institutes training of residents and fellows under master surgeons likely is equally excellent in either country, but trainings in microsurgical skills differ greatly in general in the two countries. I believe that both countries would benefit from being aware of these differences in emphasis. In observing a young surgeon who skillfully performs a free flap transfer or a complex multiple digital replantation in China, one should not assume he or she is equally skillful in tendon transfer or secondary reconstruction of an extensor tendon defect. When a senior resident or junior hand surgeon in the United States impresses you with a wonderful presentation and systematic explanation of a topic of classic hand surgery, you should not assume he or she would impress you similarly with dissection under a microscope.

Training background and culture are different; young residents and surgeons are more outspoken in the United States, while asian culture dictates residents and young surgeons speak less and be more silent in clinical or training settings. Some skilled surgeons in China often refrain from extensive speaking. Such cultural influences are seen not only in China but also in Japan and Korea. Understanding the differences enhances communication and exchanges across continents.

Clin Plastic Surg 44 (2017) xvii–xviii
http://dx.doi.org/10.1016/j.cps.2017.01.002
0094-1298/17/© 2017 Published by Elsevier Inc.

## CLINICAL JUDGMENT

Young surgeons in the United States often rely heavily on Doppler signal to assess vascular perfusion, while Chinese young surgeons are much less reliant on this technology. If distal tissue perfusion is good, there is no need to use Doppler, but if distal perfusion is poor (judged by capillary refill and tissue color), the vascular supply is certainly insufficient. Doppler is only useful in judging where the blood flow stops in relatively large vessels, but terminal branches do not create blood flow to make the Doppler work reliably. Chinese microsurgeons consider it a waste of time to try to detect blood flow signal at fingertip, where the capillary flow in the pulp and nailbed is so easily assessable. I see some surgeons in the United States become suspicious about the patency of blood flow in the hand, if they do not detect a signal, though the fingertips are well perfused. Many Chinese microsurgeons consider the American colleagues (especially young colleagues) too reliant on "machines" to test, neglecting more plain clinical signs to make judgments.

Judgments regarding tissue color also sometimes differ between the two countries. A certain degree of venous congestion is common in the 2 or 3 days after surgery. The color of the replanted part is not always normal within a few days after surgery; such suboptimal color could make less experienced surgeons worry, which is unnecessary.

## NUMBERS OF MICROSURGEONS AND VOLUME OF PRACTICE

The annual meeting of the American Society for Reconstructive Microsurgery currently draws around 300 attendees; though this apparently is not the total number of microsurgeons in the United States, it may provide an estimate. There are a number of excellent training centers in the United States with high volumes of elective cases or emergency microsurgical cases. The analogous Chinese microsurgery society meeting is attended by 1500 to over 1800 surgeons currently. The population of China is more than four times that of the United States. The volume of trauma-related microsurgical procedures is dramatically larger in China due to the size of the population and the resultant larger number of traumatic injuries to factory workers or farmers and traffic accidents. These differences render much greater chances for training of microsurgical skills in China.

In a very recent endeavor to pursue further microsurgical skills, Dr Reena Bhatt from Brown University spent a 6-week academic sabbatical at Shandong Provincial Hospital in Jinan, China in September and October 2016; she participated in replanting multiple digits and extremities at this single microsurgical center in 6 weeks. During these 6 weeks, this center replanted 96 digits with 1 failure. This implies that this center performs 16 digital replants in a week, or the number of such cases at her home institution over 6 to 8 years. Dr Bhatt noted that the Chinese team use brachial blocks with sedation as their preferred anesthesia in replantation. Their approach is with teams of surgeons to reduce fatigue. She recognized the immense dexterity and focus on efficient and sharp debridement with irrigation. Replantation of multi-level amputations is routine when feasible. Often free tissue transfers, including small perforator based glabrous flaps, are used immediately for soft tissue coverage as indicated. Intravenous infusion of Dextran is in routine use after replantation. The Shandong team is experienced enough to reliably predict survival of replanted digits; 95 out of 96 replanted digits survived, with the one failure predicted but attempted in a child with four finger multilevel trauma. Difficult replantation becomes a predictable surgery with their experience. This microsurgical center is now open to overseas microsurgeons for fellowship training and short-term visits for concentrated experience and training. Trainees can participate in any replantation cases on call, and multiple flap surgeries are also performed in the emergency setting.

It appears that actual working experience is the best indicator of the state of microsurgery, and certainly institutes within each country will differ. It is clear that more profound understanding will come from actual on-site visits and spending days or weeks observing surgeries (participating in surgery and performing vascular anastomoses as a visiting surgeon is permitted in China).

This featured essay is aimed to encourage microsurgeons across the Pacific Ocean—presumably in the two countries with the largest number of practicing microsurgeons—to understand each other better through initiating another level of communication and opening a new avenue of cooperative training for future generations of microsurgeons.

Jin Bo Tang, MD
Department of Hand Surgery
Affiliated Hospital of Nantong University
The Hand Surgery Research Center
Nantong University
20 West Temple Road
Nantong 226001, Jiangsu, China

E-mail address:
jinbotang@yahoo.com

# Editorial

# Development and Historical Evolution Half a Century Ago at the Dawn of Microsurgery

The Department of Orthopedics and Replantation Research Laboratory of the Sixth People's Hospital of Shanghai was at the forefront of technical innovation and development of limb and digital replantation and early microsurgery in the mid-1960s, half a century ago. This was a period when the entirety of China was isolated from the rest of the world, with revolutionary movements spreading over the entire country. Almost unbelievably, the early development of microsurgery took place during this period, unknown to the rest of the world. As a member of the earliest research team in the replantation laboratory and a member of the surgical team in the department, the author recollects some little-known facts dating back half a century that led to now-familiar techniques in microsurgery.

## ANASTOMOSING A GREATER NUMBER OF VEINS IS NECESSARY IN DIGITAL AND ARM REPLANTATION

Because swelling of the replanted arm was a major problem in the first cases in this unit, multiple small incisions were made to drain the venous blood. From the mid-1960s, attempts were routinely made to connect more veins than arteries in replanting an arm. Consequently, fewer replantation failures were caused by limb swelling. It became a rule to always connect more veins than arteries in limb replantation; such a rule was applied to digital replantation as well.

## THE ISCHEMIA TIME OF SEVERED LIMBS: COLD PRESERVATION

Prolonging the survival time of amputated limbs or digits was a central concern of the team at that time, because patients with arm amputations often could not be transported to Shanghai from far away in a timely fashion. There were very few centers in China capable of performing limb replantation at that time. Canine experiments were carried out to test whether preservation of the amputated limb at 0°C to 4°C substantially prolonged survival of a severed limb (**Figs. 1** and **2**). It was found that without cold preservation, the canine limb could not be successfully replanted after 10 hours of

ischemia. In contrast, cold preservation of the amputated canine limbs doubled and tripled the time of ischemia allowable before a successful limb replantation. The longest time for replantation for such an amputated canine limb reached 108 hours (**Fig. 3**). It was thought that if cold preservation could extend the ischemia time to over 100 hours (which translates to an entire day for a human limb), there was no need to seek further solutions: cold preservation should buy enough time for any patient to be transported to a replantation center.

A funny story relates to figuring out how to achieve cold preservation in some rural areas. In 1965, there was a phone call from a mountainous area of west Zhejiang about a farmer whose hand had been severed. How to preserve the hand for the long journey necessary? More than 100 popsicles were placed around the hand, which was wrapped in a plastic bag. After transfer to our unit 17 hours later, replantation was successful because of the cold preservation by the popsicles!

## RABBIT EAR AS A MODEL FOR EXPERIMENTING MICROSURGERY

In those early days, the best model for practicing vascular anastomosis was unclear. That was when rabbit ears came into use for practicing and researching surgical replantation (**Fig. 4**). Vascular diameters in the rabbit ear are similar to those of vessels in the fingers, and because ear tissue is thin, vascular flow could be easily visualized against lighting. Exercise of replantation in such a rabbit ear model formed the foundation for clinical success in digital replantation in 1966 and later free vascularized muscle transfer in 1973.

## ANASTOMOSIS OF VESSELS UNDER 1 MM

Higher rates of success in replanting digits were the goal in 1966, and it was thought that practicing anastomosis on vessels smaller than 1 mm could help. The rat femoral artery, with a diameter of 0.8 mm, was used. Anastomoses of 100 femoral arteries were set as the goal for each member in the team. This amount of practices ensured that

Clin Plastic Surg 44 (2017) xix–xxv
http://dx.doi.org/10.1016/j.cps.2017.01.003

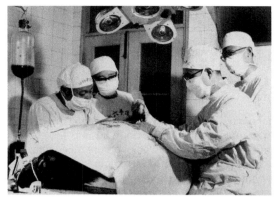

**Fig. 1.** The operative settings in the Replantation Research Laboratory in 1965 (*on the scene from left*: Zhong Wei Chen, Ling Zhang, Cheng Hua Tang, and Yong Gang Wang). (*Courtesy of* Cheng Hua Tang.)

surgeons were quite proficient in performing clinical anastomoses of vessels in the digits.

## COORDINATED EFFORTS WITH MANUFACTURERS IN DEVELOPING MICROSURGICAL INSTRUMENTS

Much effort was directed at cooperation with the Shanghai Medical Instrument Factory. At the time, there were no molds for making microsurgical needles, so workers in the factory hand-made those tiny needles. One microsurgical needle usually took 2 days of continuous labor to grind and polish under magnification. Gradually, the needle-making process was improved, and needles could be produced in batches (**Figs. 5** and **6**). After investigation into strength and smoothness of microvascular anastomosis with a variety of materials, nylon monofilaments were found the best material for suture of small vessels.

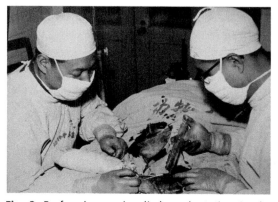

**Fig. 2.** Performing canine limb replantation in the research laboratory. (*Courtesy of* Cheng Hua Tang.)

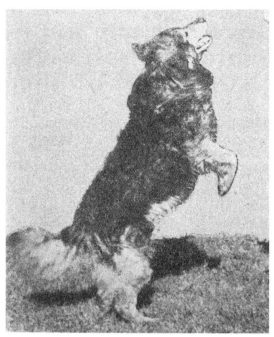

**Fig. 3.** The canine with a replanted hind limb after 108 hours of cold preservation following amputation.

## DEVELOPING A TEST FOR THE QUALITY OF VASCULAR ANASTOMOSIS

Driving the blood away from the vessels distal to the anastomosis site is a test of blood flow developed in replantation surgery in the mid-1960s. Immediate refilling of the vessel indicates excellent vascular anastomosis; slow or no refill of the vessels suggests poor or no blood flow. This method was verified first experimentally and then put into routine clinical use.

## HEAT AND LIGHT PROMOTE VASCULAR CIRCULATION AFTER REPLANTATION

After a day of experimental rabbit ear replantation in 1966, we forgot to turn off the lamp used for surgery on both ears of a rabbit and left it on overnight. The ear closer to the lamp had much better vascular perfusion than the ear on the other side. This caught our attention and prompted us to consider whether heat and light might be important for successful vascular anastomosis. Consequently, we designed an experiment to determine whether heating the replanted ear produces a significant difference, and the results were positive. Those findings led to clinical use of a lamp to warm and illuminate the replanted limb or digit.

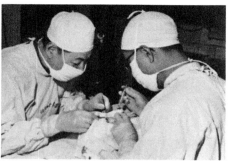 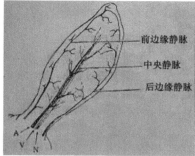

**Fig. 4.** Rabbit ear replantation (*left*) and the drawing of its arterial network (*right*). (*Courtesy of* Cheng Hua Tang.)

## ALLOGRAFT OF A CANINE LIMB

In the winter of 1966, we started experimenting on limb allotransplantation in a canine. A hind limb was transplanted from one dog to another. The survival of the allotransplanted hind limb was 2 years, without use of any immunosuppressant. At that time, less was known about immunosuppressants, which were certainly not used. The transplanted leg survived with bony fixation, connecting muscles and tendons, and vascular anastomosis. The leg functioned well, but remarkable atrophy of the leg was noted 1 year and 9 months after surgery (**Fig. 7**), the leg becoming necrotic 2 years after surgery.

## REPLANTATION SURGERY UNDER PRIMITIVE CONDITIONS

Replantation in the mid to late 1960s was performed under very primitive conditions: no operative microscope was available most of the time; surgical anastomosis was under simple magnification (using magnifying glasses) or with the naked eye. Vessels were anastomosed with

8-0, 9-0, 10-0 sutures made at great cost of time by factory workers. Thus, surgeons and factory workers worked together to design and make these fine needles and sutures in amounts sufficient for use by a limited number of surgeons. Microsurgical clamps, forceps, and needle holders were all designed during that period and put into clinical use. The surgeons all knew the workers in these instrument factories well and became friends because of frequent visits to the factories. The success rate of digital replantation was 56% in the first series of replants of 151 digits with 85 digits surviving from January 1966 to December 1971 (**Fig. 8**), mostly using primitive microsurgical tools specially made by factory workers.

## TECHNICAL PROBLEM-SOLVING AND SERVING THE PEOPLE WERE THE MAIN GOALS, WITH FEW PUBLICATIONS

As is well known, the 1960s were a period of turmoil due to the "Cultural Revolution" in China. Research institutes in many other fields of science and technology were forced to shut down. However, fortunately, research and clinical work in replantation were strongly supported and encouraged by the government and consistently had the

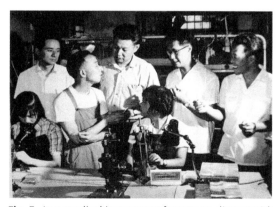

**Fig. 5.** In a medical instrument factory, to discuss with the workers producing microsurgical needle and sutures (*back row from left*: Joseph Bao, Zhong Wei Chen, Cheng Hua Tang, and Hegao He). (*Courtesy of* Cheng Hua Tang.)

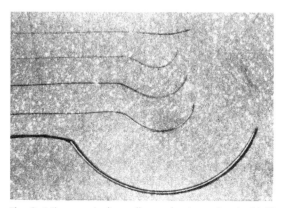

**Fig. 6.** Microsurgical needles and sutures (up to 11-0) made at that time. (*Courtesy of* Cheng Hua Tang.)

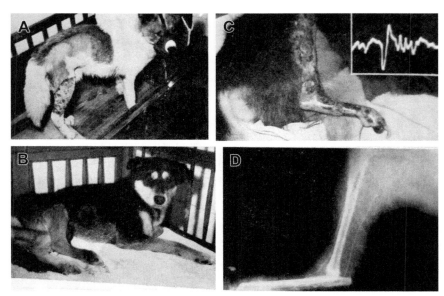

**Fig. 7.** Canine limb allotransplantation, survived 2 years. (*A*) 2 weeks after transplantation. (*B*) 3 weeks after surgery. (*C*) 1 year and 9 months after surgery. EMG examination detected muscle contraction potential, but the limb had remarkable atrophy and skin ulcerations. (*D*) Angiography indicated integrity of major vessels, though the limb became necrotic.

support of the hospital and the medical community in China as well. The Sixth People's Hospital established the Research Laboratory for Replantation of Severed Limbs in 1965, which was fully economically supported by the hospital; staff was designated, and appropriate settings were provided for experimental replantation as well as histological and biochemical assessments. The hospital had professional medical photographers take operative pictures of patients and experiments; all first-hand clinical materials were preserved. The Laboratory was located in a two-story building in the hospital. We conducted investigations answering pressing clinical questions at that time and looking into fundamental techniques of microvascular surgery. The highest objective of the period was to devote oneself to the people and not to be

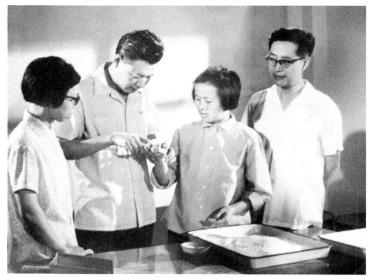

**Fig. 8.** Clinical follow-up of a patient after digital replantation (*from left*: Drs Shi Qin Shi, Zhong Wei Chen, the patient, Dr Cheng Hua Tang). (*Courtesy of* Cheng Hua Tang.)

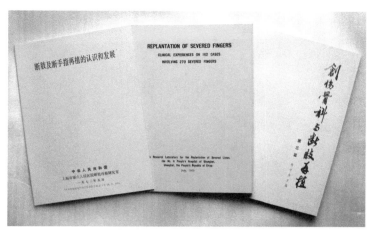

**Fig. 9.** Reprints of publications made at that time, without investigators' names, instead authored by "Research Laboratory for Replantation of Severed Limbs", and a book in the Chinese language. (*Courtesy of* Shanghai Science and Technology Press, Shanghai, China; with permission.)

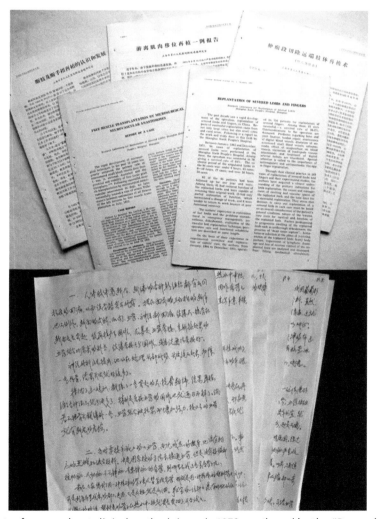

**Fig. 10.** The reprints of papers about clinical methods in early 1970s, authored by the "Research Laboratory" and preserved by the author (*upper*). The early experimental replantation and microsurgery were not published at that time, as the author recollected in a memoir about early day practice and experiments on microsurgery (*lower*).

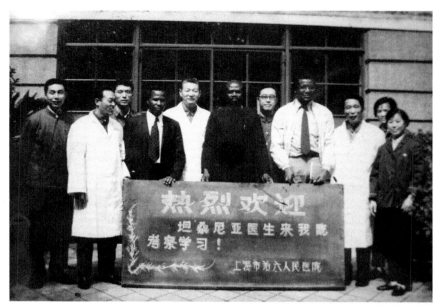

**Fig. 11.** Posing at the main gate of the hospital building together with a group of overseas visitors, with a welcome sign (*from left*: 2nd, Hegao He; 5th, Zhong Wei Chen; 7th, Cheng Hua Tang; 9th, Yan Wang).

selfish. Therefore, solving practical clinical problems was an acceptable goal. However, publications by the department and laboratory were rare, because all Chinese-language journals virtually stopped publication, and communication with colleagues outside China did not exist. Such a harsh environment imposed many hardships and frequently interfered with work order in late 1960s. Nevertheless, surgeons were able to concentrate on solving problems encountered in replantation surgery and developing essential microsurgical techniques with little consideration of reward to themselves and no pressure to publish. Laboratory results with clinical implications were tested or simply applied directly in the clinic, followed by observation and summary of outcomes. Only a few publications were made during this period and without authors' names. Instead, they were credited to the "Research Laboratory for Replantation of Severed Limbs," and some were written but not published at all (**Figs. 9** and **10**). Though few or no academic conferences existed in China during the period, surgeons from all over the country and surgeons from other countries could come to learn the techniques in later years, and surgeons in the team were often invited to perform replantations in other hospitals in other cities, which all helped popularize the techniques of replantation and microsurgery in the field's infancy. From the 1960s to the 1970s, books on replantation and microsurgery were published in an effort to popularize the new techniques of

replantation and microsurgery and later to visitors from abroad (**Fig. 11**).

The mid to late 1960s was a fertile period in the development of arm and digital replantation and many essential techniques that would later be called *microsurgery*. Microsurgery was an

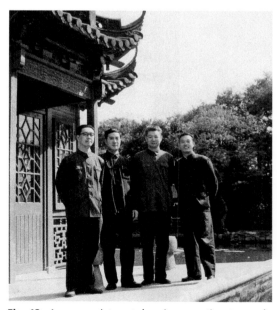

**Fig. 12.** A group picture taken in an outing to a suburban park of Shanghai on April 24, 1966 (*from left*: Cheng Hua Tang, Zhong Jia Yu, Zhong Wei Chen, and Hegao He). (*Courtesy of* Cheng Hua Tang.)

unfamiliar terminology that began emerging at that time, though otolaryngologists started to use operating microscopes in surgery as early as 1920s. Microvascular surgery was explored and microvascular anastomosis was experimented with and attempted in 1960s only in some regions, such as America, Japan, Australia and Europe; yet opportunities of communication were few. These teams explored this unknown field inquisitively. Only later did experience from different continents merge and complement each other. I was fortunate to be on the team led by the late Dr Zhong Wei Chen, and I recall that the relationship among the team members was intimate. Every member lived very close to the hospital. I clearly remember when Dr Chen was unable to finish surgery and go home, he gave me the keys to his apartment; my bedroom was in the hospital, where everybody could get in with common keys. They rode bicycles on the street together and went on outings to parks together during holidays (**Fig. 12**). I recall that one of us left a bicycle unlocked in a busy street to go to another city to operate, and came back to find the bicycle was still there days later. Though it definitely required teamwork and strenuous effort, all the team members (knowingly or unknowingly) became pioneers in microsurgical techniques, with Dr Chen undoubtedly the leader, foremost inventor, and greatest contributor to the field. Fifty years later, some of those on the team have already passed away. To represent the efforts of those involved, I have tried to include photographs of as many members of the early teams as possible, and share them with the members who today still treasure memories of the days of inventing and pioneering half a century ago. We all are happy to see microsurgery grow and flourish, with equipment and a scope of clinical applications unimaginable 50 years ago.

Note: Dr Cheng Hua Tang was a member of the earliest team in the Research Laboratory for Replantation of Severed Limbs (Dr Chen was the chief) and a member of the surgical team in the mid to late 1960s. With Dr Chen leading the efforts, Cheng Hua Tang arranged and executed the studies in the Laboratory in that period. He later was the vice chair of the Department of Orthopedics and chief of the Replantation Research Laboratory, Extremity Microsurgery Institute, The Sixth People's Hospital, Shanghai. In his eighties, he lives a happy life, still seeing patients three days a month. He is among the few early investigators of microsurgery in the 1960s still able to provide fascinating accounts of those pioneering activities started half a century ago.

Cheng Hua Tang, MD
Suite 14, Floor 6, Number 2
120 Long, Guanlong Road
Shanghai 200061, China

E-mail address:
jinbotang@yahoo.com

# A Global View of Digital Replantation and Revascularization

Jin Bo Tang, MD[a],*, Zeng Tao Wang, MD[b], Jing Chen, MD[a],
Jason Wong, MBChB, PhD[c]

## KEYWORDS

- Digital replantation • Revascularization • Wide-awake surgery • Tissue defects in the hand
- Complex hand trauma

## KEY POINTS

- Survival rates of digital replantation vary in different regions and countries, and Asian surgeons see more challenging cases and have developed some unique methods.
- Replantation of multiple digits in one or both hands can follow a structure-by-structure method or a digit-by-digit method. For replanting all 10 digits, 3 or 4 teams should be organized.
- Flow-through flaps, often venous flaps, can be taken from the distal forearm or lower extremity to repair defects of soft tissues and arteries. A pedicled digital artery flap from the adjacent digit can also repair tissue defects and supply blood to the replanted digit.
- Replanting a multilevel severed digit, a digit in a newborn or young child, or a digit amputated distal to the distal interphalangeal joint is challenging, but attempts are routinely made in Asian hospitals. A dry replantation technique can be used in a multilevel severed digit, which reduces surgical time.
- Local anesthesia can be used for digital replantation; local anesthesia with epinephrine for digital replantation has been used in selected cases.
- A few extremely difficult digital replantations illustrate how surgeons have challenged themselves in pushing the limits of microsurgery in salvaging amputated digits.

## INTRODUCTION

The early development of microsurgical techniques was built largely upon attempts and refinements of replanting the arm, hand, or digits. Half a century later, replantation techniques are mature, but globally variations or differences are seen in indications for deciding whether to pursue replantation and difficulties that microsurgeons would like to address. This review offers an analysis and global view on indications, current practices, and various other considerations about digital replantation and presents some of the most difficult and challenging cases to illustrate some of the technical triumphs of microsurgery (not necessarily functional triumphs).

To prepare this article, the lead author invited a panel of distinguished experts on replantation to join him in assembling materials: J.B.T. provided views of current indications, views, and collected success rates of digital replantation from colleagues or reports from different regions

The authors have nothing to disclose.
[a] Department of Hand Surgery, Affiliated Hospital of Nantong University, Nantong, Jiangsu, China; [b] Department of Hand and Foot Surgery, Shandong Provincial Hospital Affiliated to Shandong University, Jinan, Shandong, China; [c] Department of Plastic and Reconstructive Surgery, The University of Manchester, Manchester, UK
* Corresponding author. Department of Hand Surgery, Affiliated Hospital of Nantong University, 20 West Temple Road, Nantong 226001, Jiangsu, China.
E-mail address: jinbotang@yahoo.com

Clin Plastic Surg 44 (2017) 189–209
http://dx.doi.org/10.1016/j.cps.2016.11.003
0094-1298/17/© 2017 Elsevier Inc. All rights reserved.

of the world, especially North America and Asia, and summarized the materials from the panelists; Z.T.W. collected from Chinese colleagues some of the most unusual and challenging digital replants; J.C. summarized reports on 10-digit replantation from the Chinese literature and presented his cases of digital replantation; and J.W. reported on the approach to wide-awake digital replantation in selected patients. This collective effort was intended to offer a global update on this common and yet often challenging area of microsurgery.

## DIGITAL REPLANTATION: WHETHER TO UNDERTAKE AND HOW MUCH EFFORT TO EXPEND?

Replantation of a clean-cut amputation in the proximal half of a single digit is a well-established procedure. The indications are well described, and the essential methods are straightforward, without fundamental differences across regions. There are established principles for more complex and difficult amputations. However, in real-world practice, surgeons in different regions or different units of a given region or country execute these well-documented principles differently and are strongly affected by patients' desires and surgeons' skills, in deciding whether or how to replant. What the authors have learned in collecting materials for this article is striking. The patients' attitudes and surgeons' efforts are so diverse that surgeons in one country may actually have difficulty imagining what decisions and procedures are like in other countries:

1. Most individuals who have an amputated digit would wish for the digit to be replanted. However, when only a single digit was amputated but local tissue conditions are unfavorable and injuries are somewhat complex, European people and Americans of European heritage appear more easily accepting of not having a replantation or accepting ray amputation. If similarly complex injuries occurred in an Asian patient, the patient is usually more eager to have the digit replanted and much less willing to accept surgery to terminalize or ray amputation. Consequently, hand surgeons in the East tend to attempt much more complex replantation.
2. Most contraindications in textbooks are not real-world contraindications in the practice of many surgeons in the East. Often, the only contraindications in their practice are poor general conditions of the body and severe crush to the distal part of the digit. Replantation of distal

fingertips, or in a very young child, or of amputation at 2 levels of a digit, or of 3 or more digits of one hand, is common. Eastern surgeons frequently challenge their own replantation capability, and some become very proficient at replantation as a result of frequently having to push the technical limits of microsurgery upon the request of patients. Many western surgeons would not attempt replantation given the above conditions.

3. The survival rate of finger replantation in the United States is currently 61%, and thumb replants have a survival rate of 74%.[1] Replantation in the United States is performed in all academic medical centers and some major regional hospitals, with well-established microsurgical centers seeing higher-than-average survival rates. In the United Kingdom, replantation success can vary from 20% to 70% depending on the centers and the seniority of surgeon performing the procedure.[2] In eastern Asian countries such as China, Japan, and Korea, the survival rate of digital replantation is generally greater than 70% to 80%. Replantation in China is often performed in midlevel local hospitals (eg, county hospitals may have excellent microsurgical teams), with replant survival rates equal to those in academic centers. In the East, replantation survival rates of 60% to 70% are considered low.
4. Improved health and safety standards in the United Kingdom have significantly reduced the number of cases being performed. For example, 20 years ago, surgeons in Chelmsford performed 46 cases over a 2-year period, and more recently, only 25 cases were performed in over a 5-year period with no change in indication.[2] The industrial environments are the primary source of amputated digits in the East; hence, the frequency of injury in general is far greater than in the Americas and Europe. It is often seen that, in a midlevel hospital (eg, a county hospital) in China, surgeons handle 2 to 3 digital replants each month and replant more than 30 digits a year; some larger centers perform replantations almost every day. In contrast, most academic medical centers in the United States have only 1 or 2 digital replantation surgeries in a month, and one hand surgeon may only replant 1 or 2 digits each year. Consequently, practice volumes and the experience of the surgeons are dramatically different, although they all are microsurgeons or are microsurgery trained. In the United States, high-volume hospitals are defined as having more than 20 replants per year, and high-volume surgeons are those who perform

more than 5 replants a year.[1] For a Chinese surgeon, high volume would mean at least 20 replants per year.

5. Microsurgical operation room settings, microsurgical instruments, and sutures in the West and the East are very similar.
6. The quality of assistant surgeons and the nursing team varies considerably among replant surgerical centers. For example, in most hospitals in the United States—except in well-established centers for microsurgery—because assistants to the attending surgeon who performs replantation do not have ample exposure to replantation, responsibility rests heavily or solely on the attending surgeon. In the East, commonly 2 surgeons with microsurgical skills—one with extensive experience and another similar or less experienced—work together on the case, including replantation, and the nurses are more frequently on a replantation surgical team. In Europe, theater assistants for microsurgery require specific qualifications beyond a basic theater nurse before they can assist in operations. Therefore, the availably team to assist in microsurgery in Europe is significantly diluted.
7. Restrictions in working hours are different in different regions. The European Union working time directive is restrictive on working hours, which means junior trainees have less exposure to these emergency operations or are not required to train for the totality of the operation, providing them with even less exposure and experience to these cases. In contrast, such restriction does not exist in Asia. In the emergency operative settings, the trainees in the United States have no working hour restriction.
8. In any regions or countries, in well-established and busy microsurgical centers, postoperative care nurses are always experienced. Because of a great number of such busy centers and popularization of microsurgery into midlevel hospitals in China, postoperatively patients are monitored by nurses especially experienced in microsurgical cases with experience in judging and recording digital circulation. Major centers have independent hand or microsurgery wards with a hand or microsurgical nurse team. A 2 weeks' stay in hospital after surgery is common in Japan, Korea, and China. In contrast, the patient is discharged dramatically sooner in the United States.

In recent years, it has been suggested that decentralization in performing replantation might be a cause of the decline in survival rates of the replants in the United States over the past 10 years.[1]

Between 2002 and 2005, the survival rates for thumb and finger replants reached a peak of 83% and 69%, respectively, considered the result of centralization.[1] In well-established centers in the United States, surgeons perform more difficult replantation.[2–6] In the general hospital settings, residents and postoperative monitoring expertise are not as vigorous as in large microsurgical centers, staff are not sufficiently trained for efficient replantation surgery or aftercare. Surgeons are not prepared for extremely challenging cases.

Attitudes of patients regarding integrity of digits of the hand are different. Several publications have highlighted such differences between the United States and Japan, and Japanese surgeons preferred replantation despite agreeing that functional outcomes were suboptimal, which because of Japanese cultural beliefs.[3–5] No studies have yet compared China to the United States or Japan. Nevertheless, Chinese society does not associate loss of a finger with gang membership, as is the case in Japan.[3] From the authors' experience with patients in China and the United States, Chinese patients have more difficulty accepting not having replantation or undergoing ray amputation.

Regarding prevalence of training, not many orthopedic-trained hand surgeons in the West perform microsurgery regularly and most microsurgeons are plastic surgeons, whereas in the East, a significant number of hand surgeons from orthopedic backgrounds would be well versed in microsurgery. In Europe, the availability of severe limb salvage expertise is patchy. In the United Kingdom, major trauma centers try to address this need. However, not all plastic surgery centers are directly available at major trauma centers. In Germany, a severe hand surgery alliance has been organized to focus replantation services into a few expert centers.[7] This model is slowly being adopted in other European centers.[7] Resource factors include availability of a microsurgical team, microsurgical equipment, and high-quality nursing care that is essential to monitoring the viability of the replanted digit, which ultimately dictates success. The distance away from a microsurgical unit ultimately dictates the likelihood of the patient being offered replantation.

## TEN-DIGIT REPLANTATION

Replanting all 10 digits of both hands is challenging. In 1986, Ge and colleagues[8] reported the survival of all 10 replanted digits of a 20-year-old woman after 31 hours of ischemia. Successful replantation of all amputated digits is a considerable technical challenge. The authors found in the Chinese literature 21 patients with successful replantation of all 10 digits in mainland China over the last 30 years.[8–28]

Of these 21 patients, the youngest was 18 years old and the eldest was 45. The longest and shortest ischemia before re-establishing blood flow were 44 and 13.5 hours, respectively. The longest operative time was 34 hours (performed by 3 surgeons), and the shortest was 7 hours (by 4 teams of 8 surgeons).

### The Teams

The experience in China indicates that for such severe traumatic cases as amputation of all 10 digits of both hands, at least 3 teams of surgeons are necessary, working on the proximal stumps in both hands and the amputated distal digits simultaneously, to avoid surgeon fatigue. If possible, 4 or more teams would be better. The dorsal veins, bilateral digital arteries, and bilateral nerves are marked with 9-0 nylon suture in the distal and proximal stumps of all 10 digits during debridement for ease of later repairs.

### Two Methods: Structure-by-Structure and Digit-by-Digit

Brachial plexus anesthesia was used in most of these cases. To reduce operative time, digits were replanted using the *structure-by-structure method*, that is, performing bony fixation and tendon repairs *in all digits first* without using an operating microscope, followed by later vascular anastomosis under a microscope (**Fig. 1**). The operative time with

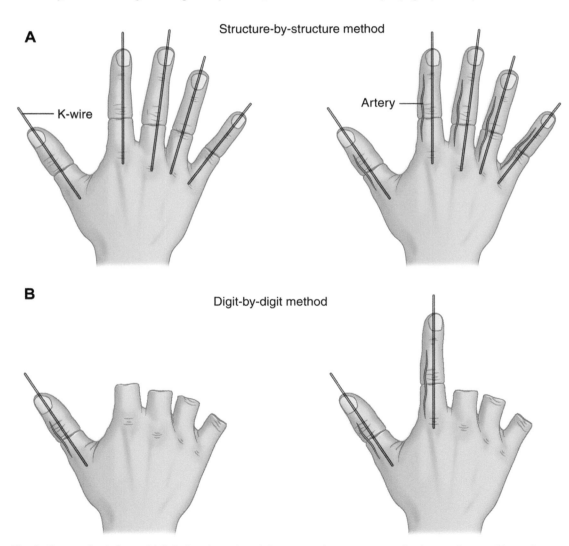

**Fig. 1.** Two methods for multidigital replantation: (*A*) Structure-by-structure method. Completion of bony fixation and tendon repairs first in most or all digits, then vascular anastomosis of these digits altogether under microscope. (*B*) Digit-by-digit method. Completion of replantation of one digit, then move to replant the next digit.

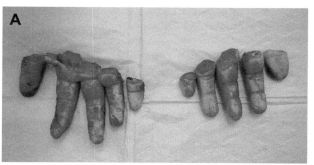
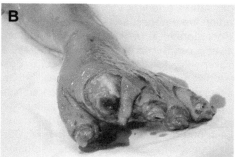

**Fig. 2.** A 35-year-old woman had 10 digits of both hands amputated. (*A*) The amputated 10 digits of the patient. (*B*) The left hand proximal digital stumps. Two teams of surgeons replanted the digits with the structure-by-structure method. (*Courtesy of* Shusen Cui, MD.)

this method in the 3 cases reported by Xie and colleagues[15] was relatively short: 9.5, 6.8, and 7.5 hours, respectively. The structure-by-structure method was used in 11 patients, for all of whom the entire operative time was less than 10 hours. One such case is illustrated in **Figs. 2** and **3**.

Replantation of digits in 10 other patients was by the *digit-by-digit method*, that is, preserving amputated digits in a refrigerator at 4°C and taking them out one by one as replantation of each digit is completed (see **Fig. 1**). The average operative time of these 10 cases was 19.5 hours (range: 7.5–33.5 hours).

In most cases, phalanges were fixed by one longitudinal Kirschner wire (K-wire) or 2 crossed K-wires. All flexor digitorum profundus tendons, flexor pollicis longus tendons, and extensor tendons were repaired, with the modified Kessler method except in one case with a double right-angle suture repair and in another case with the Tsuge method. The bilateral proper digital nerves of each digit were repaired, except that in 5 cases,

not all of the bilateral digital nerves were repaired in all digits. Liu and colleagues[16] reported that no dorsal vein was available for anastomosis in an amputated thumb, but a volar vein in the pulp was found to be healthy enough. The thumb was treated by venous arterialization and nail extraction and was free of venous crisis. Wang and colleagues[18] anastomosed all 20 proper digital arteries of the 10 digits and 40 veins for 10 digits with the goal of increasing replant survival.

### Dealing with High Incidence of Vascular Crisis

Incidence of vascular crisis during or after surgery was high. Crisis occurred in 33% of cases and typically occurred between 1 hour to 4 days after surgery, and surgical exploration was performed immediately.[8–28] In 3 patients, 3 or more attempts at surgical exploration and reanastomosis or vein grafting were necessary to deal with the vascular crisis.[10,25,27] Depending on the findings during exploration after

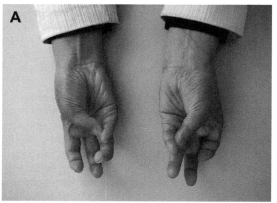
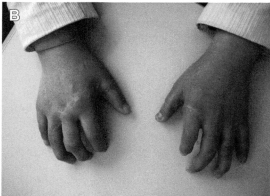

**Fig. 3.** (*A*) Volar views of the replanted digits 1 year later. (*B*) Dorsal view of the replanted digits on year later. (*Courtesy of* Shusen Cui, MD.)

replantation, artery or vein reanastomosis or vein grafting were necessary.

Postoperatively, antibiotics, anticoagulants, and antivasospasm medications were administered intravenously for 5 to 7 days. Specific dosages were given in the reports of 2 cases.[8,28] Ge and colleagues[8] administered an intravenous infusion of penicillin for 5 days, low-molecular-weight dextran 500 mL twice a day for 6 days, and oral aspirin 500 mg 3 times daily for a week. Xie and colleagues[28] used intravenous infusion of second-generation cephalosporins for a week, intramuscular injection of papaverine 30 mg 6 times daily for a week (then reduced to 30 mg 3 times a day for 4 days), intravenous infusion of low-molecular-weight dextran 500 mL twice daily for 9 days, and continuous intravenous infusion of saline 500 mL with heparin sodium 12,500 U 24 hours for 11 days.

### Postoperative Rehabilitation

Passive and active motion of joints began 4 to 6 weeks after surgery in most cases, when K-wires were removed. However, reports do not offer detailed rehabilitation protocols. Cong and colleagues[21] used an electronic heating apparatus to relieve swelling and alleviate pain in the first 2 weeks, and passive and active motion of joints began at 4 weeks. Constant force was applied to maintain passive flexion and extension of joints during a steam bath twice each day for an hour. Isometric and isotonic contraction of forearm and hand muscles was performed during active finger motion exercises.

### Follow-up

Outcomes after follow-up more than 1 year were reported in 3 cases,[18,21,23] despite that all authors reported that both hands of these patients have functionality in grasping and hold, or writing. Wang and colleagues[18] reported that at 14 months, active motion was 70° and 40° at the metacarpophalangeal (MP) and the interphalangeal (IP) joints of the left thumb, respectively, and 70° and 35° at the MP and IP joints of the right thumb, respectively. The index, middle, ring, and little fingers could move for 220°, 210°, 205°, and 200°, respectively, in the left hand, and 200°, 210°, 205°, and 200°, respectively, in the right hand. Cong and colleagues[21] reported that at 1 year after surgery active motion of the left thumb was 130° and right thumb was 140°, and finger motion ranged from 200° to 240°. Ou and colleagues[23] reported that active motion of the left thumb was 65° and right thumb was 80°. The finger motion ranged from 115° to

260° at 7-year follow-up. Two reports described tenolysis in 10 digits at 4 to 6 months after replantation.[13,16]

## DIGITAL REPLANTATION WITH LOCAL TISSUE DEFECTS

Local segmental crush injuries to the digits are common in digital amputation. In most cases, bony shortening and debridement of the crushed tissues ensure good quality of the vessels for anastomosis. However, if avulsion involves a large area of soft tissue or soft tissue or bone is missing, it is necessary to graft tissues to repair the defects. If segmental vascular defects are also present, a flow-through flap or a composite tissue transfer serving as flow-through tissue is a common way to solve this problem.

A few methods used for such conditions are given (**Fig. 4**): (1) a venous flap as a flow-through flap to repair the soft tissue defect and to reconstruct the vessels; (2) a free flap from the arm or lower extremity to cover the soft tissue defect; (3) a pedicled flap from the adjacent digit, such as a pedicled digital artery flap, to restore arterial blood flow to the amputated digit; (4) an iliac bone graft to fill a defect in the phalanx; and (5) a toe joint transfer with a plantar or dorsal skin flap to reconstruct a missing joint and soft tissues in the hand. The authors provide illustrations of the "flow-through" flap procedures in **Figs. 5–7**.

A venous flap from forearm as flow-through flap: (1) The volar part of the distal forearm offers a good and easily accessible donor site for a venous flap. (2) The cutaneous nerve in the venous flap is used as a nerve graft to the digital nerve defect site. (3) The flap is reversed to avoid venous valves that would preclude blood flow and is used to bridge the digital artery defect. (4) A major vein in the flap is chosen for anastomosis with the digital artery in the amputated distal finger part and the digital artery in the proximal stump. (5) The cutaneous nerve is sutured to repair the digital nerve defect. (6) It is of course important to confirm blood flow and skin closure and to avoid compressing the venous flap through the use of light dressings.

A pedicled digital artery flap from adjacent digit: (1) A flap is outlined and dissected in the lateral aspect of the adjacent finger according to the size of soft tissue defects in the amputated digit. (2) The digital artery is ligated distally, and the flap is harvested based on the digital artery pedicle. A wide (2–3 mm) pedicle ensures good venous return of the flap. (3) The pedicle is dissected proximally to the bifurcation of the common digital artery and rerouted to the amputated digit. (4) The distal end

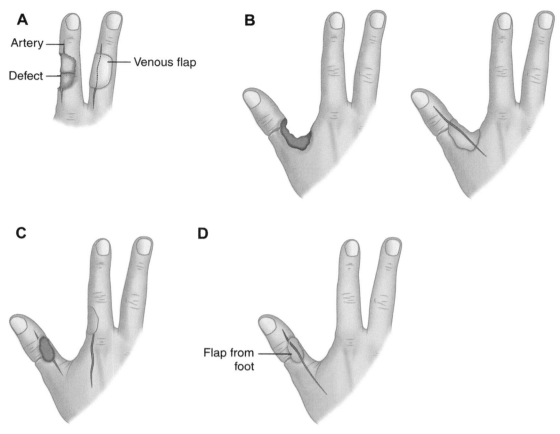

**Fig. 4.** Common methods of a soft tissue defect with a vascular defect. (*A*) Soft tissue defect with a digital artery defect, reconstructed with a venous flap, often taken from the distal forearm to repair both digital artery and the soft tissue. (*B*) Soft tissue and digital artery defects at the base of the thumb or the first web. A venous flap can be used. (*C*) Similarly, if the defects are in the proximal thumb, the pedicled digital artery flap from the index finger can be used. (*D*) The soft tissue and digital artery can also be repaired with a free flap from a foot.

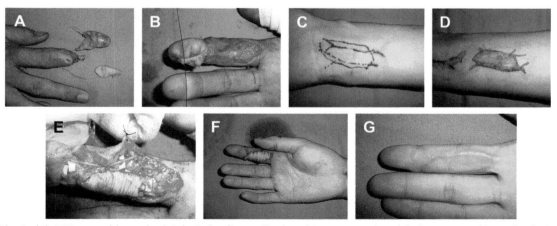

**Fig. 5.** (*A*) A 30-year-old man had right index finger distal avulsion amputation. (*B*) There was a skin and soft tissue defect of 2 × 3.5 cm on the palmar aspect of the middle phalanx level. (*C*) A venous flap was designed from the distal forearm. (*D*) The flap was harvested. (*E*) The venous flap was anastomosed both distally and proximally to the distal arteries. (*E*) Completion of flap transfer. No vascular crisis or venous congestion after surgery. (*F, G*) Appearance 1 year after surgery. (*Courtesy of* Xiao Zhou, MD.)

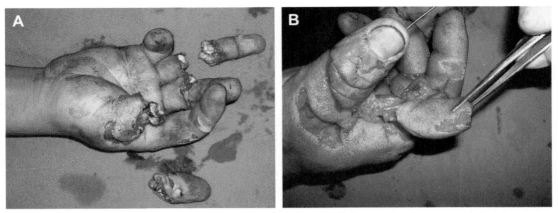

**Fig. 6.** For a case of complete thumb amputation, with soft tissue defect, a digital artery pedicled flap can be harvested to repair the soft tissue defects of the thumb and to establish blood supply to the amputated thumb. (*A*) A case of amputation of the right thumb and middle and ring fingers. (*B*) There was a soft tissue defect and digital artery defect in the thumb. The index finger was not injured, so a digital artery pedicled flap was harvested from the index finger to repair tissue defect and arterial loss of the thumb during thumb replantation. (*Courtesy of* Xiao Zhou, MD.)

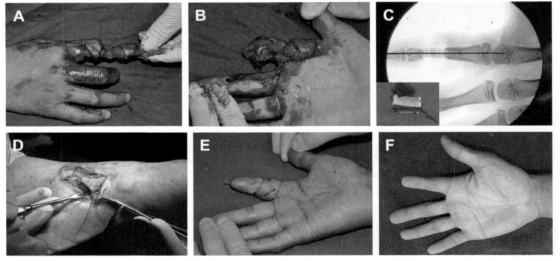

**Fig. 7.** A 13-year-old boy had right index finger incomplete amputation with only flexor tendon connected. The distal part had no blood supply. Bilateral digital arteries and nerves are crushed, with proximal interphalangeal joint (PIP) destruction resulting in a bony defect. (*A*) Volar view after injury. (*B*) Dorsal view after injury. (*C*) An iliac bone was grafted to repair the bone defect. (*D*) A venous flap was harvested from the plantar foot as a flow-through flap. Through a separate incision in the foot, the lateral cutaneous nerve was harvested to reconstruct the defect in the digital nerve. (*E*) The replanted finger and the free flap survived after surgery. (*F*) Appearance after 1 year. (Editorial comments from Jin Bo Tang, MD: *According to the authors, because of severe crush to the finger, the digital artery was crushed; there was no guaranteed blood supply to the distal finger part and no blood supply was noted distally. The team decided to harvest a venous flap to supply the blood to the distal part. Practically, vascular spasm of a crushed digital artery may resolve after surgery and may supply blood to the distal part. However, adding a flow-through flap is a guaranteed approach to deal with this type of injury. In fact, like this team, surgeons in many units in China anastomose bilateral digital arteries to enhance survival rate and reduce cold intolerance of the finger. The surgeons dealing with this case also harvested cutaneous nerve for digital nerve repair on one side, although the digital nerve on the other side was intact after being crushed. Use of a venous flap and a nerve graft is thus justified. However, if the digital artery on the other side was judged to have blood supply, and only a soft tissue defect needed to be dealt with, an easy way is a skin substitute—such as coverage with Integra—even when a part of the tendon is exposed, to avoid a free flap transfer.*) (*Courtesy of* Li Shan Zhang, MD.)

of the digital artery in the flap is anastomosed to the digital artery of the remaining portion of the amputated digit. (5) The skin is closed and noncompressive dressings are applied.

*A free flap transfer from a foot and bone grafting*: (1) Iliac bone is harvested first to fill the bony defect of the digit with longitudinal fixation using a K-wire. (2) A flap—either an arterial flap (from dorsal foot) or a venous flap (from plantar foot)—is harvested. (3) A segment of the extensor hallucis longus or brevis tendon and lateral cutaneous nerve of the foot can be harvested to repair the defects of extensor tendons and digital nerve if necessary. (4) The flap is transferred to the digit as a flow-through flap, and the nerve is reconstructed with the graft. (5) The skin is closed and noncompressive dressings are applied over the flap.

## DIGITAL REPLANTATION IN A WIDE-AWAKE SURGICAL SETTING

For the past half century, anesthesia for digital replantation in China has been brachial anesthesia with the patient wide awake during the entire procedure. A vessel loop is applied to the base of a digit or a tourniquet to the upper arm if necessary. Local anesthesia is the customary choice for replanting a digit in some hospitals in tidy amputation of a single digit or a fingertip that is clean.

Lidocaine 5–10 mL, 1% is injected into the digital sheath cavity (not around the digital nerve or artery to avoid compression), plus local infiltration to the stump (**Fig. 8**). Because the patient is awake, they can provide feedback about the pain level, and local anesthesia can be supplemented anytime. In fact, for decades almost all microsurgical procedures in the hand in China, including digital replantation, have been done with the patient awake, but epinephrine was not used locally.

Adding epinephrine to local anesthesia in the hand for a bloodless or less bloody surgical field is recognized as being safe,[29,30] but using epinephrine in the context of vascular repair microsurgery is considered a contraindication.[29,31] The wide-awake local anesthesia, no tourniquet approach allows the surgeon to assess active motion of the hand during operation.[32] Based on observations of pulsatile blood flow from the digital arteries using this technique for other hand operations, one author (J.W.) and his colleagues challenged this belief by performing replantation and revascularizations using epinephrine in local anesthesia.

### Why Would We Want to Do This?

Although performing a revascularization under local anesthesia would seem to make the

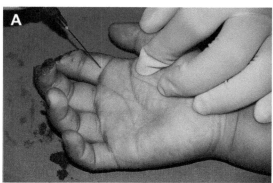

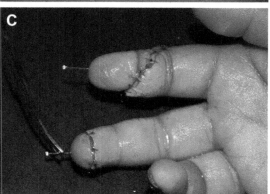

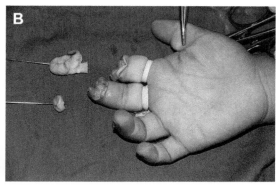

**Fig. 8.** Injection of local anesthesia into digital flexor sheath tunnel to achieve distal anesthesia for replantation performed by Lin Feng Liu, MD. (*A*) Injection. (*B*) Finger tourniquet applied during the surgery. (*C*) Immediately after surgery.

procedure more challenging, however, there are patients who would prefer surgery by local anesthesia and some patients whereby general anesthesia would be considered too great a risk. In some centers where microsurgery is routine and surgeons have expertise in wide-awake surgery, it is acceptable.

The experienced surgeon should be very comfortable with microvascular digit salvage and be prepared to carry out a range of procedures using the wide-awake technique. Familiarity is best gained through flexor tendon or digital nerve repairs, whereby repairing damage to the associated single digital vessel injury may be used as training. The wide-awake surgical approach was used by one of the authors (J.W.) and colleagues in 12 patients. Three cases are presented in **Figs. 9–11**.

### Understanding the Pharmacology

The use of epinephrine in the context of compromised vascular flow appears counterintuitive without a clear understanding of the dynamics of injected epinephrine. Lidocaine and epinephrine injected into digits reduce digital blood flow after 5 to 10 minutes, and the digital flow returns to normal after 1 hour.[33] The half-life of adrenaline in plasma is only 11 minutes, although the local effects in tissue are longer lasting.[34] In contrast, anesthesia with a combination of lidocaine with 1:100,000 epinephrine can last 10 hours,[35] which has certain implications in the case of microvascular surgery. First, provided the replantation

takes longer than an hour, the authors debride the stump, find the vessels, and perform bone fixation; vasoconstriction should have no impact on the arterial flow to the digit at subsequent vascular anastomosis. In other words, vasoconstriction by epinephrine is not likely to be a problem to the anastomosed digital artery or veins. Second, because this combination of anesthesia can last the entirety of the replantation surgery, use of epinephrine in the context of replantation is not as counterintuitive as it might seem. In addition, phentolamine reverses vasoconstriction in 5 seconds when given as a local injection.[36]

### Awareness of the Zone of Trauma

Because the effects of epinephrine on blood flow to the digits in replantation and revascularization are transient, the issues around blood flow actually have more to do with the extent of trauma. The mechanisms of injury dictate how extensive this traumatized zone is, which requires careful judgment before embarking on salvage.

The mechanisms of digital amputation are typically either sharp, crush, or avulsion. The traumatized zone is smallest with sharp injuries and greatest with avulsions but can vary depending on the degree of energy transfer. Similar to Jackson's zones of viability,[37,38] the zone of trauma can progress or resolve depending on local blood flow. The longer the period of warm ischemia, the greater the extent of tissue necrosis and thus more likely the progression to failure. As in conventional

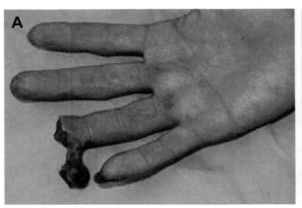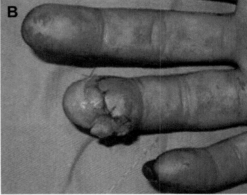

**Fig. 9.** A 21-year-old man injured his ring finger. (*A*) Skin bridge was still intact but was amputated completely and devascularized. All arteries disrupted distal to tip with only central pulp digital artery seen. (*B*) The patient wished to have the procedure done with the lowest anesthetic risk and was not fasted; given the options, he agreed to have the procedure under wide-awake anesthesia. At the level of the distal palmar crease, 1% lidocaine and 1:200,000 epinephrine infiltration were used with "hole-in-one" digital infiltration. The ulnar digital artery was identified and vein graft from volar forearm was harvested and anastomosed to the central artery. Flow was acceptable despite using adrenaline. As no venous anastomosis was performed, the tip went on to be congested and kept bleeding from the tip wound edge for several days until venous drainage was reestablished. The tip went on to heal uneventfully and survived completely.

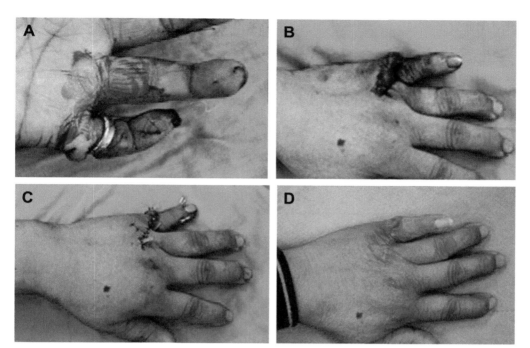

**Fig. 10.** A 63-year-old woman suffered from a ring avulsion of the left little finger after it being caught in heavy machinery. (*A*) Only the volar skin and radial digital nerve were intact. (*B*) Infiltrated at the distal palmar crease were 5 mL of 1% lidocaine and 1:200,000 epinephrine, and the incarcerated ring was removed. (*C*) The fractured proximal phalanx was fixed with 2 K-wires, followed by repair of the flexor and extensor tendons, both digital arteries, one dorsal vein and ulnar side digital nerve. (*D*) At 6 months, the alignment of the digit. As wide awake was offered, the patient accepted the procedure, whereas she would have declined it under general anesthesia. This case illustrates that it can change the patient attitude toward merits of surgery.

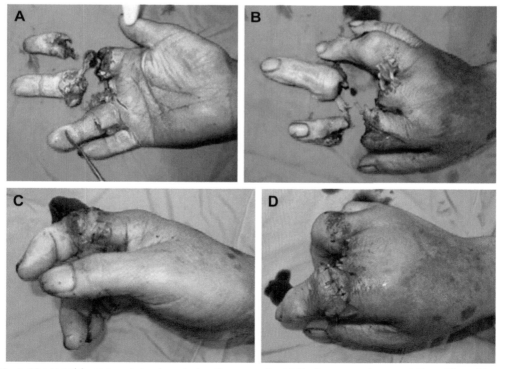

**Fig. 11.** A 48-year-old man sustained an index finger and middle finger crush amputation. The wide-awake setting was used in the replanation. (*A*) Volar view of the amputated two fingers. (*B*) Dorsal view of injury. (*C*) Immediately postoperative view of the repaired index finger. (*D*) Volar view of repaired index finger. The decision to only salvage one digit was made in discussion with the patient on the table at the time of surgery. This case illustrates how patient involvement in the surgical procedure can help aid the surgical decision process.

revascularization and replantation, these factors have to be taken into account, and nonviable tissue must be debrided and vascular repairs performed on healthy vessels. In order to achieve this, shortening the bone of the amputated digit is the simplest primary way to facilitate debridement and soft tissue repair. However, when the digit cannot be shortened, liberal use of vein helps reconnect vessels.

### Surgical Techniques

Surgery itself starts with a standard local infiltration technique, using 1% lidocaine and 1:200,000 epinephrine. Typically 5 mL is administered at the midline of the damaged digit distal to the palmar crease and a further 2 mL in the midline of the site to be dissected. The authors routinely premark veins on the wrist or forearm and reserve 3 mL of local infiltration for vein harvest if required. A temporary tourniquet can be applied to facilitate a quicker dissection but is not used routinely.

Surgery then follows the approach used for digital salvage performed most frequently by the surgeon. The authors' preferred technique order of repair is: debridement, identification of structures and trimming of vessels to the healthy vascular intima, bone fixation (shortening and compression where possible), tendon repairs, arterial repair, and venous repair after flow is re-established. It is critical to ensure strong pulsatile flow from the artery after a heparin flush and check the flow after careful anastomosis. The authors routinely flush out the amputated part with heparinized saline to minimize the risk of thrombosis. Vein grafts are harvested from the wrist and are usually required if primary digital shortening is not performed. It is important to hydrodilate the vein to allow for constrictions, twisting, and holes to be identified in the vein graft.

Furthermore, the graft length necessary for bridging the vessel defect can be more accurately made when the vein is filled with fluid. Anastomosis of the vein graft is usually to the distal vessel first, then onto the proximal vessel, so that the re-establishment of flow does not ever remain static. The nerve is repaired after vascular repair, followed by skin closure.

### Postoperative Care

None of the patients who have had wide-awake replantation by the author (J.W.) needed conversion to general anesthesia. Pushing oral fluids and allowing the patient to ambulate postoperatively do not appear to be detrimental to the circulation of the digits. Careful monitoring is required to ensure the digit remains perfused after surgery with observation every 30 minutes for the first 12 hours, followed by hourly observations for the next 12 hours. This schedule is best monitored by nurses with microsurgical expertise in a high-dependency unit setting. Patients are monitored for 48 hours and then stepped down to a regular ward.

## EXTREMELY CHALLENGING DIGITAL REPLANTATION

It is reasonable to believe that Chinese surgeons deal with more patients with extremely challenging digital replantation, considering that China has the largest population (20% of the world population); machine-related workplaces are common, and Chinese surgeons are willing to challenge themselves to a "fine sewing job" in the most difficult hand repairs. Some of these cases indeed push the limit of tissue repairs possible by the most skilled of hands. A few such cases from China are presented here.

### Replantation of 17 Digital and Palm Segments of a Hand

In December 2006, He JE, Xie SQ, Zhang HF, Hang YG, and their team members treated an 18-year-old girl who suffered severance of 5 digits and the palm of her right hand into 17 segments (**Fig. 12**).

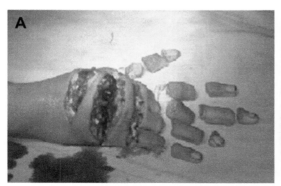
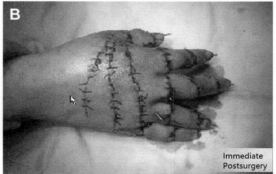

**Fig. 12.** Severances of a palm and 5 digits into 17 segments of an 18-year-old girl. (*A*) After injury. (*B*) Immediately after surgery. (*Courtesy of* Jian Xi Hou, MD.)

The severance occurred at 5 levels from the distal metacarpal bone to the thumb or fingertips. Responding to the urgent request of her family, 7 hand surgeons were assembled and divided into 4 teams to replant all amputated parts.

*Teams 1 and 2* performed bony fixation and vascular anastomosis at each of 3 transection levels in 4 digits using the *dry replantation* technique, that is, connection of any 2 distal segments together with vascular anastomosis and bony fixation in the bloodless field and no blood flow in the vessels (**Fig. 13**). The dry replanting technique is widely used in China to connect any 2 distal segments of a digit that is severed at 3 or more levels. Phalanges were shortened not more than 2 to 3 mm at each severance level to maximize digital length. Each digit was immobilized with one K-wire longitudinally, and 1 or 2 digital arteries were anastomosed in each digit. Two veins

were anastomosed at each of these junctions in each digit.

Surgeons in *team 3* replanted segments at the most proximal severance level. Surgeons in *team 4* reattached the distal digital parts assembled by teams 1 and 2 to the replanted parts prepared by team 3, with vascular anastomosis and nerve repair and tendon repairs, in the order from thumb to index, middle, ring, and little fingers (see **Fig. 13**).

A total of 59 vascular anastomoses were performed in this hand, including 26 anastomoses of 3 common digital arteries and 10 proper digital arteries at different cut levels, and 33 anastomoses in multiple veins on the dorsal digits and palm. A total of 27 repairs were made at the common or proper digital nerves among the 5 digits. They reported that extensor tendons were repaired with a figure-8 method, and flexor

**A**  Teams 1 and 2

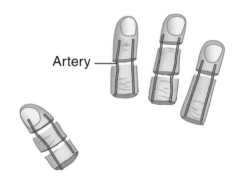

Artery

**B**  Team 3

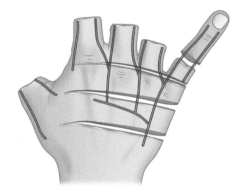

**C**  Team 4

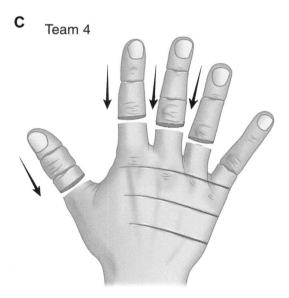

**Fig. 13.** Teamwork in replanting this case. (*A*) Connection of the distal segments of the thumb, index, middle, and ring finger with bony fixation, extensor tendon repairs, and vascular anastomosis by teams 1 and 2. (*B*) Connection of the proximal segments with vascular anastomosis and skin closure by team 3. (*C*) Putting the distal and proximal replanted parts together with bony fixation, extensor tendon repair, vascular anastomosis, and skin closure by team 4.

tendons were also repaired. Total surgical time was 21 hours.

Postoperatively, the patient was placed in a dorsal plaster with intravenous anticoagulation therapy. On the second and third days, venous congestion was found in the thumb, middle, and ring fingers. Small incisions were made in the thumb and fingertips to allow blood to drain from day 3 to 8 to relieve venous congestion, and low-dose heparin was used intravenously. The venous crisis resolved at day 8 after surgery. To treat partial necrosis of the thumb tip and middle fingertip, they were debrided and covered with a pedicled flap from the lower abdomen, with complete flap survival. The K-wire in the thumb was removed at postoperative day 35, and the K-wires in the fingers were removed at day 60. Hand therapy then began to improve finger motion. Tenolysis and finger joint releases were necessary 2 or 3 years after replantation. Functional recovery at 8 years is shown in **Fig. 14**.

This is obviously an extreme case of digital replantation. In each finger, at least one artery had to be connected at 3, 4, or 5 levels, which was a technical challenge. After surgery, tenolysis in some digits was required, and stiffened finger joints were released. With active involvement in therapy, the patient gained function of these digits and had thumb pinch, finger extension, and partial active finger flexion. She could write, hold, grip, and pinch using the replanted hand.

### Simultaneous Severance at the Digit and Palm

A 20-year-old man had his right index and middle fingers completely severed and his palm severed as well. Yang WL and his team replanted the amputated parts. The second and third metacarpal bones were shortened by 4 mm and the proximal phalanges of the index and middle fingers were shortened by about 3 mm. The digital arteries at the palm were anastomosed directly, but bilateral digital arteries of 2 fingers were anastomosed with vein grafting, and flexor digitorum profundus tendons were repaired. The superficialis tendons were resected. In each

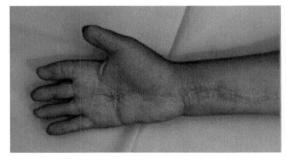
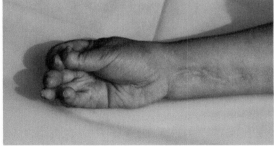

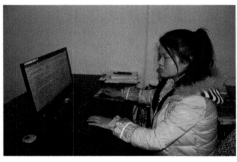
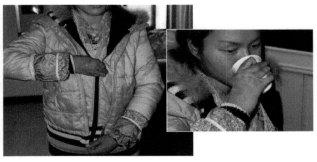

**Fig. 14.** Follow-up 8 years after surgery. (*A*) Function of the hand. (*B*) Use of the hand in daily life. (Editorial comments from Jin Bo Tang, MD: *The surgeons on this surgical team presented surgical details and earlier follow-up in Injury Extra 2014;45:41–44. They followed this patient again recently and sent the pictures in (A) for inclusion. I think this is one of most difficult and challenging digital replantations I have ever seen. It is hard to imagine the replanted digits could survive and can function to a certain extent. This is the result of extremely coordinated teamwork, and the vast amount of vessel and nerve repairs in a single case is just hard to believe. The postoperative rehabilitation was well executed, which contributed greatly to the regained function.*) (*Courtesy of* Jian Xi Hou, MD.)

finger, 4 veins were anastomosed at the dorsal palm, and 3 dorsal veins were anastomosed in each of the 2 fingers. Bilateral digital nerves were repaired directly in both fingers. Active finger flexion and extension were noted during follow-up (**Fig. 15**).

## Replantation of Fingertip of Newborn

Replanting the digits of infants and toddlers is very challenging. During cesarean section, the left index finger of a newborn was severed at the distal interphalangeal (DIP) joint level on March 9, 2013. The newborn was brought to the operating room for replantation 30 minutes later, and replantation surgery by Lei YW and Li L began 1 hour after his arrival and lasted for 2.5 hours (**Fig. 16**). Phalanges were not shortened, and the bones were fixed with longitudinal insertion of a 25-G injection needle from the fingertip. The DIP joint capsule was repaired

with 6-0 nylon sutures. The extensor and flexor tendons were repaired with figure-8 repair using 6-0 nylon sutures. Under an operating microscope with ×12 magnification, the ulnar-side digital artery was found and anastomosed, and 2 dorsal veins were anastomosed with 12-0 sutures, 3 stitches for each vessel. Then, the radial-side digital artery was found and anastomosed with 4 stitches of 12-0 sutures. Bilateral digital nerves were also sutured. Normal capillary refill and color in the replanted tip were confirmed. The newborn was placed on hibernation therapy in the newborn intensive care unit with anticoagulation therapy. On postsurgical day 2, venous congestion was noted. Suture stitches for skin closure were removed partially, and cotton swabs were used to add gentle pressure to the fingertip and release to help venous return. The color of the replanted tip became normal at day 4, and the needle for bony fixation was removed 2 weeks after surgery. Follow-up

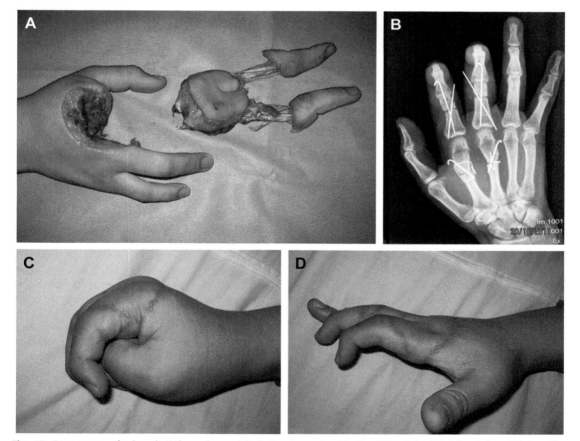

**Fig. 15.** Severances of a hand at the palm and 2 digits at proximal to the PIP joints. (*A*) After injury. (*B*) A radiograph shows bony fixation. (*C*) Flexion of the hand during follow-up after 1 year. (*D*) Extension of the hand. (*Courtesy of* Wu Li Yang, MD.)

A

B

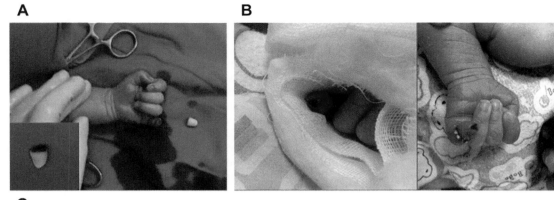

C

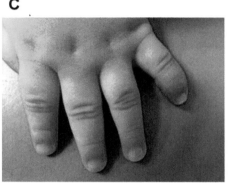

Fig. 16. Replantation of a newborn. (*A*) The little finger amputated at the level of the distal interphalangeal joint several minutes after birth. (*B*) The replanted little finger in the first week (*left*) and second week (*right*) after surgery. (*C*) 8 months after surgery. (*Courtesy of* Jin Liang Zhang, MD.)

6 months after surgery revealed excellent cosmetics and normal vascular circulation of the finger (see **Fig. 16**).

Replanting fingertips, multiple digits, digits in young children, or a digit severed at 2 levels are also challenging, but considered more routine than the examples presented above (**Figs. 17–19**). A digit with most of its structures attached but no blood supply needs revascularization (which is not replantation), but such a digit is usually handled similarly to a replantation with regard to vascular anastomosis. Restoration of blood flow in one digital artery on a digit is usually sufficient. The authors illustrate revascularization of a finger with unique methods after tissue avulsion of all fingers of a hand (**Fig. 20**).

## SOME ESSENTIAL CONSIDERATIONS AND FUTURE PERSPECTIVES

Although classic knowledge and methods are not the core of this article, several points essential to all replantation surgeries, regardless of geographic regions and expertise levels of operators, are brought to the attention of readers:

1. Recognizing the possibility of survival of the distal finger (ie, distal to the finger DIP joint or through nail). The potential of the body in nourishing the distal fingertip is amazing, especially in young children. In children, direct suture of the amputated distal fingertip has 40% to 50% chance of survival without anastomosing vessels.[39,40] Suture the distal fingertip back directly if you are unable to find vessels and perform anastomosis. Do not discard the distal part! In children or young or middle-aged adults, the tip heals amazingly well in many cases, but direct suture of the distal part is most disappointing in the elderly.

2. Smoking, local tissue crush or avulsion, and advanced age are 3 major risk factors for failed digital replantation. The patient should be prohibited from smoking after surgery, and patients older than 70 years should not be considered candidates for digital replantation in most situations. Conditions such as avulsion, localized crush, or tissue defect are unfavorable; how to deal with them is a key in replanting a digit, a test to a surgeon's skills.

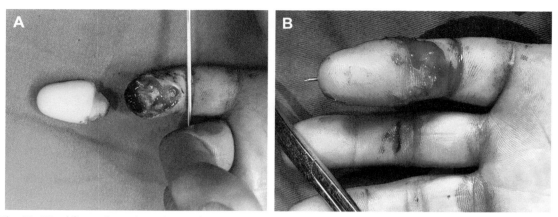

**Fig. 17.** Distal fingertip replantation at the DIP joint level of the right index finger of a 57-year-old man (surgery performed by Jing Chen, MD). (*A*) Before surgery. (*B*) During surgery right after anastomoses of one digital artery and one volar vein. One K-wire was used to fix the digital bones after trimming the bone stumps for 3 to 4 mm. The replant survived without events after surgery.

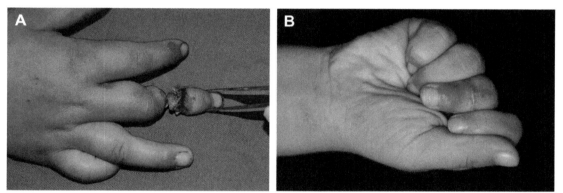

**Fig. 18.** Replantation of the right middle finger of a 4-year-old girl with anastomosis of one artery and one vein and repairs of bilateral digital nerves (performed by Jing Chen, MD). (*A*) Before surgery. (*B*) 5 months after surgery.

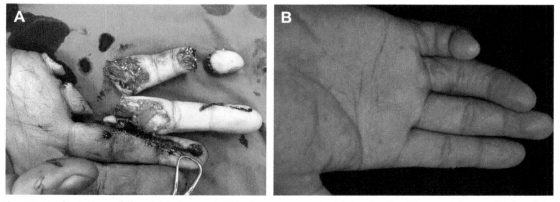

**Fig. 19.** Replantation of the right ring and little fingers severed at 2 levels of a 56-year-old man. At the distal amputation level of the little finger, one digital artery and one vein were anastomosed (performed by Jing Chen, MD). (*A*) Before surgery. (*B*) 6 months after surgery.

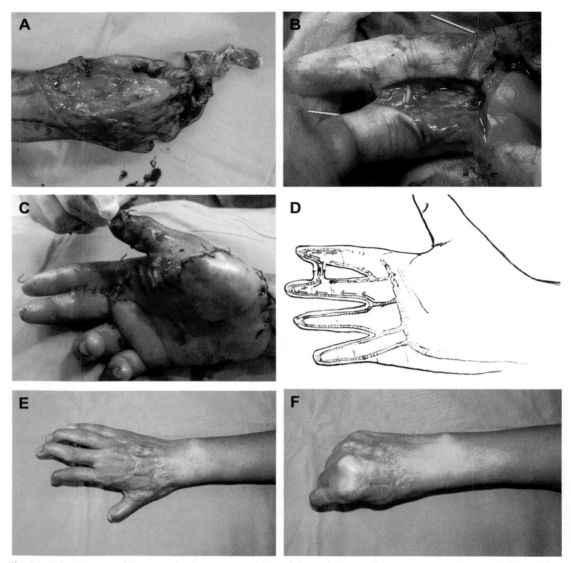

**Fig. 20.** (*A*) A 38-year-old woman had massive avulsion of the soft tissue of the right hand. Thumb, index, middle fingers had no skin and subcutaneous tissue coverage. The index finger had no arterial supply. (*B*) Therefore, a digital artery in the middle finger was taken to reconstruct the blood supply in the index finger. (*C*) Skin closure after anastomosis of the digital artery. (*D*) A drawing showing the arterial blood flow in the fingers. Six weeks later, the pedicle between the index and middle finger was cut and both index and middle finger had good blood supplies and survived well. (*E, F*) The hand seen 1.5 years after surgery. (*Courtesy of* Yi Ming Cai, MD.)

3. Anastomosis of bilateral digital arteries and 3 veins is urged for an amputated digit if the patient lives in a cold region; in Northern China, repair of bilateral arteries of a digit is popular because cold intolerance of the digit is often a problem. Anastomosis of bilateral digital arteries and 3 veins would also increase the chance of replant survival and decrease the impact of vascular crisis of any vessels.

4. Skin substitutes are available. It is wise to use them to ease the tension of a skin closure, avoid compression to repaired vessels, or reduce surgical time and complexity of grafting tissues.

5. Be prepared for exploration and reanastomosis during the first few days after replantation. Exploration and reanastomosis are keys to improve digital survival rate. Timely exploration, release of local compression, reanastomosis of vessels, or grafting a vein to replace a

thrombosed artery is also key to increase survival rate.

In reports, survival rates of replants have been usually presented. It is true that the success of a replantation surgery is judged according to survival of the replant. However, many do not describe the functional status of a digit or a hand. The replanted digits often have decreased touch sensation (or lack it completely), stiffness, marked cold intolerance, and poor cosmetic appearance, similar to a digit after soft tissue, bone, nerve, or tendon repairs.[41–48] The above problems are the reasons terminalization of the single digit is also a common practice when the patient has been fully informed about the risks of re-exploration, stiffness, nerve pain, cold intolerance, secondary surgery, and time off work.[49–52] These problems are the challenges and future targets in improving true success in replanted digits.

Because replantation surgery is extremely expertise-dependent, we suggest that level of expertise of the surgeons be included into future reports on this subject.[53–55] There has been a growing number of reports including the information about the expertise levels, particularly when the reports are about a difficult procedure or analysis of success and failure rates.[56–58] With the inclusion, the outcomes can be interpreted along with expertise levels of the surgeons and success rate and functional outcomes of replantation analyzed against expertise levels of the surgeons.

## SUMMARY

The survival rates of digital replantation range from 65% to 85% in most countries. Asian surgeons tend to challenge themselves more often in performing very complex and difficult digital replantations. The tissue defects in the traumatized zones of a digit may be repaired with a venous flap from the forearm, a pedicled digital artery flap, or a free flap from the foot to serve as a flow-through flap. Straightforward single-digit amputations can be replanted with the patient wide awake, with local anesthesia, and with epinephrine injection to the digits without use of a tourniquet. The authors have introduced a few new methods for extremely challenging cases, such as *a structure-by-structure method* for replanting multiple digits of a hand and a *dry (bloodless) replantation technique* for replanting a digit severed at 2 or more levels. Multiple surgical teams and microsurgical expertise among all team members are essential for such cases.

## ACKNOWLEDGMENTS

We acknowledge the following expert replantation surgeons who provided their insight and cases that are included in this review: J. Chen, MD, Affiliated Hospital of Nantong Unviersity, Jiangsu; Wu Li Yang, MD, Changde Orthopedic Hospital, Hunan; Shusen Cui, MD, Jinan Japan-China Friendship Hospital of Jinin University, Jinin; Jian Xi Hou, MD, Renji Traumatology and Microsurgery Hospital, Zhengzhou, Henan; Li Shan Zhang, MD, Lin Feng Liu, MD, Shandong Provincial Hospital, Jinan; Yi Ming Cai, MD, Shanghai Sixth People's Hospital, Shanghai; Xiao Zhou, MD, Wuxi Ninth People's Hospital, Jiangsu; Jin Liang Zhang, MD, Sunde Heping Surgical Hospital, Fushan, Guangdong, China. The contributors' names are also printed in the figure legends.

## REFERENCES

1. Hustedt JW, Bohl DD, Champagne L. The detrimental effect of decentralization in digital replantation in the United States: 15 years of evidence from the national inpatient sample. J Hand Surg Am 2016;41:593–601.

2. Breahna A, Siddiqui A, Fitzgerald O'Connor E, et al. Replantation of digits: a review of predictive factors for survival. J Hand Surg Eur Vol 2016;41:753–7.

3. Shauver MJ, Nishizuka T, Hirata H, et al. Traumatic finger amputation treatment preference among hand surgeons in the United States and Japan. Plast Reconstr Surg 2016;137:1193–202.

4. Nishizuka T, Shauver MJ, Zhong L, et al. A comparative study of attitudes regarding digit replantation in the United States and Japan. J Hand Surg Am 2015;40:1646–56. e1–3.

5. Mahmoudi E, Swiatek PR, Chung KC, et al. Racial variation in treatment of traumatic finger/thumb amputation: a national comparative study of replantation and revision amputation. Plast Reconstr Surg 2016;137:576e–85e.

6. Haas EM, Volkmer E, Holzbach T, et al. Optimising care structures for severe hand trauma and replantation and chances of launching a national network. Handchir Mikrochir Plast Chir 2013;45: 318–22.

7. Sears ED, Chung KC. Replantation of finger avulsion injuries: a systematic review of survival and functional outcomes. J Hand Surg Am 2011;36:686–94.

8. Ge J, Zhu XZ, Wang Z, et al. A report of survival of all replanted 10 digits of a patient. Chin J Hand Surg 1986;2:44–6.

9. Wang CQ, Cai JF, Fan QS, et al. A case of successful replantation of completed severed ten digits of both hands. Medical Journal of Chinese People's Liberation Army 1988;13:141.

10. Cai LF, Xin CT, Tian LJ, et al. Complete survival of re-planted ten digits. A case report. Chin J Microsurg 1990;13:234–5.

11. Li QT, Zhang CQ, Yang KF, et al. Successful replan-tation of completed severed 10 digits in a case. Chin J Hand Surg 1995;33:283–4.

12. Ou YF, Deng JQ, Peng YG, et al. Report of a case of successful replantation of 10 digits. Chin J Micro-surg 1996;19:78.

13. Yang RG, Zhou MW, Chen Z, et al. A case of replan-tation of 10 digits of both hands in a deaf. Chin J Hand Surg 1998;14:246.

14. Xie ZR, Liang M, Yin L. Successful replantation in ten digits of both hands of a patient. Chin J Microsurg 1998;21:247.

15. Xie CP, Zhao DS, Zhang W, et al. Three cases of suc-cessful replantation of ten-digit amputation. Chin J Microsurg 1999;22:61.

16. Liu XY, Zhen P, Ge BF, et al. Survival of replantated ten digits with crush injuries in a case. Chin J Micro-surg 2000;23:31.

17. Zhao HR, Deng WX, Liu BH, et al. Successful replan-tation of ten-digit amputation of a case. Chin J Hand Surg 2000;16:228.

18. Wang ZT, Li J, Chen FS, et al. A case of replantation in ten-digit amputation with anastomosis of 60 ves-sels. Chin J Hand Surg 2001;17:69.

19. Zhu JK, Liu ZW, Chen JF, et al. Survival of replanted ten digits after complete severance. Chin J Practical Hand Surg 2001;15:252–3.

20. Xie ZR, Yin L, Liang M. Follow-up results of function of replanted ten digits. Chin J Microsurg 2003;26:141–2.

21. Cong HB, Sui HM, Wang ZM, et al. Successful replantation of ten amputated digits of both hands. Chin J Microsurg 2002;22:239.

22. Wang CB, Bao YS. Report of a case of successful replantation of completed severed 10 digits. Chin J Microsurg 2004;27:202.

23. Ou YF, Peng YG, Weng YH, et al. Long-term follow-up of functional outcomes of replanted ten digits. Chin J Microsurg 2003;26:301–2.

24. Liu JY, Fan XH, Zhuang FF. A case of successful replantation of completed severed 10 digits of both hands. Military Medical Journal of Southeast China 2006;8:17.

25. Cui SS, Li R, Li CY, et al. Survival of replantation in amputated ten digits with comminuted frac-tures and ecchymosis. Chin J Microsurg 2009; 32:173–4.

26. Cong HB, Sui HM, Wang ZM, et al. Ten-digit replan-tation with seven years follow-up: a case report. Microsurgery 2010;30:405–9.

27. Wang XY, Su WJ, Chen L, et al. Successful replanta-tion of amputated ten digits in a patient. Chin J Mi-crosurg 2012;35:9.

28. Xie WY, Zhang XS, Chen XZ, et al. Successful replantation in amputated ten digits of a case

and review of literature. Chin J Microsurg 2014; 37:504–7.

29. Lalonde D, Bell M, Benoit P, et al. A multicenter pro-spective study of 3,110 consecutive cases of elec-tive epinephrine use in the fingers and hand: the Dalhousie Project clinical phase. J Hand Surg Am 2005;30:1061–7.

30. Ilicki J. Safety of Epinephrine in digital nerve blocks: a literature review. J Emerg Med 2015;49:799–809.

31. Hutting K, van Rappard JR, Prins A, et al. Digital ne-crosis after local anaesthesia with epinephrine. Ned Tijdschr Geneeskd 2015;159:A9477.

32. Lalonde D, Martin A. Epinephrine in local anes-thesia in finger and hand surgery: the case for wide-awake anesthesia. J Am Acad Orthop Surg 2013;21:443–7.

33. Sylaidis P, Logan A. Digital blocks with adrenaline. an old dogma refuted. J Hand Surg Am 1998;23: 17–9.

34. Gu X, Simons FE, Simons KJ. Epinephrine ab-sorption after different routes of administration in an animal model. Biopharm Drug Dispos 1999; 20:401–5.

35. Green D, Walter J, Heden R, et al. The effects of local anesthetics containing epinephrine on digital blood perfusion. J Am Podiatr Med Assoc 1992;82:98–110.

36. Hinterberger JW, Kintzi HE. Phentolamine reversal of epinephrine-induced digital vasospasm. How to save an ischemic finger. Arch Fam Med 1994;3: 193–5.

37. Jackson DM. The diagnosis of the depth of burning. Br J Surg 1953;40:588–96.

38. Chen L, Chiu DT. Spiral interrupted suturing tech-nique for microvascular anastomosis: a comparative study. Microsurgery 1986;7:72–8.

39. Butler DP, Murugesan L, Ruston J, et al. The out-comes of digital tip amputation replacement as a composite graft in a paediatric population. J Hand Surg Eur Vol 2016;41:164–70.

40. Cheng L, Chen K, Chai YM, et al. Fingertip replanta-tion at the eponychial level with venous anasto-mosis: an anatomic study and clinical application. J Hand Surg Eur Vol 2013;38:959–63.

41. Kwon GD, Ahn BM, Lee JS, et al. Clinical outcomes of a simultaneous replantation technique for ampu-tations of four or five digits. Microsurgery 2016;36: 225–9.

42. Ma Z, Guo F, Qi J, et al. Effects of non-surgical fac-tors on digital replantation survival rate: a meta-anal-ysis. J Hand Surg Eur Vol 2016;41:157–63.

43. Panattoni JB, De Ona IR, Ahmed MM. Recon-struction of fingertip injuries: surgical tips and avoiding complications. J Hand Surg Am 2015; 40:1016–24.

44. Prucz RB, Friedrich JB. Upper extremity replanta-tion: current concepts. Plast Reconstr Surg 2014; 133:333–42.

45. Sun YC, Chen QZ, Chen J, et al. Prevalence, characteristics and natural history of cold intolerance after the reverse digital artery flap. J Hand Surg Eur Vol 2016;41:171–6.

46. Chen QZ, Sun YC, Chen J, et al. Comparative study of functional and aesthetically outcomes of reverse digital artery and reverse dorsal homodigital island flaps for fingertip repair. J Hand Surg Eur Vol 2015;40:935–43.

47. Liodaki E, Xing SG, Mailaender P, et al. Management of difficult intra-articular fractures or fracture dislocations of the proximal interphalangeal joint. J Hand Surg Eur Vol 2015;40:16–23.

48. Tang JB, Blazar PE, Giddins G, et al. Overview of indications, preferred methods and technical tips for hand fractures from around the world. J Hand Surg Eur Vol 2015;40:88–97.

49. Tang JB, Elliot D, Adani R, et al. Repair and reconstruction of thumb and finger tip injuries: a global view. Clin Plast Surg 2014;41:325–59.

50. Lee SH, Jang JH, Kim JI, et al. Modified anterograde pedicle advancement flap in fingertip injury. J Hand Surg Eur Vol 2015;40:944–51.

51. Usami S, Kawahara S, Yamaguchi Y, et al. Homodigital artery flap reconstruction for fingertip amputation: a comparative study of the oblique triangular neurovascular advancement flap and the reverse digital artery island flap. J Hand Surg Eur Vol 2015;40:291–7.

52. El-Diwany M, Odobescu A, Bélanger-Douet M, et al. Replantation vs revision amputation in single digit zone II amputations. J Plast Reconstr Aesthet Surg 2015;68:859–63.

53. Tang JB. Re: Levels of experience of surgeons in clinical studies. J Hand Surg Eur Vol 2009;34:137–8.

54. Tang JB. Outcomes and evaluation of flexor tendon repair. Hand Clin 2013;29:251–9.

55. Tang JB, Giddins G. Why and how to report surgeons' levels of expertise. J Hand Surg Eur Vol 2016;41:365–6.

56. Storey PA, Goddard M, Clegg C, et al. Pyrocarbon proximal interphalangeal joint arthroplasty: a medium to long term follow-up of a single surgeon series. J Hand Surg Eur Vol 2015;40:952–6.

57. Mattila S, Waris E. Unfavourable short-term outcomes of a poly-L/D-lactide scaffold for thumb trapeziometacarpal arthroplasty. J Hand Surg Eur Vol 2016;41:328–34.

58. Sletten IN, Hellund JC, Olsen B, et al. Conservative treatment has comparable outcome with bouquet pinning of little finger metacarpal neck fractures: a multicentre randomized controlled study of 85 patients. J Hand Surg Eur Vol 2015; 40:76–83.

# Exploring New Frontiers of Microsurgery
## From Anatomy to Clinical Methods

Zeng Tao Wang, MD[a],*, You Mao Zheng, MD[b],
Lei Zhu, MD[c], Li Wen Hao, MD[a], Ya Bin Zhang, MD[d],
Chao Chen, MD[a], Li Feng Xia, MD[d], Lin Feng Liu, MD[e]

## KEYWORDS

- Microsurgery • Anatomy • Vasculature of flaps • Vascularized joint transfer • Miniflap
- Perforator flap

## KEY POINTS

- This article describe anatomic studies of the hand to develop new microvascular flaps, including the cutaneous branch network system of the lateral side of the finger, the anatomic relationship between the cutaneous branches of the proper digital artery and proper digital nerve, and the anatomy of perforator arteries in the thenar region.
- The article presents our experience in clinical applications of 8 miniflaps for hand reconstruction.
- The article describes findings and discusses the anatomy and clinical use of several flaps, including the dorsalis pedis flap, the medialis pedis vascular network flap, and the lateral pedis vascular network flap.
- The article describes our experience of vascularized free toe joint transfer, and presents our method to improve the range of active motion following toe joint transplant.

## INTRODUCTION

Over the past decades, the authors have sought to explore new frontiers in microsurgery to improve functional and aesthetic outcomes following microsurgical reconstruction of the hand. Our approach has been multidirectional toward this goal. This article outlines our efforts and describes how novel microsurgical ideas and procedures can be developed based on a more profound understanding of anatomy and functionality of the donor site tissue used in tissue transfer.

This article discusses 4 topics: (1) anatomic study of the hand for developing new flaps; (2) application of miniflaps from the hand, including clinical experience with 8 unique flaps in the hand; (3) anatomic and clinical discussion concerning several flaps from other parts of the human body; (4) our methods and outcomes in vascularized free toe joint transfer.

## ANATOMY OF THE HAND FOR DEVELOPING NEW FLAPS

Choosing the hand region as a flap donor site for the repair of soft tissue hand defects can offer better function and appearance following reconstruction.[1–5] However, these surgeries may damage

The authors have nothing to disclose.
[a] Department of Hand and Foot Surgery, Shandong Provincial Hospital, Shandong University, 324 Jingwu Road, Jinan 250021, Shandong, China; [b] Department of Hand and Foot Surgery, Enze Hospital of Taizhou Enze Medical Center (Group), No. 1 Tongyang Road, Luqiao District, Taizhou 318000, Zhejiang, China; [c] Department of Hand and Foot Surgery, Qilu Hospital of Shandong University, 107 Wenhuaxi Road, Jinan 250012, Shandong, China; [d] Department of Hand and Foot Surgery, The Fourth People's Hospital of Shanxi Province, 512 Xianningdong Road, Xian 710043, Shanxi, China; [e] Department of Hand Surgery, Weinan Hand and Foot Surgery Hospital, 150 Laocheng Road, Weinan 714000, Shanxi, China
* Corresponding author.
E-mail address: wzt@sdu.edu.cn

major vessels of the hand during flap harvest. To address this concern, the investigators have explored the use of miniflaps from the hand and wrist regions to repair tissue defects in the hand since the year 2000. In exploring these miniflaps, our goals were to (1) limit the size of donor sites to allow direct closure; (2) carefully elevate flaps, preserving major vessels and nerves; and (3) better match the flap and recipient site's skin color and texture.

### Lateral Cutaneous Arterial Network of the Fingers

Several dorsal cutaneous branches arise from the proper digital artery at the proximal and middle phalanges.[6–8] These dorsal cutaneous branches are 0.1 to 0.3 mm in diameter and form a vascular chain through which ample blood flows. The dorsal cutaneous branches travel from lateral to dorsal along the finger, arborizing into smaller secondary branches and then into ascending and descending branches. These branches connect to neighboring vessels to form a chain of cutaneous branches covering the lateral aspect of the finger (**Fig. 1**). This network of cutaneous vessels allows the design of pedicle flaps without the need to sacrifice the digital artery in fingers when surgeons confirm abundant blood supply through the network.

### Anatomic Relationship Between Cutaneous Branches of Digital Artery and Digital Nerve

The proper digital artery accompanies the proper digital nerve in the finger and lays deep to the proper digital nerve. The number of cutaneous branches running volar to the proper digital nerve is usually greater than those dorsal to the nerve (**Fig. 2**). Very rarely, more cutaneous branches of the digital artery travel dorsal to the digital nerve rather than volar to it.

When harvesting a miniflap, 1 side of the cutaneous branches is sacrificed in order to preserve the proper digital nerve. By carefully identifying all cutaneous branches from the proper digital artery, surgeons should ligate the side with fewer cutaneous branches during dissection to preserve a more robust blood supply to the flap (**Fig. 3**).

### Anatomy of Perforator Arteries in the Thenar Region

The perforator arteries in the thenar region originate from several distinct vascular sources. These perforator arteries can travel through 3 different muscular septa, creating longitudinal cutaneous branch network systems of the thenar soft tissue. One such septum exists between the radial side of the extensor pollicis brevis and the first metacarpal bone, where several cutaneous branches from the first dorsal metacarpal artery often exist (**Fig. 4**). Another septum between the abductor pollicis brevis and flexor pollicis brevis contains 1 to 3 cutaneous branches that arise off the superficial branch of the radial artery and the princeps pollicis artery and their arterial connection (**Fig. 5**). At the ulnar side of the superficial head of the flexor pollicis brevis, a rather large cutaneous branch originats off the superficial palmar arch, connecting to vessels of the radial proper digital artery of the index finger or from the princeps pollicis artery (see **Fig. 5**).

## MINIFLAPS FROM THE HAND

Soft tissue deficits often result in traumatic finger injuries. The authors believe that the best reconstructive option for these soft tissue defects in the finger, especially the fingertip or pulp, is a

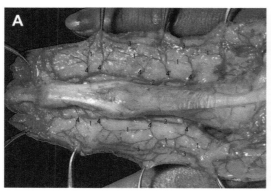
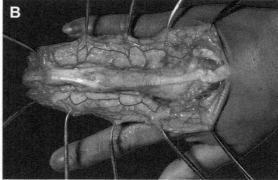

**Fig. 1.** Numbers and location of dorsal cutaneous branches from the digital artery. (*A*) 1, dorsal cutaneous branches; 2, proper digital artery and nerve; 3, dorsal digital vein; 4, dorsal cutaneous branches. (*B*) In the same specimen shown in *A*, the dorsal cutaneous branches is highlighted with red ink showing continuity of the network along the entire length of the finger. Though in most fingers this network is large, the network is small in some fingers. (*Courtesy of* Zeng Tao Wang, MD.)

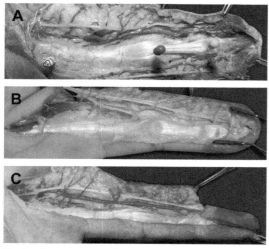

Fig. 2. The anatomic relationships between cutaneous branches of proper digital artery and proper digital nerve. (A) Numbers of cutaneous branches passing volar to the proper digital nerve exceed those along the deep aspect. (B) Cutaneous branches volar and dorsal to the digital nerve are equal in numbers; (C) rarely cutaneous branches dorsal to the digital nerve are more numerous than those volar to the digital nerve. (*Courtesy of* Zeng Tao Wang, MD.)

regional or free flap from the hand or wrist. Various miniflaps harvested from the hand have been reported for smaller soft tissue defects of the hands. The pedicled homodigital flap remains a common option for fingertip defect.[9] Omokawa and colleagues[10,11] described the anatomy and clinical use of a hyothenar flap transfer for fingertip reconstruction. Kim and colleagues[12] reported fingertip reconstruction using a hypothenar perforator flap. Kamei and colleagues[13] published 2

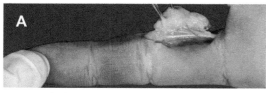

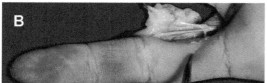

Fig. 3. (A) The side with fewer cutaneous branches from the digital artery is volar to the digital nerve. (B) The branches volar to the digital nerve were divided. (*Courtesy of* Zeng Tao Wang, MD.)

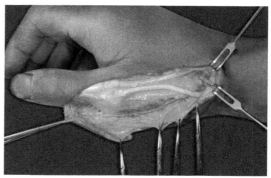

Fig. 4. The first dorsal radial metacarpal artery bifurcates from the radial artery in the anatomic snuff box running in this septum and giving off several cutaneous perforators. (*Courtesy of* Zeng Tao Wang, MD.)

cases of free thenar flaps pedicled on the superficial palmar branch of the radial artery for reconstruction of soft tissue defect in the hand. Omokawa and colleagues[14] went on to describe the vascular and neural anatomy of the thenar region in further detail. Iwuagwu and colleagues[15] introduced the use of free thenar flap based on the deep (main) branch of the superficial palmar branch of the radial artery. Zhu and colleagues[16] used digital artery perforator flaps in fingertip reconstruction. This article presents our experience in using 8 types of miniflaps from the hand and wrist to repair defects in the fingers and thumb.

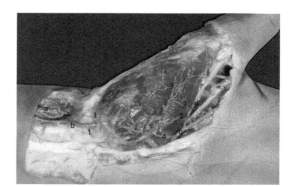

Fig. 5. Arterial supplies in the thenar area. a, radial artery; b, superficial palmar branch of the radial artery; c, superficial palmar arch; d, communicating branch between the superficial palmar arch and princeps pollicis artery; 1, cutaneous branches of the superficial palmar branch of the radial artery; 2, cutaneous branches from communicating branch between superficial palmar arch and princeps pollicis artery; 3, cutaneous branch perforating between abductor pollicis brevis and flexor pollicis brevis; 4, cutaneous branch of the superficial palmar arch. (*Courtesy of* Zeng Tao Wang, MD.)

### Digital Artery Cutaneous Branch Network Flap

A digital island flap pedicled on the proper digital artery is easy to harvest, but this procedure sacrifices a proper digital vascular bundle.[17–19] In 2006, the authors designed a flap on the lateral side of the proximal phalanx based on the vascular network of dorsal cutaneous branches off the proper digital vessels (**Fig. 6**). The axis of the flap lies along the midlateral line of the finger. To protect the vascular network on the lateral side of the finger, the authors include fascia with a width of 5 to 10 mm around the pedicle. Before flap harvest, the authors routinely test clamping major branches from the digital artery to the flap to ascertain that blood supply from neighboring branch network to the flap is sufficient. If the authors find the blood supply from the network is insufficient, the authors either abandon this type of the flap, or instead harvest the flap as a free flap based on a main branch that is clamped, or the authors harvest this flap based on the digital artery. The authors had to change the surgical plan in 20% of our patients. Preoperatively the authors could rule out 10% of fingers, which have no good network based on ultrasound or angiography. In other words, in 30% of the fingers, the arterial network flap cannot be harvested. The flap was transferred distally to cover soft tissue defects in the finger. The sensory nerve branch innervating the flap was coapted to the distal stump of the proper digital nerve.

Preoperative ultrasound or angiography can help rule out the fingers which have no reliable branch networks. However, plan changes based on intraoperative test clamping of the vessels to the flap are important. This flap could be harvested in about 70% of the fingers in our patients, in which blood supply through the network was reliable.

The authors applied this flap technique in 55 cases of finger pulp or nail bed loss associated with exposure of distal phalanx bone or the insertion site of the flexor digitorum profundus (FDP) tendon. This flap was introduced by the lead author (Wang ZT), and a coauthor (Zheng YM) performed most of the procedures presented here. Postoperative follow-up for these patients ranged from 6 to 12 months. Partial necrosis of the flap occurred in 2 cases (3.6%), and the wounds in these 2 cases healed with local debridement and regeneration with granulation tissue. All of the other patients recovered well from the procedure, with an acceptable appearance and texture of the flaps. Static 2-point discrimination on the flaps ranged from 8 to 12 mm at the time of follow-up. The donor site and clinical outcomes have proved to be identical to the digital artery island flap; however, both proper digital arteries of the finger are spared by using the digital artery cutaneous branch network instead of the proper digital artery for vascular supply.

This flap is illustrated in a 22-year-old man with a soft tissue and nail bed defect of the left index finger. A digital artery cutaneous branch network flap off the radial index finger was planned (**Fig. 7**A). The flap, based on the vascular network of dorsal cutaneous branches off the proper digital artery, was raised and transferred to the cover nail bed defect (**Fig. 7**B, C). A follow-up at 6 months after surgery showed that the flap survived completely with a hypertrophic linear scar at the donor site (**Fig. 7**D, E).

### Free Digital Artery Perforator Flap

The main disadvantage of a digital artery pedicle flap is the required sacrifice of 1 digital artery. This disadvantage can be overcome by using a flap based on the cutaneous branch network of the digital artery. The key to success in the cutaneous branch network flap is the meticulous identification of cutaneous branch connections. Both digital artery pedicle flaps and digital artery cutaneous branch network pedicle flaps leave a visible surgical scar between flap recipient site and donor site. A limitation of the 2 flaps is that they cannot be used to reconstruct soft tissue defects within the proximal phalangeal region.

Based on our anatomic studies, the diameter of the 2 major dorsal cutaneous branches of the proper

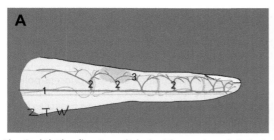
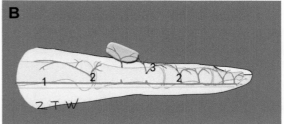

**Fig. 6.** (A) The flap is pedicled with a series of digital artery cutaneous branches: 1, proper digital artery; 2, cutaneous branches from proper digital artery; 3, digital artery cutaneous branches. (B) The flap is elevated and transferred distally.

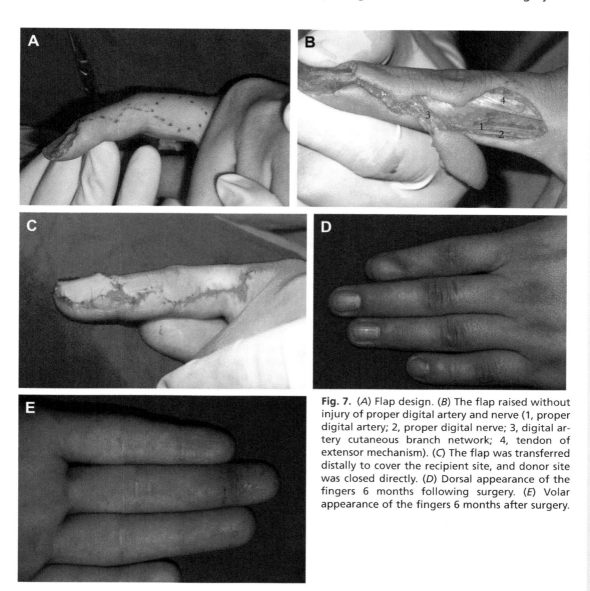

Fig. 7. (A) Flap design. (B) The flap raised without injury of proper digital artery and nerve (1, proper digital artery; 2, proper digital nerve; 3, digital artery cutaneous branch network; 4, tendon of extensor mechanism). (C) The flap was transferred distally to cover the recipient site, and donor site was closed directly. (D) Dorsal appearance of the fingers 6 months following surgery. (E) Volar appearance of the fingers 6 months after surgery.

digital artery is 0.1 mm to 0.3 mm at their origins where they bifurcate off the proper digital artery (see **Fig. 1**). A free flap based on cutaneous branch arteries and dorsal finger vein drainage can be designed with vascular anastomoses performed using 12-0 sutures (**Fig. 8**).[6] Since 2009, the authors have performed 30 cases using free digital artery cutaneous branch flap transfer. Most of the procedures were performed by coauthors (Zhu L and Hao LW) based on an idea from, and the first few procedures performed by, the lead author. The flap sizes ranged from 1.8 × 0.9 cm to 3 × 2 cm. All flaps survived well, without vascular complications. Prolonged mild flap edema was observed in 9 cases

until up to 6 months following surgery. All edema eventually subsided in the flaps, restoring a better flap to recipient site match, which continued to improve as time progressed.

This technique was shown in a 35-year-old man presenting with a fingertip defect in the right index finger. A digital artery perforator flap off the radial side of the middle finger was outlined (**Fig. 9**A). Dissection of the flap began along the dorsal finger and progressed palmarly, exposing the digital artery as well as its perforators (**Fig. 9**B). The flap was raised and transferred to cover the soft tissue defect of the fingertip (**Fig. 9**C, D). The flap survived with a mild bulky appearance at 3 years follow-up.

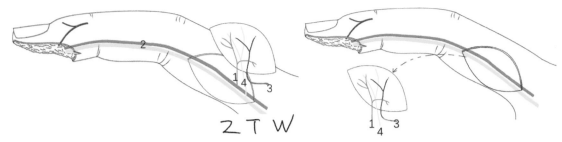

**Fig. 8.** The design of free digital artery perforator flap: 1, cutaneous branches originated from proper digital artery (pedicle); 2, proper digital artery and nerve; 3, dorsal digital vein; 4, branch of proper digital nerve.

### Free Superficial Palmar Branch of the Radial Artery Flap

The superficial palmar branch of the radial artery gives off several cutaneous branches that supply the radial palmar skin before entering the abductor pollicis brevis muscle. These cutaneous branches have connections with other cutaneous branches in the thenar region, allowing larger flaps to be designed based on the superficial palmar branch of the radial artery (see **Fig. 5**). A free flap can be raised based on the superficial palmar branch of the radial artery (**Fig. 10**), which can be anastomosed to the proper digital artery, or can be used to repair a digital artery defect as a flow-through flap. Depending on the specific needs, the flap can be designed with varying sizes, locations, and shapes. An example of this clinically advantageous flexibility in flap design is seen in soft tissue reconstruction of the finger. For defects on the dorsal finger, a flap can be raised proximal to the transverse wrist crease out of the glabrous palmar skin, providing a better skin match to the dorsal finger skin. In contrast, for defects of the volar glabrous skin, a flap can be raised distal to the transverse wrist crease. In addition, lateral finger defects can be reconstructed using a flap design centered on transverse wrist crease to include both skin types along with the natural transition.

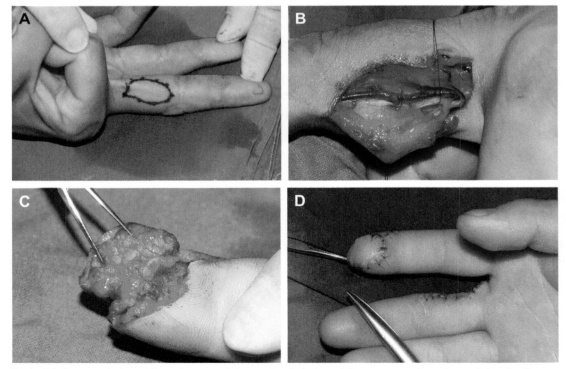

**Fig. 9.** (*A*) Flap was designed from the area of the proximal phalanx. (*B*) A cutaneous branch supplying the flap was identified. (*C*) The cutaneous branch was anastomosed to the proper digital artery. (*D*) Immediately after surgery.

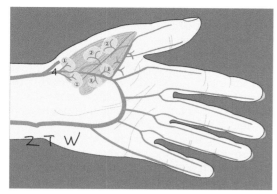

**Fig. 10.** Design of several flaps in the thenar area (1, cutaneous branches from superficial palmar branch of the radial artery; 2, cutaneous branches emerge between the abductor pollicis brevis and flexor pollicis brevis; 3, cutaneous branches from the superficial palmar arch; 4, superficial palmar branch of the radial artery).

The surgical team led by a coauthor (Zhang YB) applied this flap technique in 33 cases from June 2003 to June 2015. Venous insufficiency of the transferred flap occurred in 1 case, which was salvaged with immediate exploration and revision of the vein anastomosis. Partial necrosis occurred in another case, which healed with local debridement and ingrowth of granulation tissue to the necrotic area. Thirty cases were followed and showed acceptable cosmetic outcomes.

This flap was illustrated in a 37-year-old man who had soft tissue loss over the lateral distal phalanx of the left thumb associated with exposure of distal phalanx. The authors designed a flap based on the superficial palmar branch perforators of the radial artery. The flap was harvested by first incising the proximal margin of the flap, taking care to identify and preserve the superficial venous drainage system. Next, the flap was elevated to identify the superficial palmar branch of the radial artery while preserving the cutaneous perforators. Afterwards, the free flap was harvested and transferred to the recipient site. The superficial palmar branch of the radial artery was anastomosed to a proper digital artery and the superficial vein was anastomosed to a dorsal thumb vein under an operating microscope. The flap provides good skin coverage to the defect site, which can be seen at 6 months after surgery (**Fig. 11**).

### Free Midthenar Flap

In the midthenar area, cutaneous vascular branches emerge between the abductor pollicis

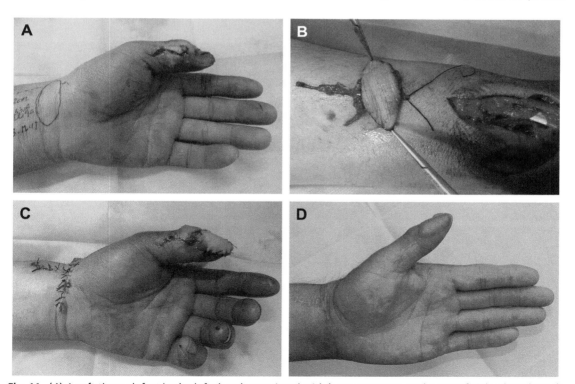

**Fig. 11.** (*A*) A soft tissue defect in the left thumb associated with bone exposure, and a superficial palmar branch of radial artery flap outlined at the proximal radial palm region. (*B*) The flap was raised. (*C*) The free flap was transferred to cover the soft tissue defect. The flap donor site was closed directly. (*D*) Good appearance of the flap coverage site and donor site 6 months after surgery.

brevis and flexor pollicis brevis (see **Fig. 5**). The diameter of these cutaneous branches is larger than 0.2 mm, and superficial veins in this region are abundant. The authors have designed flaps that are supplied by a cutaneous artery and drained by superficial veins (see **Fig. 10**). The authors applied this approach in 9 cases from November 2007 to January 2015 with no flap losses.

One such case was a 27-year-old man who presented with a soft tissue defect over the ulnar aspect of the distal interphalangeal joint of the left small finger, with the FDP tendon and the distal phalanx exposed (**Fig. 12**A). Cutaneous arterial branch locations in the muscle septum between the abductor pollicis brevis and flexor pollicis brevis were identified by Doppler examination preoperatively. The authors designed a thenar flap centered on these identified cutaneous arteries (**Fig. 12**B). Flaps were harvested by first incising along the ulnar margin of the flap, identifying 1 to 2 superficial veins and dissecting an appropriate length of these veins to serve as the flap drainage vessels. Through an incision in the proximal margin, the sensory nerve branches to the flap were also identified and divided with enough length. Second, dissection was continued deeper until the fascia of the superficial head of the flexor pollicis brevis was reached, then the flap was

undermined radially in the prefascial plane over the flexor pollicis brevis muscle until reaching the septum between the abductor pollicis brevis and the flexor pollicis brevis muscles. Third, cutaneous branch perforators in the septum were carefully identified, then dissected free deeper for a longer pedicle and larger vessel diameter (**Fig. 12**C). Fourth, the cutaneous artery branch was ligated and the flap freed. Fifth, the flap was transferred to the recipient site and microvascular anastomoses performed between the cutaneous arterial branch of the flap to the digital artery and between the superficial veins of the flap to the superficial veins of the finger (**Fig. 12**D). The sensory nerve was coapted with the proximal stump of the ulnar proper digital nerve. The 2-year follow-up image shows complete survival of the transferred flap with a good cosmetic appearance. Static 2-point discrimination of the flap was 11 mm.

## Free Ulnar Thenar Flap

The superficial palmar branch of the radial artery becomes the radial superficial palmar arch after passing beneath the abductor pollicis brevis. Several cutaneous branches of larger diameter come from the superficial palmar arch and can be used in free flap design (see **Figs. 5** and **10**).

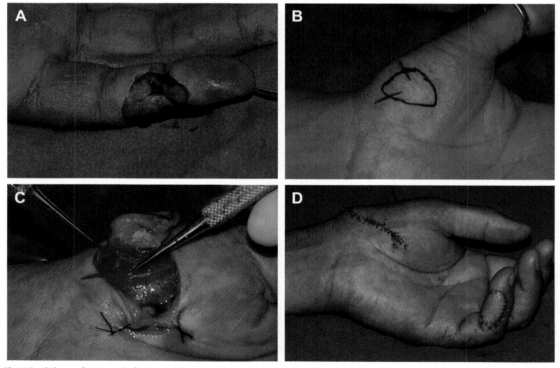

**Fig. 12.** (*A*) A soft tissue defect over the volar aspect of the left little finger with tendons and joint exposure. (*B*) Flap design. (*C*) Exposure of the flap pedicle (based on a cutaneous arterial branch). (*D*) Donor site was closed directly.

Because the recurrent branch of the median nerve is also situated in this area, raising a flap based on cutaneous branch perforators from the superficial palmar arch requires extra care to avoid nerve injury. The authors also recommend limiting the size of flaps from this location in order to allow direct closure of the donor sites.

The authors (Zheng YM and his team) applied this flap technique in 9 patients from May 2009 to March 2015 with no flap losses. Here the authors present the technique in a 20-year-old man who sustained a finger pulp injury of his left middle finger associated with exposure of the distal phalanx and the insertion of the FDP tendon. The authors designed a cutaneous branch flap from the proximal ulnar thenar region of about 2 × 2.5 cm (**Fig. 13**A).

First, the authors incised the proximal radial margin of the flap, identifying 1 to 2 superficial veins and dissecting an appropriate length of these veins to serve as the flap drainage vessels. A sensory nerve to the flap was also identified and preserved (**Fig. 13**B).

Second, the incision was extended distally and dissection was carried down to the fascia of the superficial head of the flexor pollicis brevis and then undermined ulnarly in the prefascial plane over the flexor pollicis brevis muscle.

Third, the cutaneous branch arterial perforators from the superficial palmar arch were carefully identified. The authors incised the ulnar margin and elevated the flap supplied by the cutaneous branch originating from the superficial palmar arch and drained by the superficial veins (**Fig. 13**C, D).

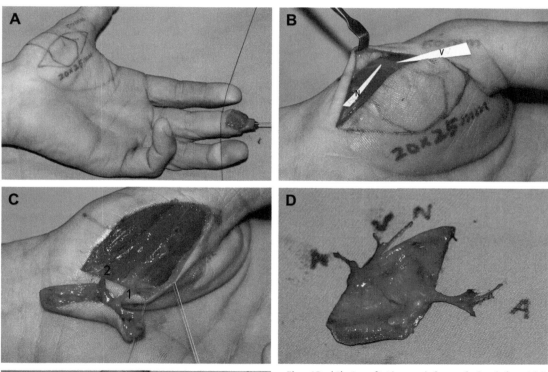

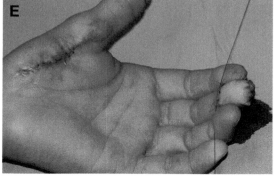

Fig. 13. (*A*) A soft tissue defect of the left middle finger with exposure of the bone and the FDP tendon. Preoperative flap design. (*B*) A superficial vein (*V*) and sensory nerve (*N*) were identified. (*C*) The flap was elevated and showed 2 cutaneous arteries: 1, a cutaneous artery from superficial palmar arch; 2, a cutaneous artery issued from abductor pollicis brevis. (*D*) Flap was harvested. (*E*) Completion of the flap transfer.

Fourth, the flap was transfer to the recipient site and vascular anastomoses were performed under an operating microscope (**Fig. 13**E). At 6 months' follow-up, the flap showed an excellent cosmetic appearance and static 2-point discrimination of 11 mm.

### Free First Dorsal Radial Metacarpal Artery Flap

The first dorsal radial metacarpal artery branches from the radial artery in the anatomic snuff box and runs under the extensor pollicis brevis tendon heading distally along the radial border of the first metacarpal. It delivers several cutaneous branches to the skin of the radial thenar region. This artery can be used in a pedicled flap design (**Fig. 14**A). The superficial venous system is robust in the thenar territory, providing adequate drainage through an often easily identified vein (**Fig. 14**B). There are 3 sensory nerves in this region: the superficial branch of the radial nerve (**Fig. 14**B), the terminal branch of the lateral antebrachial cutaneous nerve, and the superficial thenar sensory branch of the median nerve. The long axis of the flap is designed along the radial border of the first metacarpal bone, around the dorsal and volar skin junction. Similar to the superficial palmar branch of the radial artery flap, flaps can be raised to include varying amounts of glabrous and dorsal hand skin depending on the needs of the recipient sites.

This flap was applied in 23 clinical cases in the lead author's unit from March 2007 to March 2015. Arterial insufficiency of the transferred flap occurred in 1 case and was salvaged with immediate exploration and revision of the arterial anastomosis. All the other flaps survived completely. One such case is a 30-year-old man with soft tissue injury over the radial aspect of the distal left thumb associated with exposure of the distal phalanx. The authors designed a free first dorsal radial metacarpal artery flap to repair the defect (**Fig. 15**A).

First, flap harvesting was begun by incising the dorsal margin of the flap, identifying 1 or 2 superficial veins, and dissecting an appropriate length of these veins to serve as the flap drainage vessels (**Fig. 15**B).

Second, dissection was continued deep along the ulnar side of the extensor pollicis brevis tendon, identifying the first dorsal radial metacarpal artery and 2 sensory nerve branches to the flap (**Fig. 15**C). The 2 sensory nerves are branches of a nerve from the superficial branch of the radial nerve (**Fig. 15**B).

Third, the authors incised the volar skin margin of the flap and dissected dorsally along the prefascial plane (**Fig. 15**C, D).

Fourth, the vessels were divided, and the free flap was transferred to cover the thumb defect. The proximal stump of the radial proper digital artery of the thumb was anastomosed with the first dorsal radial metacarpal artery of the flap, and another cutaneous artery (originated from the palmar superficial branch of the radial artery) of the flap was anastomosed to the distal stump of the radial proper digital artery of the thumb to improve survivability. The vein from the flap was anastomosed with a dorsal digital vein. The cutaneous nerves of the flap were coapted with the radial proper digital nerve (**Fig. 15**E, F). At 6 months' follow-up, the flap had a good appearance with a static 2-point discrimination of 10 mm.

### Cutaneous Branch Perforator Flap Based on the Radial Proper Digital Artery of the Thumb

At least 1 cutaneous branch emerges from the radial proper digital artery of the thumb at the first metacarpal neck region (**Fig. 16**A). After branching from the radial proper digital artery of

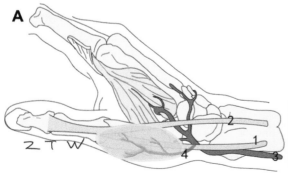
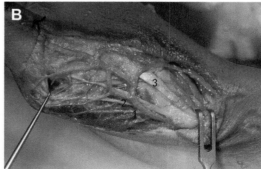

**Fig. 14.** (*A*) The first dorsal radial metacarpal artery flap: 1, extensor pollicis brevis; 2, extensor pollicis longus; 3, radial artery; 4, the first dorsal radial metacarpal artery (pedicle). (*B*) The superficial veins and sensory nerves in area of the first dorsal radial metacarpal artery flap: 1, superficial veins; 2, sensory nerve of the flap; 3, extensor pollicis brevis.

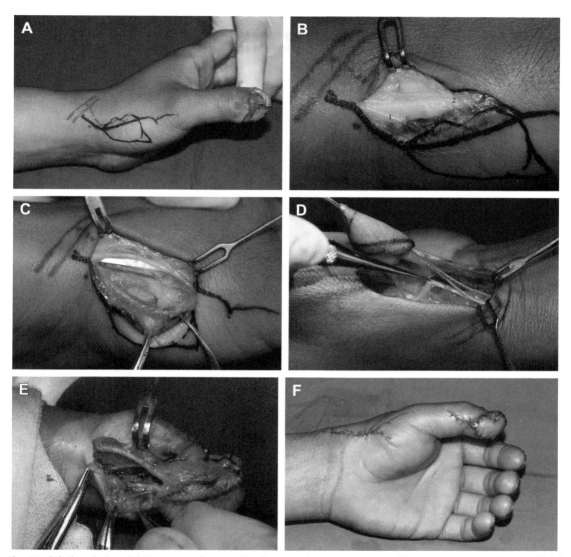

**Fig. 15.** (*A*) Flap design. (*B*) Exposure of a superficial vein and cutaneous nerve (1, cutaneous nerve; 2, superficial vein). (*C*) Exposure of the first dorsal radial metacarpal artery. (*D*) Vessels and nerve were isolated proximally. (*E*) Anastomosis of the pedicle vessels and nerve to those in the recipient site. (*F*) Flap coverage in the recipient site.

the thumb, the cutaneous branch runs in the septum between the abductor pollicis brevis muscle and the neck of the first metacarpal bone. Then, this cutaneous branch gives off several branches supplying the flexor pollicis brevis muscle and the first metacarpophalangeal joint. Terminal branches supply the skin on the distal radial thenar region (see **Fig. 16**A). With this anatomic knowledge, a cutaneous branch flap can be designed on the distal radial thenar skin. The cutaneous branch can be isolated to its origin from the radial proper digital artery to achieve a longer, larger-diameter pedicle facilitating microvascular anastomoses (**Fig. 16**B, C).

One coauthor (Zhang YB) and his team applied this flap technique in 19 cases from July 2007 to January 2015 based on the lead author's idea for flap design. There were no flap losses. A case of a soft tissue defect over the radial aspect of the distal phalanx on the left index finger associated with bone exposure in a 31-year-old man is presented here. The authors designed the distal radial thenar skin flap based on a cutaneous branch vessel from the radial proper digital artery of the thumb at the first metacarpal neck region. Flap harvesting techniques were performed as follows:

First, the authors incised the volar margin of the flap. The incision was deepened until the abductor

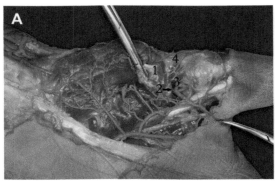

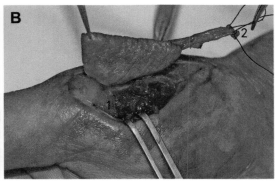

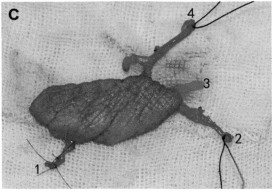

**Fig. 16.** (*A*) The perforator artery runs at the radial side of neck of the first metacarpal area over the abductor pollicis brevis muscle (1, abductor pollicis brevis muscle; 2, radial proper digital artery of thumb; 3, perforator artery on the radial side of neck of 1st metacarpal area; 4, neck of 1st metacarpal bone). (*B*) A flap was harvested based on a perforator artery from the radial proper digital artery of the thumb (1, perforator artery from the radial proper digital artery of the thumb; 2, superficial vein). (*C*) The vessels (*1, 2,* and *4*) and the nerve (*3*) of this flap.

pollicis brevis muscle was reached and then dissection continued dorsally along the fascial plane over the abductor pollicis brevis until reaching the septum between the abductor pollicis brevis muscle and the neck of the first metacarpal bone.

Second, the authors carefully identified the cutaneous branch vessel originating from the radial proper digital artery of the thumb to be used as the flap pedicle.

Third, the authors incised the dorsal margin of the flap, identifying 1 to 2 superficial veins and dissecting them to an appropriate length for venous

drainage for the flap and a sensory nerve and its branches innervating the flap. The sensory nerve branches to the flap were also identified and divided with enough length.

Fourth, the incision was deepened to reach the extensor pollicis brevis tendon and then dissection continued volarly over the extensor pollicis tendon until reaching the septum between the abductor pollicis brevis muscle and the neck of the first metacarpal bone.

Fifth, the authors ligated the cutaneous branch at its origin to achieve a longer and larger-diameter vascular pedicle (**Fig. 17**A).

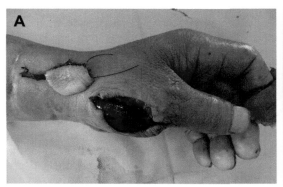

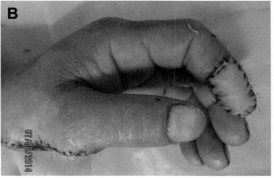

**Fig. 17.** (*A*) The flap was raised. (*B*) A soft tissue defect of the index finger was repaired with transfer of the free flap.

Sixth, the authors elevated the flap and transferred it to the recipient site. Vascular anastomosis was performed under an operating microscope (**Fig. 17**B). The sensory nerve of the flap was coapted with the stump of the proper digital nerve. The 6 months' follow-up showed complete flap survival and an acceptable cosmetic appearance. Static 2-point discrimination on the flap was 10 mm.

### Dorsal Radial Carpal Perforator Flap

The dorsal radial carpal skin is supplied by cutaneous perforators originating from the radial artery and dorsal carpal branch of the radial artery (**Fig. 18**). Using superficial veins as the main drainage system for this skin, it can be elevated and transferred as a free flap. From March 2012 to March 2015, 1 coauthor (Liu LF) and his colleagues designed this flap and applied it in 8 fingers. All flaps survived well, without vascular complications.

One such case with this flap is a 31-year-old woman who had soft tissue loss over the dorsal aspect of the distal phalanx in the left ring finger associated with exposure of the distal phalanx. The authors designed a cutaneous branch perforator flap centered over the dorsal radial carpal area (**Fig. 19**A). Flap harvesting techniques were performed as follows:

First, the authors incised the skin margin of the flap. A superficial vein was identified and cut at an appropriate pedicle length. Second, the incision was deepened to expose the cutaneous perforator emerging from the radial artery (**Fig. 19**B). Third,

the cutaneous perforator artery was divided at an appropriate pedicle length, and the flap was fully raised (**Fig. 19**C) and transferred to the recipient site. Fourth, the authors performed vascular anastomosis and the defect was covered (**Fig. 19**D). Fifth, the donor site was closed primarily (**Fig. 19**E). A 1-year follow-up, there was complete flap survival with good cosmesis (**Fig. 19**F).

### Challenges of These Miniflaps

Using these miniflaps from the hand for vascularized free tissue transfer is a microsurgical challenge. Although these flaps have merits, as described earlier, the disadvantages of miniflaps for soft tissue reconstruction in fingers are that the pedicle is short; the diameter of the artery is less than 0.3 mm, making preoperative vascular evaluation difficult; cutaneous branches are tiny and easily injured during flap elevation; there is a steep learning curve; the anastomoses are difficult, requiring technical skill and special instruments (**Figs. 20** and **21**); and flaps are limited in size. The authors use a 12-0 monofilament suture and a 20× microscope, and make 4 interrupted stitches to suture an artery of a diameter of 0.3 mm and 6 stitches for an artery of a diameter of 0.5 mm. The reasons for our high success rate with these miniflap procedures are that all procedures are performed by experienced microsurgeons, 0.3-mm arteries less often spasm, and the flaps are small so collateral circulation from the recipient site is easily established separate from the anastomosis of the vascular pedicle.

The authors have found postoperative edema of some of the transferred flaps, which lasted for a few days. This edema resolution may indicate reestablishment of collateral circulation promoting flap survival even if the anastomosed vessels become partially occluded. All these miniflap transfers were performed by a microsurgeon who regularly performs microsurgical tissue transfer (level of expertise, ≥III according to a grading method of expertise level[20,21]). The authors have found this to be an important factor to ensuring successful transfer. In addition, the authors cannot exclude the possibility of survival of these tissue flaps as a graft, even if the vascular connection fails after anastomosis.

The authors also acknowledge that some of the tissue defects treated with these flaps might heal with regeneration of the skin and subcutaneous tissues without flap transfer. These flaps in our series are for clinicians who want to challenge themselves with difficult small free vascularized tissue transfers. The authors have shown that such procedures are feasible and are regularly used by our teams.

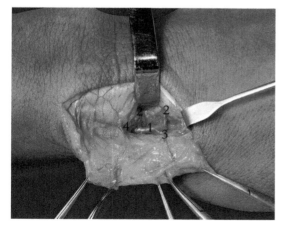

**Fig. 18.** Blood supply in the radial side of the wrist area: 1, radial artery; 2, dorsal carpal branch of the radial artery; 3, cutaneous branch of the radial artery; 4, radial styloid recurrent branch of the radial artery. (*Courtesy of* Zeng Tao Wang, MD.)

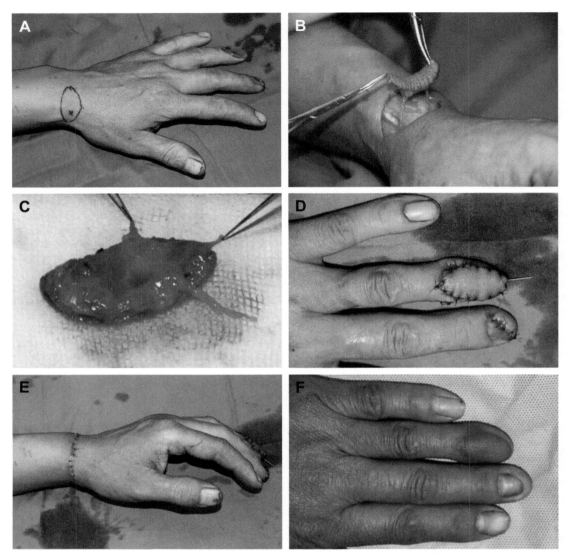

**Fig. 19.** (*A*) A soft tissue defect over the dorsal aspect of the distal phalanx in left ring finger with bone exposure. A flap was designed from the wrist area. A cutaneous arterial branch was identified based on Doppler signals and marked as shown. (*B*) The flap was raised. (*C*) The pedicle of the flap is shown (artery, a cutaneous branch originated from the radial artery; vein, a superficial vein). (*D*) The flap was transferred to cover the soft tissue defect. Blood circulation of flap is good. (*E*) Flap donor site was closed directly. (*F*) One year after surgery.

## ANATOMIC AND CLINICAL VIEWS ON FLAPS
### Dorsalis Pedis Flap Sparing the Deep Fascia

The appearance and function of dorsalis pedis skin are approximate for reconstruction of the hand. It is an ideal donor site for the repair of dorsal wounds of the hand or fingers.[22–27] However, the extensor tendon at the donor site is exposed after the dorsalis pedis flap is raised, leading to a high failure rate of skin grafts. Along with other frequent complications (eg, nonhealing or prolonged wound, soft tissue infection,

osteomyelitis, skin graft adhesion to bone and tendon with frequent skin breakdown, and cold intolerance), clinical applications of the dorsalis pedis flap are limited. The reason for the failure of skin grafts at the donor site is that the typically described dissection for the flap includes the deep fascia of the dorsal foot leaving only a slim peritenon.

The authors think that this traditional technique removes too much soft tissue, which can be preserved while still avoiding damage to the flap and dorsalis pedis neurovascular pedicle. The main

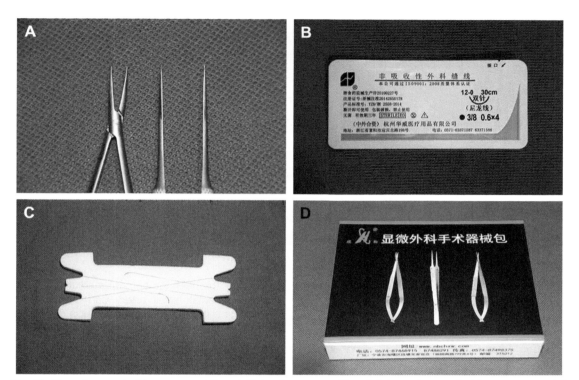

**Fig. 20.** The microsurgical instruments (*A*) and 12-0 nylon sutures (*B* and *C*) in a microsurgical instrument set (*D*) used in the surgeries in the lead author's unit. The forceps and needle holders are the same as are used in suturing vessels of diameters greater than 0.5 mm.

cutaneous perforators from the dorsalis pedis artery branch within 1 to 2 cm of the base of the first intermetatarsal space and pass through the deep fascia toward the skin. The authors have modified the method of our dorsalis pedis flap harvest to reflect this. The authors first incise the flap along the lateral margin, keeping the deep fascia intact. Then the authors dissect the dorsalis pedis flap in the plane superficial to the deep fascia of the foot until the first intermetatarsal space. At this point the authors incise the deep fascia longitudinally along the inside edge of the second metatarsal between the extensor hallucis brevis muscle and the first dorsal interosseous muscle. The authors expose the dorsalis pedis artery and its branches and dissect between the dorsalis pedis artery and the underlying soft tissue of the first intermetatarsal space (**Figs. 22** and **23**). With this technique, the deep fascia is preserved, facilitating skin graft survival at the donor site.

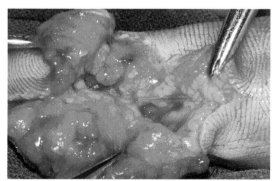

**Fig. 21.** Artery anastomosis of a free digital artery perforator flap in a fingertip. The arterial caliber of the flap is 0.3 mm, and the caliber of the recipient artery (the distal stump of digital artery) is 0.4 mm.

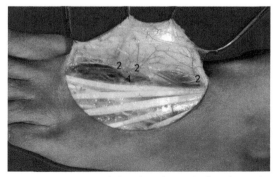

**Fig. 22.** Dissection of the dorsalis pedis flap from the superficial of the deep fascia to the space between the first and second metatarsal bases: 1, dorsalis pedis artery; 2, cutaneous branches. (*Courtesy of* Zeng Tao Wang, MD.)

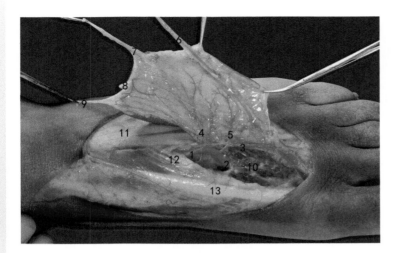

**Fig. 23.** Exposure of the dorsal pedis artery (marked as 1) and its branches (2–5) and veins (6–9) and dissection between the dorsalis pedis artery and the gap of the first and second metatarsal bases (2 and 10) and extensor tendons (11–13). (*Courtesy of* Zeng Tao Wang, MD.)

## Medialis Pedis Vascular Branch Network Flap

The medialis pedis flap is based on the deep branch of medial plantar artery,[28–31] but the blood supply to the skin in this flap consists of 5 branches. Listed from proximal to distal, these branches are the medialis pedis artery, anterior medial malleolus artery, medial branch of the deep branch of the medial plantar artery, medial tarsal artery, and medial branch of the first plantar metatarsal artery (**Fig. 24**). The 5 branches have an extensive intervascular network longitudinally along the region between the abductor hallucis muscle, the tarsal bone, and the first metatarsal bone. Each of the 5 branches can sufficiently supply the skin of this flap through this vascular network of the medialis pedis artery. Therefore, any of these 5 branches can be used as a vascular pedicle for this flap. For example, the medial branch of the first plantar metatarsal artery can be used to design a flap to repair a defect of the distal foot (**Fig. 25**). The medialis pedis artery can be used as the pedicle to transfer the flap to cover a defect of the heel; the anterior medial malleolus artery or medial tarsal artery can be used as pedicle for a flap transferred to repair a defect on the medial ankle or dorsal foot.

## Lateral Pedis Vascular Branch Network Flap

The blood supply of the lateral pedis flap consists of 6 branches. Listed from proximal to distal, these vessels are the lateral marginal artery of the foot, lateral marginal terminal branch of the peroneal artery, perforator from the lateral plantar artery, anterior lateral malleolar artery, lateral tarsal artery, lateral perforator emerging beneath the fifth metatarsal base, and lateral perforator emerging beneath the fifth metatarsal neck (**Fig. 26**). The 6 branches have an extensive intervascular network longitudinally along the lateral pedis muscle and bone interspace. Each of the 6 branches can supply the lateral pedis skin through the lateral pedis vascular network. Each of the 6 branches can be used as the supplying pedicle in flap design, either local.

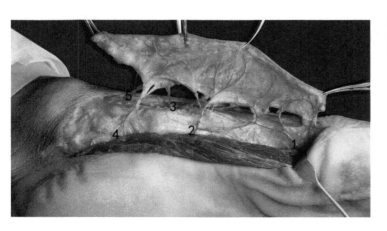

**Fig. 24.** Blood supply to the medialis pedis skin contains 5 branches (marked as 1–5). (*Courtesy of* Zeng Tao Wang, MD.)

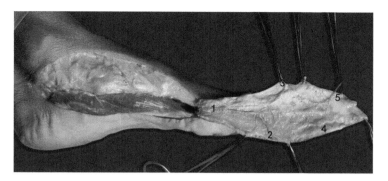

Fig. 25. Each of the 5 branches (marked as 1 to 5) can be used as the pedicle to design flaps. The tibial branch of the first plantar metatarsal artery can be used as the pedicle of a flap to reconstruct the front foot. (*Courtesy of* Zeng Tao Wang, MD.)

The authors used the modified dorsalis pedis flap in more than 40 patients over the past 10 years. The authors found the modification decreased donor site morbidity. This vascular branch network flap from the foot has been used in 20 patients. The authors found this flap feasible, but in 3 patients the authors gave up the plan of using this flap during harvest because of insufficient arterial supply to this flap.

## VASCULARIZED FREE TOE JOINT TRANSFER

Vascularized proximal interphalangeal (PIP) joint transfer from the second toe to the finger has been used for decades in the PIP joint reconstruction of the hand, with reports of mixed outcomes with regard to active range of motion (ROM) in the transferred joints.[32–36] The range of motion of the PIP joint in the second toe is from 0° to 5° extension to 75° flexion. However, the motion of the PIP joint in the finger is from 0° extension to 110° flexion; 40° more than that in the toe. Moreover, the ROM of a transferred toe PIP joint decreases considerably over time postoperatively, being about 40° (ranging from 24° to 60°).[32,34,37]

From 1997 to 2012, the authors performed 159 vascularized toe PIP joint transfers (159 patients) to fingers. The authors could only follow 67 patients thus far, because some of the patients lost contact and some refused to be followed or moved out of the region. At an average follow-up of 16 months (13 months to 5 years), the average active ROM of the transfer joint was more than 70°.

The surgical steps for the toe joint transfer are as follows:

1. Donor harvest. The PIP joint is harvested with one side of the proper digital artery and nerve as the neurovascular pedicle from the second toe (**Fig. 27**). One or 2 dorsal digital veins are dissected and divided with enough length to be used as the drainage veins. A 1 × 0.5 cm skin paddle is harvested with the joint as a monitoring paddle of blood supply, as well as to decrease the tension of skin closure at the recipient site. The flexor and extensor tendons were harvested with sufficient length.
2. Recipient site. A midlateral incision is made in the recipient finger. The toe PIP joint is then transferred to the finger and inserted between

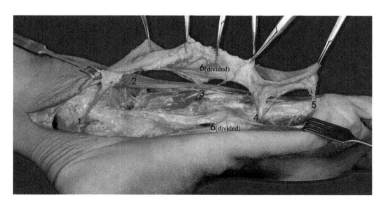

Fig. 26. The blood supply of the lateral pedis skin contains 6 branches (marked as 1–6). (*Courtesy of* Zeng Tao Wang, MD.)

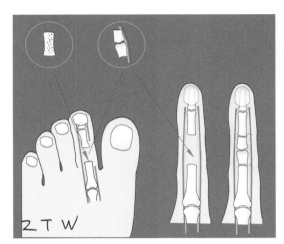

**Fig. 27.** The PIP joint of the second toe is transferred to the finger, and an iliac bone graft is inserted into the donor site.

the proximal and middle phalanges of the finger. Excess bone of the finger phalanges is resected. If there is a bony deficit, iliac bone grafts are inserted into the gaps. Internal fixation is achieved by longitudinal insertion of a Kirschner wire (1.0-mm diameter) in almost all patients except in a few patients with a mini-plate. The artery, nerve, veins, and tendons are connected with corresponding structures in the finger. The skin paddle of the toe joint is sutured with skin of the finger. The recipient hand is immobilized using a dorsal splint post-operatively. If the monitoring paddle is located on the dorsal surface, a volar splint is used instead.

3. Donor site closure. An iliac bone graft is inserted into the gap in the toe after harvest of the PIP joint of the toe and fixed with Kirschner wire. Continuous splinting is applied to the donor foot for 8 weeks.

## Postoperative Care

The recipient hand is immobilized using a splint after the operation. At the third postoperative week, the splint is removed during the daytime, and the patient is instructed to perform active flexion and extension exercise of the fingers and wrist. Careful attention must be paid to prevent the Kirschner wire from breakage. The purpose of rehabilitation in this period of time is to strengthen the muscles of the hand, reduce stiffness of transferred joints, and promote bone healing. The splint is applied at night. The splint and Kirschner wire are removed at 6 weeks after the operation, followed by active and passive

exercises of the fingers. The passive ROM exercise of the reconstructed PIP joint is performed with a goal of reaching 20° to 30° of hyperextension and the maximal achievable flexion in next a few months (**Fig. 28**).

## Secondary Wedge Osteotomy

About two-thirds of the patients achieved hyperextension of the PIP joint after therapy. In these patients, the authors performed a volar wedge osteotomy in the proximal phalangeal neck or middle phalangeal base to turn the excess hyperextension into increased flexion as shown in **Fig. 28**. Postoperative care is the same as in the PIP joint transfer protocol. The radiographs showing the osteotomy and internal fixation in a case and follow-up are shown in **Fig. 29**. In the other patients, the authors did not perform the wedge osteotomy, because the PIP joints either failed to have sufficient range of motion or the joints did not have hyperextension after rehabilitation.

## Tenolysis

Tenolysis is needed if tendon adhesion is severe, which was necessary in 15 patients in our case series. A Z-plasty may be needed in cases with severe scar contracture.

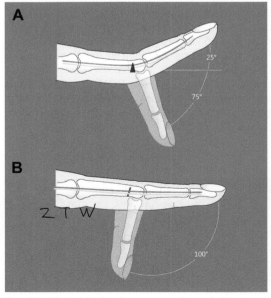

**Fig. 28.** (A) Achieving hyperextension of the transferred toe PIP joint is a goal of rehabilitation after the joint transfer. (B) An osteotomy is performed in the proximal phalangeal neck, to turn the hyperextension of the transferred toe joint to digital flexion.

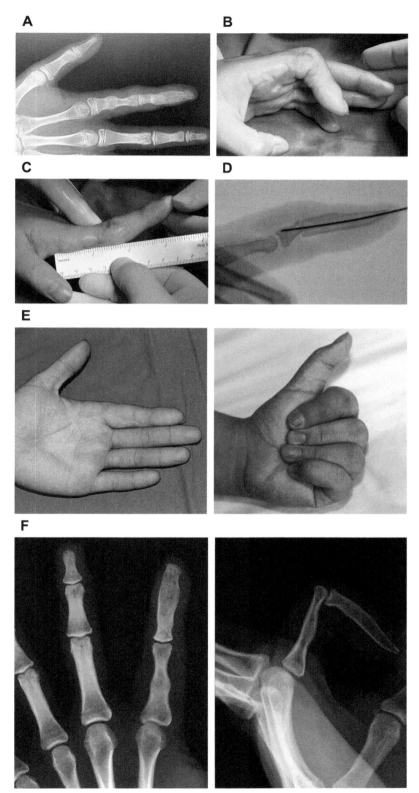

**Fig. 29.** (*A*) A radiograph showing postoperative bony healing of the transferred toe PIP joint to the left index finger of a 15-year-old male patient. (*B, C*) Active flexion of the transferred joint reached 70° and hyperextension reached 25° after rehabilitation exercise. (*D*) Intraoperative radiograph of osteotomy. (*E* and *F*) At 5-year follow-up, full flexion and extension of the joint. (*F*) Radiographs showing normal articular structures and bone healing.

## Complications in Our Patients

Nine (5.7%) of the patients who had neurovascular free toe joint transfer developed complications 3 month to 2 years following surgery. There were 2 types of complications: bony absorption and osteoarthritis. Bony absorption occurred within 6 months following the operation, leading to joint structure collapse and severe joint instability. The main factor leading to bone absorption was probable articular damage from Kirschner wire fixation. There are 2 factors that can increase this damage when fixing a joint using a Kirschner wire: repeatedly penetrating the articular surface and excessive rotation speed of the pin. Excessive rotation speed of the Kirschner wire can create heat, leading to surrounding tissue damage. Osteoarthritis mostly occurred more than 6 months from the time of surgery. There are 2 possible causes of the osteoarthritis. One is that the nerve of the vascularized joint did not adequately heal or was improperly repaired. Another cause for this joint deterioration is inappropriate postoperative exercise (the bony structure of the toe joint determines that the flexion degree cannot be increased by exercise, but some patients do excessive passive flexion exercise and cause rupture of the ligaments of the PIP joint) or excessive use of the reconstructed joint. The authors often noted delayed union of the bone in transferred toe joints. Therefore, the authors had to prolong bone fixation with a Kirschner wire upto or over 3 months. In 3 patients, nonunion developed, which required repeated bone graft and ultimately had poor motion of the transferred joints.

## Key Points to Achieving a Greater Range of Digital Motion

The following key caveats that the authors have found to increase the final ROM of the transferred toe joints should be emphasized: (1) the joint should be fixed in full extension when performing internal fixation because flexion degree is more valuable than extension degree for a transferred toe joint, and (2) passive extension exercise must be designed to achieve hyperextension so that a wedge osteotomy can be performed to turn the hyperextension range to increased flexion. The investigators also consider that digital extensors and flexors should be powerful, which is the prerequisite for active ROM exercise; and the surrounding tissues should be healthy and soft with less scar, to permit a good return of joint motion and to prevent joint contracture or stiffness.

## ACKNOWLEDGMENTS

The authors appreciate valuable review and comments from Dr Daniel Kwan, Assistant Professor of Plastic Surgery, Rhode Island Hospital, and The Alpert Medical School of Brown University, Providence, Rhode Island.

## REFERENCES

1. Ozcanli H, Cavit A. Innervated digital artery perforator flap: a versatile technique for fingertip reconstruction. J Hand Surg Am 2015;40:2352–7.
2. Wong M, Kiat DT, Sebastin SJ, et al. Heterodigital vascular island flap for simultaneous resurfacing and revascularization of digits. Ann Plast Surg 2009;62:34–7.
3. Pham DT, Netscher DT. Vascularized heterodigital island flap for fingertip and dorsal finger reconstruction. J Hand Surg Am 2015;40:2458–64.
4. Lee SH, Jang JH, Kim JI, et al. Modified anterograde pedicle advancement flap in fingertip injury. J Hand Surg Eur Vol 2015;40:944–51.
5. Wang H, Chen C, Li J, et al. Modified first dorsal metacarpal artery island flap for sensory reconstruction of thumb pulp defects. J Hand Surg Eur Vol 2016;41:177–84.
6. Erken HY, Akmaz I, Takka S, et al. Reconstruction of the transverse and dorsal-oblique amputations of the distal thumb with volar cross-finger flap using the index finger. J Hand Surg Eur Vol 2015;40:392–400.
7. Zhang G, Ju J, Li L, et al. Combined two foot flaps with iliac bone graft for reconstruction of the thumb. J Hand Surg Eur Vol 2016;41:745–52.
8. Mitsunaga N, Mihara M, Koshima I, et al. Digital artery perforator (DAP) flaps: modifications for fingertip and finger stump reconstruction. J Plast Reconstr Aesthet Surg 2010;63:1312–7.
9. Atasoy E, Ioakimidis E, Kasdan ML, et al. Reconstruction of the amputated finger tip with a triangular volar flap. A new surgical procedure. J Bone Joint Surg Am 1970;52:921–6.
10. Omokawa S, Yajima H, Inada Y, et al. A reverse ulnar hypothenar flap for finger reconstruction. Plast Reconstr Surg 2000;106:828–33.
11. Omokawa S, Ryu J, Tang JB, et al. Anatomical basis for a fasciocutaneous flap from the hypothenar eminence of the hand. Br J Plast Surg 1996;49:559–63.
12. Kim KS, Kim ES, Hwang JH, et al. Fingertip reconstruction using the hypothenar perforator free flap. J Plast Reconstr Aesthet Surg 2013;66:1263–70.
13. Kamei K, Ide Y, Kimura T. A new free thenar flap. Plast Reconstr Surg 1993;92:1380–4.
14. Omokawa S, Ryu J, Tang JB, et al. Vascular and neural anatomy of the thenar area of the hand: its surgical applications. Plast Reconstr Surg 1997;99:116–21.

15. Iwuagwu FC, Orkar SK, Siddiqui A. Free superficial palmar branch of the radial artery flap for the reconstruction of defects of the volar surface of the digits, including the pulp. Plast Reconstr Surg 2013;131: 308e–9e.

16. Zhu L, Kou W, Hao L, et al. Repairing fingertip defect by transplanting flap nourished with cutaneous branches (8 cases report). Shandong Med J 2009; 49:21–3.

17. Usami S, Kawahara S, Yamaguchi Y, et al. Homodigital artery flap reconstruction for fingertip amputation: a comparative study of the oblique triangular neurovascular advancement flap and the reverse digital artery island flap. J Hand Surg Eur Vol 2015;40:291–7.

18. Han SK, Lee BI, Kim WK. The reverse digital artery island flap: an update. Plast Reconstr Surg 2004; 113:1753–5.

19. Han SK, Lee BI, Kim WK. The reverse digital artery island flap: clinical experience in 120 fingers. Plast Reconstr Surg 1998;101:1006–11.

20. Tang JB. Re: Levels of experience of surgeons in clinical studies. J Hand Surg Eur Vol 2009;34:137–8.

21. Tang JB, Giddins G. Why and how to report surgeons' levels of expertise. J Hand Surg Eur Vol 2016;41:365–6.

22. Zuker RM, Manktelow RT. The dorsalis pedis free flap: technique of elevation, foot closure, and flap application. Plast Reconstr Surg 1986;77:93–104.

23. Vila-Rovira R, Ferreira BJ, Guinot A. Transfer of vascularized extensor tendons from the foot to the hand with a dorsalis pedis flap. Plast Reconstr Surg 1985; 76:421–7.

24. Takami H, Takahashi S, Ando M. Use of the dorsalis pedis free flap for reconstruction of the hand. Hand 1983;15:173–8.

25. Su R, Mei X, Gu Y. Thumb reconstruction by second toe transfer and dorsalis pedis flap, with the use of a peroneal perforator flap to replace the skin deficit on the foot. J Hand Surg Eur Vol 2013;38:435–7.

26. McCraw JB. On the transfer of a free dorsalis pedis sensory flap to the hand. Plast Reconstr Surg 1977; 59:738–9.

27. Eo S, Kim Y, Kim JY, et al. The versatility of the dorsalis pedis compound free flap in hand reconstruction. Ann Plast Surg 2008;61:157–63.

28. Wong SS, Wang ML, Su MS, et al. Free medialis pedis flap as a coverage and flow-through flap in hand and digit reconstruction. J Trauma 1999;47:738–43.

29. Rodriguez-Vegas M. Medialis pedis flap in the reconstruction of palmar skin defects of the digits: clarifying the anatomy of the medial plantar artery. Ann Plast Surg 2014;72:542–52.

30. Chai YM, Wang CY, Wen G, et al. Combined medialis pedis and medial plantar fasciocutaneous flaps based on the medial plantar pedicle for reconstruction of complex soft tissue defects in the hand. Microsurgery 2011;31:45–50.

31. Ishikura N, Heshiki T, Tsukada S. The use of a free medialis pedis flap for resurfacing skin defects of the hand and digits: results in five cases. Plast Reconstr Surg 1995;95:100–7.

32. Tsubokawa N, Yoshizu T, Maki Y. Long-term results of free vascularized second toe joint transfers to finger proximal interphalangeal joints. J Hand Surg Am 2003;28:443–7.

33. Sun W, Chen C, Wang Z, et al. Full-length finger reconstruction for proximal amputation with expanded wraparound great toe flap and vascularized second toe joint. Ann Plast Surg 2016;77:1.

34. Squitieri L, Chung KC. A systematic review of outcomes and complications of vascularized toe joint transfer, silicone arthroplasty, and PyroCarbon arthroplasty for posttraumatic joint reconstruction of the finger. Plast Reconstr Surg 2008;121:1697–707.

35. Koshima I, Inagawa K, Sahara K, et al. Flow-through vascularized toe-joint transfer for reconstruction of segmental loss of an amputated finger. J Reconstr Microsurg 1998;14:453–7.

36. Chen SH, Wei FC, Chen HC, et al. Vascularized toe joint transfer to the hand. Plast Reconstr Surg 1996; 98:1275–84.

37. Kimori K, Ikuta Y, Ishida O, et al. Free vascularized toe joint transfer to the hand. A technique for simultaneous reconstruction of the soft tissue. J Hand Surg Br 2001;26:314–20.

# Severe Crush Injury to the Forearm and Hand
## The Role of Microsurgery

Francisco del Piñal, MD, PhD[a],*, Esteban Urrutia, MD[a,b], Maciej Klich, MD[a,c]

KEYWORDS

- Crush syndrome • Hand • Compartimental syndrome • Free flap • Hand revascularization
- Microsurgery

KEY POINTS

- Microsurgery changes the prognosis of crush hand syndrome.
- Radical debridement should be followed by rigid (vascularized) bony restoration.
- Finally, bringing vascularized gliding tissue allows active motion to be restored.

## INTRODUCTION

Severe crush injuries to the hand and fingers often carry an unavoidably bad prognosis, resulting in stiff, crooked, and painful hands or fingers. In follow-up, osteoporosis is often times seen on radiographs. A shiny appearance of the skin and complaints of vague pain may lead the surgeon to consider a diagnosis of reflex sympathetic dystrophy,[1] to offer some "explanation" of the gloomy prognosis that a crush injury predicates. Primary or secondary amputations are the common end options of treatment.

In the authors' experience, the prompt and precise application of microsurgical techniques can help alter the often dismal prognosis held by those suffering from severe crush injuries. To avoid the progression of a severely crushed hand to a useless hand, one should understand that the pathophysiology involved in the distal forearm, wrist, and metacarpal area is different from that in the fingers. Therefore, this article discusses the pathology and treatment of injuries involving the distal forearm, wrist, or metacarpal area and fingers separately.

## ACUTE CRUSH TO THE DISTAL FOREARM, WRIST, AND METACARPAL AREA OF THE HAND
### Clinical Presentations and Pathophysiology

Two striking features after a severe crush injury are

1. The affected joints tend to stiffen and the affected tendons tend to stick.
2. The undamaged structures distal to the area of injury usually get involved.

The trauma appears to have a "contagious" effect that spreads distally, similar to a fire spreading to the higher floors in a skyscraper. There is no satisfactory explanation as to why normal anatomy seemingly spared during the initial traumatic event should convert to abnormality. To most, the consequence, a frozen hand, is more devastating

The authors have nothing to disclose.
[a] Instituto de Cirugía Plástica y de la Mano, Private Practice, Hospital La Luz and Hospital Mutua Montañesa, Madrid/Santander, Spain; [b] Department of Orthopaedic Surgery, School of Medicine, Pontificia Universidad Catolica de Chile, Santiago, Chile; [c] Department of Traumatology and Orthopedics, Clinical Hospital, Warsaw, Otwock, Poland
* Corresponding author. Calle Serrano 48-1B, E-28001-Madrid, Spain.
E-mail addresses: drpinal@drpinal.com; pacopinal@gmail.com

Clin Plastic Surg 44 (2017) 233–255
http://dx.doi.org/10.1016/j.cps.2016.11.002

than the original injury, that is, a focal trauma in the forearm (**Fig. 1**).

This traumatic event will cause localized devascularization in the forearm and result in healing by fibrosis locally. These facts, however, do not explain the end result of a frozen hand, which often is very painful. The authors attempted to reveal mysterious pathophysiology of the crush syndrome of the hand, but such attempts have not been fruitful.[2]

In exploring the pathophysiology, the following questions can be posed: *What causes a healthy tendon to be unable to glide? Or a normal joint to stiffen? Or an uninjured finger to deviate?* Several factors can shoulder some of the blame: insufficient debridement, the presence of dead space that fills with debris or hematoma, unstable fixation, and poor coverage. The underlying commonality with these factors is that they contribute to the formation of an enormous amount of fibrotic

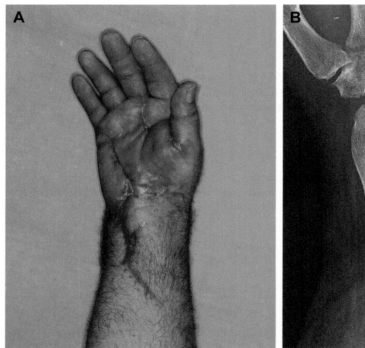

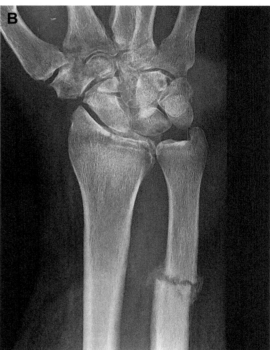

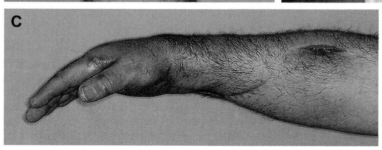

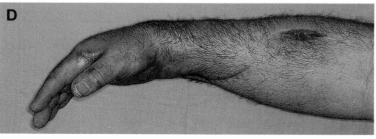

**Fig. 1.** An example of a frozen hand as discussed. (*A*) This 44-year-old man was referred 4 months after sustaining a crush injury to his forearm and wrist by a press. Parts of the wounds were left to heal by secondary intention for fear of losing the whole hand. (*B*) Malunion is present in several areas of the radius, ulna, and carpal bones. It is notable that his fingers became stiff and immobile despite being practically uninvolved. (*C*) The patient is unable to make a fist. (*D*) The patient is unable to extend the fingers. (Copyright © 2015, Francisco del Piñal, MD.)

and scarred tissue. All of them are responsible for a delay in the commencement of active motion, which leads to the loss of tendon gliding and joint stiffness. Muscle contracture, secondary to diagnosed or undiagnosed compartment syndrome, would drag the fingers into dysfunctional positions.

Within this chaotic milieu of diminished blood supply, hematoma, unstable fractures, and poor soft tissue coverage in severe crush injuries, it is easy to foresee that any contaminant could lead to one of the most dreaded complications—deep space infections. Fibrosis and contamination with or without infection result in the dismally functionless "frozen" hand. Furthermore, chronic, unremitting pain is a common component of this syndrome in its later stage. Although a handy acronym "CRPS1" (complex regional pain syndrome) could offer an easy explanation to the onset of pain, a more logical and clearer explanation is that the nerves are either unable to glide and thus causing pain without movement (neurodesis) or ischemic in the confines of heavy scarring. The discomfort is exhausting for the patient both physically and psychologically, and amputation may be needed as the endpoint treatment (**Fig. 2**).

## MANAGEMENT

With the diligent and quick application of the appropriate techniques, a surgeon can halt the progression from crush injury to frozen hand, illustrated in **Fig. 2**. It is hoped that aggressive operative management will result in a better functioning hand in the setting of an admittedly devastating injury. Management keys are to address each of the factors that lead to the poor results. Because of the complexity in the decision-making process and the technical expertise required in the treatment, it is crucial that the utmost care be undertaken by a skilled team of surgeons. With minimal variations, management focuses on addressing the 4 pillars in the listed order:

1. Debridement
2. Bone management
3. Neurovascular structures damaged
4. Soft tissue defect

### Radical Debridement

In the setting of a severe crush to the forearm and the hand, there is a large amount of devitalized or threatened tissue. The devitalized tissue is a nidus for an inflammatory response, creating a wound bed that heals primarily through the means of fibrosis. This results in a massive amount of scarring. Reducing the burden of dead or dying tissue is paramount to promoting the revascularization of bone as well as for aiding tendon gliding.

When the crush injury involves the metacarpals, one has to consider debriding the interosseous muscles should they be devascularized and/or denervated. Most of the blood supply to the interosseous muscles enters proximally,[3] and an injury to the carpal arch unavoidably impairs the arterial inflow into the deep muscles of the hand. In addition, compartment syndrome in the hand may occur with minimal clinical symptoms and remains difficult to diagnose.[4] Such compartment release should occur with low suspicion to preempt future dysfunction.

When the crush injury occurs at the carpal level, severe derangement of the carpal architecture—including floating carpal bones, disruption of the deep carpal arches, and potentially hand devascularization—can be expected. Acute hand amputation is not rare,[5] and late amputation due to deep hand infection is unfortunately common. Amputation is not surprising in this scenario, because the entire central portion of the hand is deprived of its arterial inflow, and potential interosseous muscle necrosis may occur if revascularization is needed.[2]

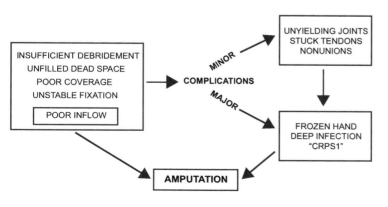

**Fig. 2.** Flowchart showing the natural progression in mismanagement of complex injuries. CRPS1, complex regional pain syndrome.

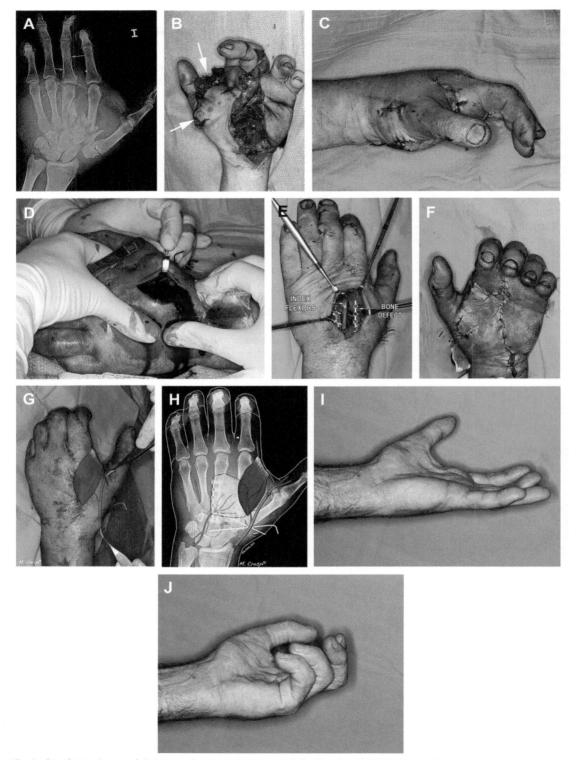

**Fig. 3.** (*A*, *B*) Massive crush injury at the central portion of the hand. Debridement and primary stabilization were carried out as an emergency. Notice that the first web space and thenar musculature (*arrows*) suffered hydraulic extrusion. The radial side of the hand had marginal blood supply, with Doppler signals in the dorsum of the thumb only. (*C*, *D*) Three days after the injury, secondary to hematoma and edema, a massively swollen "balloon"

Interestingly, simple debridement of this central devitalized tissue can lead to further problems because the dead space created may fill with blood upon release of the tourniquet.[6] This central hematoma might become secondarily infected, and if not infected, it may still lead to the formation of densely fibrotic tissue, with both carrying an ominous prognosis. The only way the authors found to manage this central dead space is with coverage with a well-vascularized free muscle flap. The muscle flap contours well to the 3-dimensional defect and changes the local environment from scar formation to well-padded, well-vascularized tissue.[6] A vascularized bone graft may be needed as a solution in selected cases (**Fig. 3**).

## Bone Injury or Defect

Typically, a crush injury does not cause simple fractures only, but rather a mixture of simple and comminuted fractures that are often characterized by cortical shattering and free cortical fragments. Primary or secondary bone loss after debridement is frequent. Furthermore, when the injury area includes a joint, the fracture may burst into small, nonfunctional pieces, making joint reconstruction impossible. Despite that specific fractures need different treatments, it is important to note, however, that achieving rigid fixation with minimally invasive techniques permits early commencement of active range of motion with tendon gliding and causes less local devascularization. In the metacarpals and phalanges, the authors usually achieve satisfactory results with the use of intramedullary cannulated screws,[7] and stable fixation is achieved in minimal time with no dissection and devascularization of the tissue (**Fig. 4**).

If minimally invasive techniques (eg, fixation with intramedullary cannulated screws) are not feasible for fracture fixation, then plate fixation is the next option. Both methods will allow for early motion, diminishing the risk of adhesions. It is not always possible to perform fixation with ideal results. When a joint has severe damage that prevents

functional recovery, it is best to replace the joint. This especially applies when the joint injury occurs in the setting of severe soft tissue injury (**Fig. 5**). Although this approach seems very aggressive, the reward is often a much better end result with overall less patient suffering and faster healing times. One should bear in mind that early rehabilitation is of the utmost benefit in *all* hand trauma cases and of even more benefit as the degree of injury increases.

Unlike crush injuries in metacarpal or phalangeal regions, major carpal injuries can rarely be fixed rigidly enough as to allow for early motion as the concomitant ligamentous injuries require prolonged immobilization times. If rigid fixation is unfeasible, then Kirschner wires and other devices are used as needed. Fortunately, at the wrist level, tendons adhesions are very forgiving, much the same as with zone III or IV flexor tendon injuries, and tolerate some delay in starting mobilization. Furthermore, with wrist immobilization, the fingers can still be allowed to move, preventing tendon adhesions at the wrist.

At the level of the distal radius, the preferred method of rigid fixation, especially with joint involvement, is with volar locking plates. When the fracture involves the shaft of the radius, multiple, shattered, devascularized fragments are commonly seen.

Very severe crush injuries often require a wide, and often both dorsal and volar, approach to appropriately manage the bony injury. This, in turn, creates an increased need for flap coverage. Although this may be a potential drawback, liberal usage of free tissue transfer will often benefit patients by virtue of the fact that the surgeon can better radically debride any tissue of dubious vascularity as well as for allowing the addition of subcutaneous tissue for better tendon gliding.

In any locations, cortical bone fragments devoid of periosteal connections are best debrided away and replaced with cancellous bone. This approach will speed up wound healing times without an increase in infection rates. When

hand can be seen. (*E*) The metacarpal length was restored using locking-type plates. An estimation of the size of the dead space can be inferred from the fact that the flexors are visible from the dorsal wound. (*F*) After fixation, the blood supply to the radial side of the hand was still marginal: compare the paleness of the thumb, index, and middle fingers to the pinkness of the small and ring fingers. (*G*) The extensor digitorum brevis was used to obliterate the dead space and restore pulsatile flow to the thumb, index, and middle fingers by bypassing the zone of injury from the radial artery to the princeps pollicis artery. The massive bone defect was reconstructed with a vascularized medial femoral condyle graft, including a generous component of soft tissue (*H*) (see also **Fig. 7**). (*I, J*) The patient declined further surgery that was advised to improve extensor tendon gliding (an adipofascial flap). Despite this, the patient achieved a reasonable functional status.

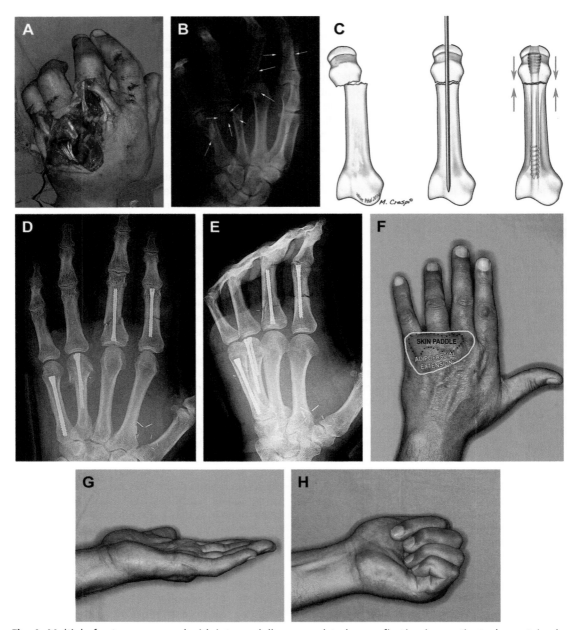

**Fig. 4.** Multiple fractures managed with intramedullary cannulated screw fixation in a patient who sustained a crush injury. (*A, B*) Soft tissue defect and extensor tendon laceration of the ring and little fingers and open fractures (*arrows*) with severe comminution of the head of the ring finger metacarpal. (*C*) Sketch summarizing intramedullary fixation with cannulated screws placed into the metacarpals. (*D, E*) The fractures were treated with a standard 3.0-mm headless cannulated screw for the index finger; a 3.0-mm antegrade screw for the comminuted middle finger; a Y strutting for the ring finger (and primary bone grafting of the defect); and a 4.0-mm-diameter screw for the small finger. (*F*) An adipofascial free flap was used for coverage to provide a gliding environment for the extensor tendons in this severe injury. One year later, minimal flap tailoring and partial hardware removal were performed. (*G, H*) Clinical result at 2 years. (Copyright © 2015, Francisco del Piñal, MD.)

the defect is large, or when there is a large area of tissue devascularization, cancellous bone grafting alone will not ensure bony union or the bony healing is delayed. The cancellous bone grafting greatly interferes with the functional outcome in the authors' experience (**Fig. 6**).

For this reason, the authors advocate early use of vascularized bone transfer, which is preferable

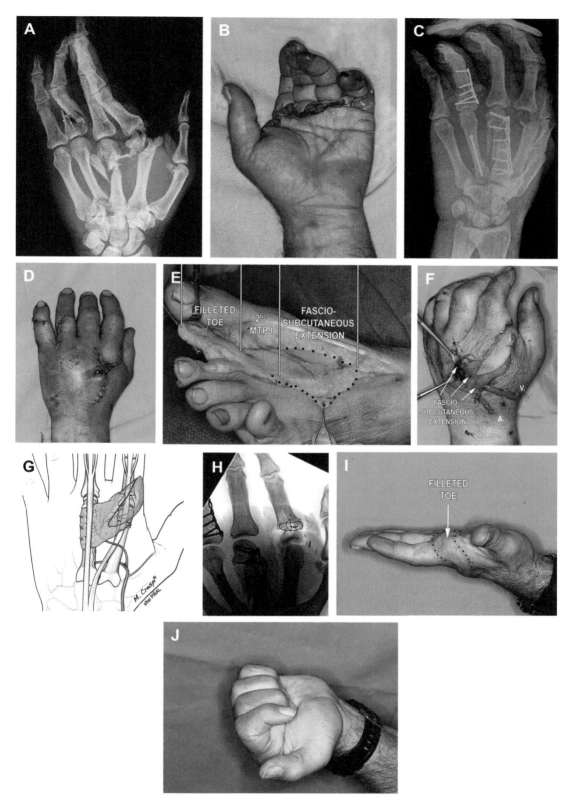

**Fig. 5.** (*A, B*) This 45-year-old heavy smoker had his central 3 fingers devascularized in a crush injury, sustaining multiple comminuted fractures. (*C, D*) Fixation and revascularization were carried out in the emergent setting. The

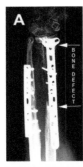
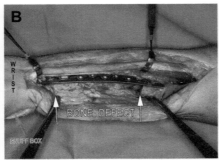
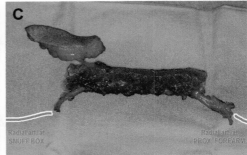

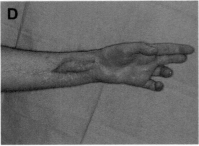
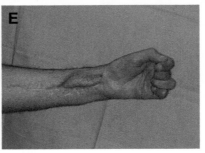

**Fig. 6.** This patient was seen 18 months after a crush injury to his hand and forearm. Two previous attempts to reconstruct the radius with nonvascularized bone had failed. The patient was wearing a splint to support his painful wrist and nearly frozen hand. (*A*) In the preoperative radiograms, a faint shadow of the bone graft could be seen. (*B*) At surgery, the bone graft, which had been replaced by scar tissue, was resected. The plate, despite being bent, was kept in place, as it was providing sufficient stability and maintained the correct length of the radius. The proximal screws in the radius were removed, the wrist distracted, and the fibula slotted into place. Noteworthy here is the lack of fat in the wrist, and the flexors crumpled together. Also, the radial artery had been damaged in the previous surgery and is now indistinguishable from the fibrotic mass. (*C*) The combined 14-cm radius and radial artery defect were reconstructed by a flow-through fibula flap. A skin paddle was also included to add fat distally and to monitor the reconstruction. (*D, E*) The generalized stiffness in the hand and wrist was already so established that only limited functional improvement, albeit painless, was achieved despite secondary tenolysis and joint release. (Copyright © 2015, Francisco del Piñal, MD.)

in this situation. Not only will vascularized bone promote rapid healing but also it will resist infection. When the defect is less than 3 or 4 cm, the authors' preferred flap is the medial femoral condyle flap (**Fig. 7**),[9] but the skin island may have variations that may make it less preferential.[10] A vascularized lateral scapular free flap can address both bone and soft tissue defects, but the skin on the back, like the iliac crest, is often too thick. The fibula has an innate problem of no guaranteed blood supply when used as small segments. In the senior

author's observation, the fibula flap only has a secondary role in treating small complex defects.

## Neurovascular

Combined injuries are often associated with major arterial injuries that if unrecognized or mismanaged may lead to primary or subacute amputation.[5,11] Typically, the radial, ulnar, and/or both carpal arches are avulsed. In this setting, emergency reconstruction is a must. The senior author

index finger metacarpophalangeal (MP) joint was beyond repair and debrided. The wounds were temporarily closed by allowing joint collapse. (*E, F*) Five days later, the soft tissue defect was re-created. A composite metatarsophalangeal joint from the second toe, including a filleted toe and a dorsal fasciosubcutaneous extension[8] flap, harvested to provide tissue to aid in gliding dorsally, was transplanted. The third metacarpal also underwent bone graft in this second stage. (*G*) Sketch showing the insetting of the flap to separate the hardware from the extensor tendon. (*H*) Intraoperative fluoroscopy. (*I, J*) Result at 6 months. No other surgery was performed nor is planned. The lack of full extension of the PIP joint is probably due to the lack of intrinsic muscles of the index finger (ie, a traumatic claw deformity) and could be corrected by a lasso-type operation. The patient is very pleased with his results and declines further reconstruction. (Copyright © 2015, Francisco del Piñal, MD.)

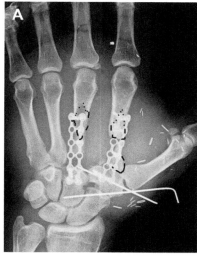

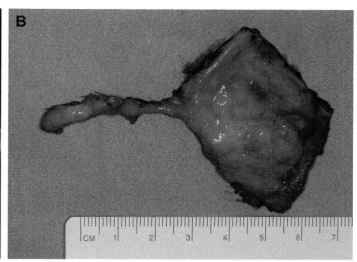

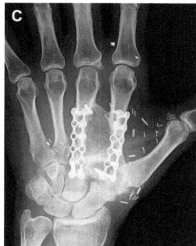

**Fig. 7.** (*A*) A large defect of two-thirds of the anterior aspect of the second and third metacarpals. The bony lengths were maintained temporarily with locking plates. (*B*) A 4 × 3 cm medial femoral condyle corticoperiosteal flap stabilized in place with 2.0-mm screws allowed the authors to span the defect and permitted immediate range of motion. (*C*) A plain radiograph 7 months after the operation (the same patient as in **Fig. 3**). (Copyright © 2015, Francisco del Piñal, MD.)

is a firm advocate for the use of arterial grafts instead of reverse vein grafts at the time of reconstructing the superficial carpal arch. It is technically much easier to suture an artery to an artery and vessel caliber discrepancy is avoided. Furthermore, the surgeon can combine the arterial graft with a soft tissue flap to help to close the dead space. As for graft patency rates, the cardiac-surgery literature, which is much more extensive, illustrates the excellent long-term patency rates of arterial grafts. Overall, the speed of surgical repair is essential in these complicated settings.

There are several sites from which to harvest donor arteries, including the deep inferior epigastric, thoracodorsal, contralateral radial artery, and descending femoral artery, with each having its advantages.[12] As most of the authors' surgeries

are carried out under regional anesthesia, the senior author prefers an artery from the dorsum of the foot[13] (when a toe transfer is not foreseen) or the deep inferior epigastric artery in the case that a toe transfer may be needed in the future (**Fig. 8**).

As opposed to the relatively high incidence of major arterial injuries, the incidence of tendons and nerve injuries is relatively low with crush mechanisms. If there is nerve damage, for the most part, the nerves are avulsed, and in these cases, the authors defer the reconstruction for some days to weeks. Tendons are repaired primarily if possible. Occasionally, the surgeon can place a silicone rod in the path of a future tendon transfer. This allows the surgeon, in a second stage, to pass a tendon graft using the rod as a guide and without risking damage to previously repaired structures. This same maneuver can be used to span nerve

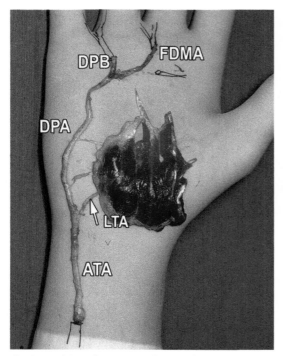

**Fig. 8.** In this cadaveric simulation, the deep plantar branch and the first dorsal metatarsal arteries are to be connected to the common digital arteries. ATA, anterior tibial artery; DPA, dorsalis pedis artery; DPB, deep plantar branch; FDMA, first dorsal metatarsal artery; LTA, lateral tarsal artery. (Copyright © 2015, Francisco del Piñal, MD.)

defects. Regarding the nerves, as mentioned before, primary defects are rare. A much more common problem, discussed later, involves a healthy nerve that secondarily becomes entrapped in scar and thus provokes "causalgic" pain.

### Defect Coverage

As a general principle, the authors avoid local flaps for defect coverage in crush injuries to minimize local tissue insult. To minimize local damage, they are staunch advocates of using the "reconstructive elevator" as opposed to the "reconstructive ladder." When a local flap is going to compromise the final result (either in function or in the speed of recovery), the authors opt for reconstruction with a free flap. Although the alternatives are numerous, in the senior author's practice, moderate defects are treated with gracilis, iliac, or lateral arm flaps. These flaps have the advantage of being near the site of injury or of causing minimal donor site morbidity. The authors have not had any problems with the use of gracilis muscle flaps for coverage in the dorsum of the hand, because this flap is both aesthetically

pleasing and it offers the tendon better excursions (**Fig. 9**). The authors do, however, try to avoid coverage with free muscle flaps if they foresee the need for secondary surgery underneath the flap. For large defects, they prefer the anterolateral thigh (ALT) *fascial* flap or an expanded gracilis (achieved by removing the outer epimysium) flap. In the experience of the senior author, the ALT flap is too thick for use in the hand, and the donor site morbidity is too significant to justify.

Another, less evident, situation where the authors have found the use of free flaps beneficial is after a severe crush trauma at the level of the carpus. Although there may appear to be good soft tissue coverage, the wound bed may be exhausted and without the ability to provide for adequate gliding of the tendons. Fat would undergo necrosis, which leads to the loss of tendon gliding. In this setting, the nerves would also have difficulty gliding, resulting in neurodesis as a source of pain. It is under these circumstances that the addition of a free adipofascial flap may have an astonishing benefit to the patient even in the patients with intact skin coverage.[14]

By the same token, "marginally surviving tissue" in major trauma will not provide the ideal environment for tissue healing. Complications, such as delayed tendon healing, adhesions, tendon rupture, delayed bone union, and nonunion, will increase dramatically. Even worse, major complications, such as deep infection or amputations, increase exponentially in the setting of marginally surviving tissue. So despite the risk of salvage, the authors strongly recommend that one pursue an aggressive stance in order to head off the spiral of complications that may ultimately lead to hand amputation (**Fig. 10**).

### TIMING

Ideally, the reconstruction should be done in one stage; however, the complexity of the injury might make it unwise to pursue all the steps in one sitting (**Table 1**). In the senior author's experience, very lengthy surgery increases the chance of making mistakes, even at the hands of expert surgeons. If at all possible, the night should be for resting. Despite the authors' indoctrination of the importance of immediate free flap coverage, they see no problems in delaying flap coverage for 24 to 48 hours and thereby having a refreshed surgical team. The authors also see no problems in performing the initial debridement and vascular reconstruction with temporary bone fixation at the time of presentation and delaying definitive closure and fracture management. In the authors'

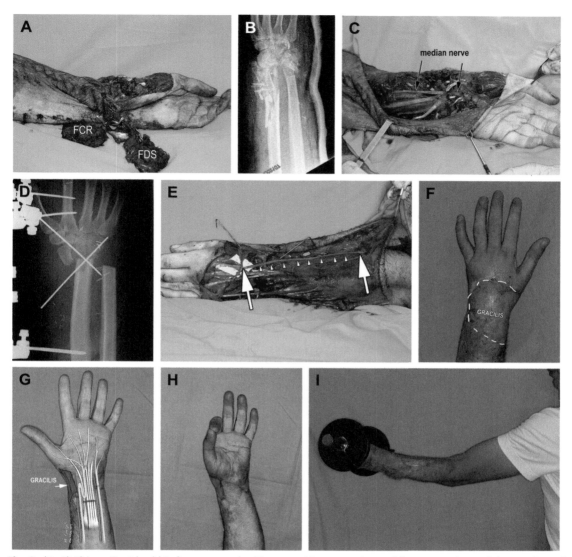

**Fig. 9.** (*A*, *B*) This patient had his forearm crushed by a machine press. Loss of flexor muscles and destruction of the wrist joint are evident. (*C*) The presence of a normal hand and the median nerve partially in continuity tipped the balance toward reconstruction. Resuscitation of hypovolemic shock was simultaneously performed by the anesthesiologist. (*D*) To allow for healthy bone healing, about 8 cm of shortening was required. This also allowed primary ulnar nerve and arterial repair. The median nerve was folded on itself. The flexor and extensor tendons were also repaired. (*E*) Despite shortening of the forearm, a 20-cm saphenous vein graft was necessary to connect the veins of the hand with a healthy vein in the elbow (*arrows*). (*F*) The dorsum of the hand, wrist, and distal forearm was covered with a skin-grafted gracilis muscle flap. (*G–I*) Limited but useful function justified the exhausting reconstructive effort. (Copyright © 2015, Francisco del Piñal, MD.)

opinion, with the use of a logical roadmap, staging the reconstruction will not alter the final results (**Fig. 11**).

## COMPLICATIONS

In the setting of major injuries, such as severe crush injuries to the forearm and the hand,

complications are to be expected. They should be handled as aggressively as the original injury; otherwise, the whole reconstruction may be marred. This applies even to seemingly "minor" problems because they can, and often will, result in a major setback. Among the more innocuous complications are delayed wound healing and nonhealing of one of the fractures. In the authors'

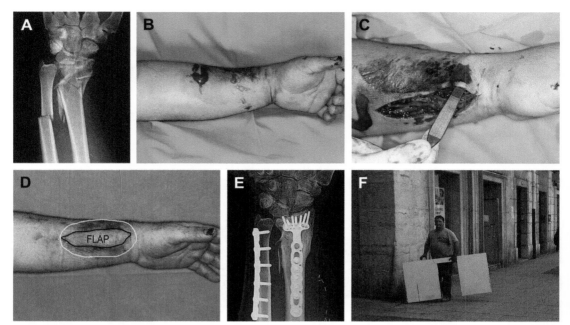

**Fig. 10.** (*A*) This patient's forearm was crushed by a brick wall, causing comminuted fractures of the radius and a shaft of the ulna. (*B*) Skin and wrist swelling is evident at 12 hours. (*C*) Release of the distal forearm compartments and hematoma evacuation were sufficient for decompression. Although local tissue was enough to cover the plates, it was insufficient to provide a healthy environment for fracture healing and tendon gliding. Note that the skin flap is paper thin. (*D*) A lateral arm fasciosubcutaneous flap was used to wrap around the bone and provide a healthy fat layer for tendon gliding. Immediate range of motion was started. The patient regained nearly normal wrist motion and 115% grip strength on his affected (dominant) hand. (*E*) A plain radiograph taken at 1 year. (*F*) The patient returned to his original occupation. He was photographed here by the senior author, who happened upon him while he was working (with patient permission). (Copyright © 2015, Francisco del Piñal, MD.)

**Table 1**
**Roadmap of management of the severe crushed hand**

| | Emergency (and Order of Care) | Second Stage(s) (3–14 d) | Later Stages (mo) |
|---|---|---|---|
| General | 1. Radical debridement | | |
| Muscle | 2a. Debride doubtful muscle<br>2b. Release compartments<br>(2c. Placement of rods) | Rods to prepare the path for tendon transfers | (If muscle loss)<br>Tendon transfers<br>Free muscle transfer |
| Bone | 3. Definitive fixation if feasible/restore length if not | • Definitive fixation if not done<br>• Vascularized bone graft (VBG)<br>• Joint transfers | Tackle delayed union with VBG |
| Tendon | 4. Primary repair when possible | Grafts | Tenolysis/gliding flaps |
| Blood | 5. Revascularize | Additional inflow if needed | |
| Nerves (rarely severed) | 6. Primary repair when possible | Nerve grafts | |
| Cover | 7. (If needed) Free flap (0–48 h) | Replace doubtful cover | |
| Amputations | (3). Replantation/ectopic replant | Toe transfers | |

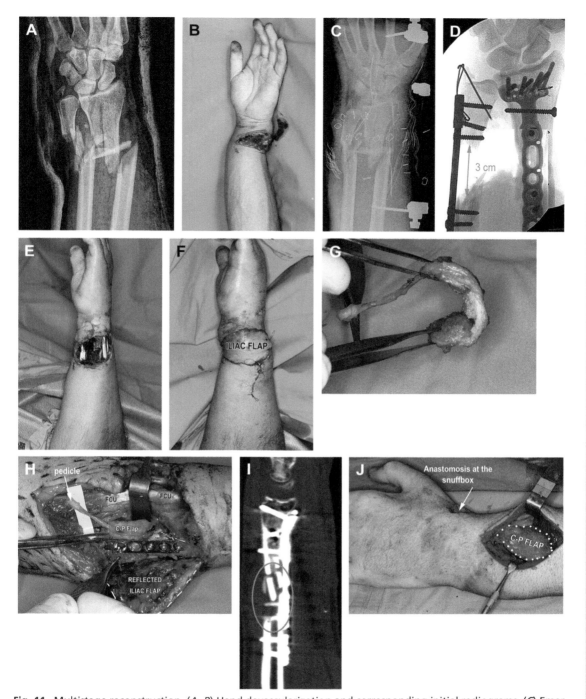

**Fig. 11.** Multistage reconstruction. (*A, B*) Hand devascularization and corresponding initial radiograms. (*C*) Emergency double bypass at the wrist with vein grafts and repair of the tendons were performed. An external fixator temporarily maintained the reduction. (*D–F*) Three days later, the radius was arthroscopically reduced and fixed with the application of a plate, but the ulna was left with a gap of 3 cm. The ulnar soft tissue defect was covered with an iliac free flap. (*G, H*) On day 13, the iliac flap was elevated and reflected ulnarly. Notice the vascular repair was protected by the flexor carpi ulnaris. A medial femoral condyle corticoperiosteal flap (C-P flap) was tailored to wrap around the defect opposite the plate. (*I*) At 6 months, the patient reported a new pain in his radius. A computed tomographic scan revealed an evolving nonunion despite primary cancellous bone grafting. (*J*) The contralateral medial femoral condyle was used as a graft to treat a nonunion of the radius, and the 2.7-mm ulnar plate was removed concomitantly. (*K, L*) Result 9.5 months after the surgery. An artistic rendering of the surgery on this patient. (*M*) The patient felt so well that, without permission, he started going to the gym 2 months later. He is shown here doing pushups in the office 9.5 months after the original trauma. He regained full range of motion. (Copyright © 2015, Francisco del Piñal, MD.)

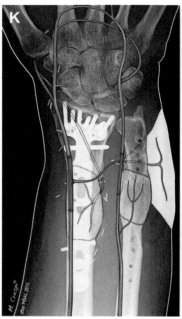
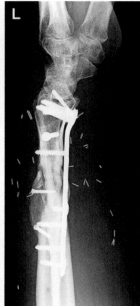
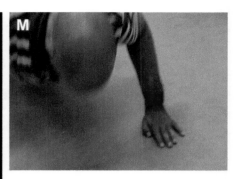

**Fig. 11.** (*continued*)

hands, such cases are *nearly always* managed with the placement of a vascularized bone graft (medial femoral condyle) (see **Fig. 11**). Some might consider this policy too radical, but a nonvascularized bone graft has no chance in the setting of devascularized tissue, which is the main feature of this syndrome.

A lack of tendon excursion is also commonly seen. Some of the patients may actually have near full passive range of motion but very little active motion. This is frequently due to the loss of fat (the gliding tissue) that occurs for several reasons, including the original trauma, surgery, or as a result of infection. Fat is extremely sensitive to traumatic damage, and the lack of fat precludes tendon sliding (see **Fig. 3**). As a preventive measure, the authors always try to include some vascularized fat surrounding their flaps when they harvest them to tackle this problem. As stated previously, the lack of fat can also contribute to pain and lack of cooperation at the time of rehabilitation.

The appearance in the immediate postoperative period of any skin flap struggling should raise *red flags*. This is going to be a source of major problems in many of the cases and should be monitored by the leading surgeon. Even if the flap ultimately survives, the "minimal" consequence will be that the fat underneath the ischemic flap will die, worsening the gliding environment for the tendons in the area. However, this complication is minor compared with

the most common, which is a deep wound infection. In the senior author's experience, most cases of deep infection have been the consequence of "minor" tissue flap ischemia, which, in time, leaves devascularized bone exposed and sets the stage for a deep infection. One has to understand that small amount of nonfractured bone may be of no consequence in any other scenario, but in the setting of a crush injury, that "bit of bone" is devascularized and has minimal resistance to infection. The infection then spreads and results in major catastrophe unless aggressive measures to replace the flap are taken (**Fig. 12**). Seemingly overly aggressive attitudes may salvage the patient from a poor outcome (**Fig. 13**).

## MANAGEMENT OF ACUTE CRUSH TO THE FINGERS

Crushed finger injuries, although often less severe, may portend considerable disability and morbidity, and thereby, become a greater surgical challenge. The "minor" variants in this subgroup consist of finger injuries where the skin envelope is preserved yet the arterial supply has been interrupted (**Fig. 14**). This can be due to either direct injury to the vessel by a bone spike or an arterial avulsion as a result of the vessels being tethered by the local fascia or side branches. Major clues that would lead one to suspect vascular impairment are phalangeal

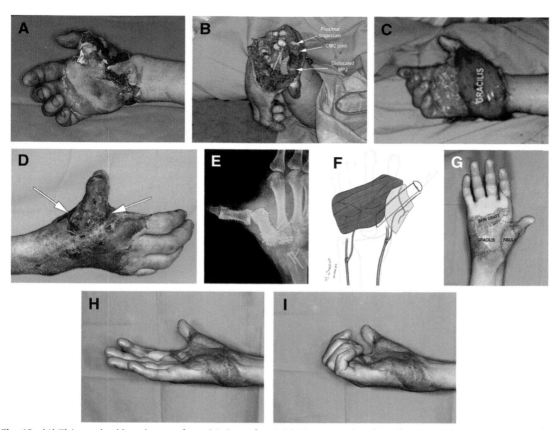

**Fig. 12.** (*A*) This crushed hand was referred 6 days after initiating care elsewhere for impending amputation after a hot press injury. The palm suffered a third-degree burn. (*B*) Emergency debridement gives a better view of the severity of the initial injury. Notice that the thumb is actually hanging by a minimal skin bridge. The MP joint is dislocated. All could be repositioned but were marginally vascularized. (*C*) After debridement, which included the entire proximal carpal row, the thumb was revascularized and a free gracilis was used for coverage. The confluence of the gracilis and the healthy native tissue over the first metacarpal showed signs of delayed healing (*arrows*), which was expected to heal by secondary intention and thus was managed conservatively. (*D*) Over the ensuing weeks, a "minor" infection that began on the "minimally" exposed first metacarpal resulted in a major deep infection with multiple draining sinuses around the thumb (*arrows*) and destruction of the thumb metacarpal, the MP joint (whose reconstruction had failed), the proximal phalanx, the carpometacarpal joint, the trapezium, and half of the trapezoid. All of the prior reconstruction had to be excised (marked in *red dots* in *E*). Fortunately, the wrist could be spared during the debridement, and some motion was preserved. (*F*) A fibular osteocutaneous flap spanned the defect of the thumb and helped clear the infection while also resulting in an immobile thumb. The deleterious effects of delaying range of motion in the rest of the hand can also be appreciated in these pictures (*G–I*). (Copyright © 2015, Francisco del Piñal, MD.)

fractures with longitudinal fractures lines, fractures with significant displacement, color changes, tingling, and numbness. Fingers with vascular insufficiency should be immediately explored and revascularized because amputations have been reported. In most cases, repair of one of the digital arteries restores the flow and solves the problem.[15]

In the intermediate setting of a crushed finger, the skin envelope and/or the bone may be beyond repair. In the best case scenario,

shattered cortical bone heals very slowly. By the same token, delayed bone healing has a major impact on ultimate digital function. At a minimum, comminuted phalangeal fractures require adding cancellous bone graft to speed up healing. Not infrequently, and despite fixation and bone grafting, healing might not occur. For such cases, a vascularized phalanx may solve the problem through a one-stage surgery.[16] Bear in mind, however, that some range of motion almost always will be lost. Furthermore, crush injuries in

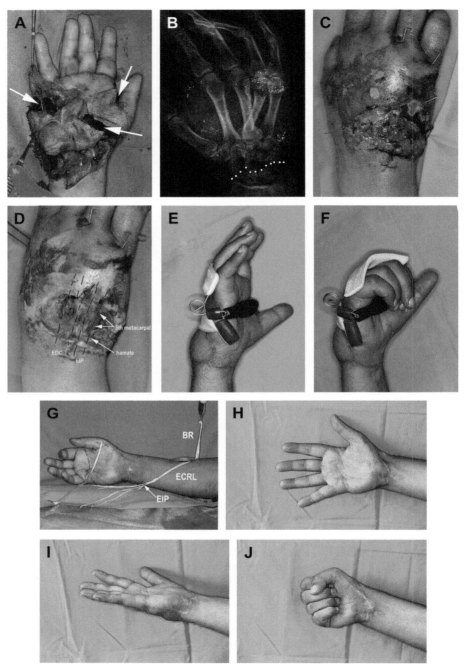

**Fig. 13.** (*A*) This 35-year-old man sustained a crush to his hand and wrist. In addition to the extrusion of the intrinsic musculature (*arrows*), all flexors and most of the extensor tendons were also severed. The radial and ulnar artery and median and ulnar nerves were also divided. All structures were repaired primarily, and blood flow was restored to the hand. (*B*) The patient also had perilunate (*dots*) and carpometacarpal (3–5) dislocations, which attest to the severity of the injury. Only Kirschner wires were used for fixation. (*C*) At 10 days after surgery, there was viable granulation tissue intermingled with marginally viable skin flaps and unstable skin grafts, threatening to expose the distal carpal row and metacarpal bases. (*D*) Very reluctantly, the senior author decided to explore this recently revascularized hand. The wounds were debrided, leaving the bone and repaired tendons exposed, and a free lateral arm flap was inset to provide healthy tissue. (*E*–*G*) An anticlaw splint was worn, and at 7 months, the function of intrinsic muscles were replaced with tendon transfers in the usual fashion for ulnar-median nerve palsy (extensor carpi radialis longus tendon grafts to intrinsic muscles, brachioradialis tendon to the lateral sesamoid, and extensor indicis properius tendon to the abductor pollicis brevis). (*H*–*J*) Function at the 18-month follow-up visit. This patient illustrates the importance of being aggressive to prevent deep infection and the need to plan out the stages to be used in the reconstruction. (Copyright © 2015, Francisco del Piñal, MD.)

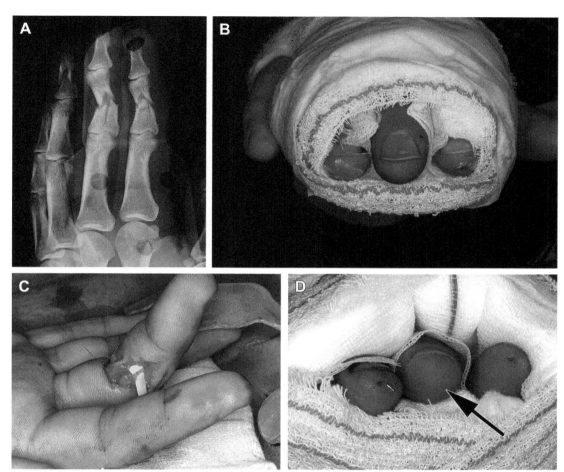

**Fig. 14.** This patient sustained a crush injury to his fingers 28 hours before consultation. Bluish discoloration, tingling, and numbness prompted him to seek a second opinion. (*A*) The radiological hallmarks of a crushed finger with vascular compromise can be seen on the preoperative radiograms (longitudinal splitting, widening, and major displacement). (*B*) Bluish discoloration on the middle finger is evident. (*C*) The artery was exposed on one side and repaired. (*D*) Compare the color of the middle finger (*arrow*) in (*B*). (Copyright © 2015, Francisco del Piñal, MD.)

the area of the proximal phalanx can entail destruction of the pulley system. The authors have yet to find a satisfactory solution to this latter problem. Many of those cases end up with severe flexion contractures or amputation. Nevertheless, in select cases, the authors have had some success to this gloomy problem by transferring toes (**Fig. 15**).

In the authors' hands, major soft tissue loss of the fingers is best solved with the use of thin, pliable, free flaps. Their preferred free flaps for digital defect coverage are neurocutaneous flaps taken from the side of the toes, usually the tibial side of the second toe.[17] Not only does this flap provide top soft tissue cover for fingers but also provides a vascularized nerve and artery for flow-through reconstruction (**Fig. 16**).

In their most severe forms, crushed fingers have barely identifiable structures and are obviously beyond reconstruction. Apart from the possibility of replantation of some spare parts, the only other sound alternative is a free toe transfer. The authors recommend the liberal use of toe transfers in all patients, even in aged patients, provided they are fit and without serious comorbidities. This practice pattern is based on the positive experience of the senior author when toe transfers have been performed (through December of 2015, the senior author has done 420 toe-to-hand transfers with 3 failures).[18,19] In cases where a single finger is amputated proximal to the proximal interphalangeal (PIP) joint, the authors recommend ray amputation. This recommendation is based on 2 key facts. First, a replanted finger amputated proximal to the PIP joint

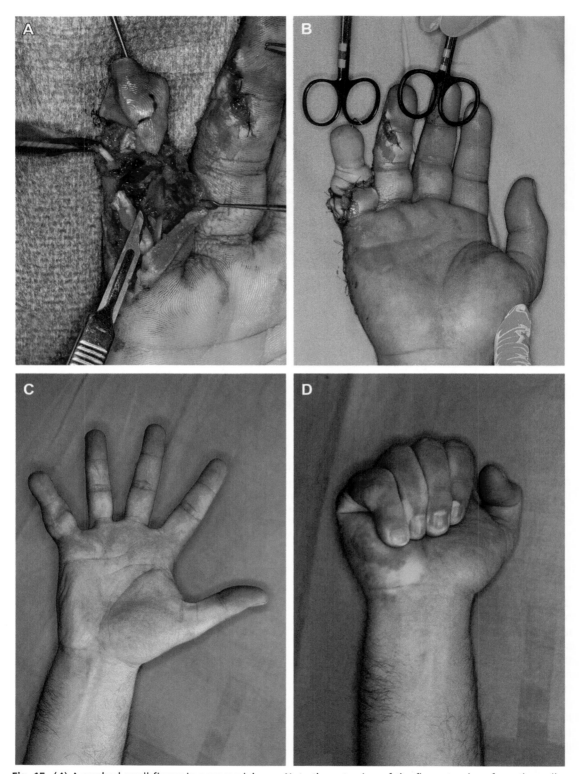

**Fig. 15.** (*A*) A crushed small finger in a young laborer. Note the extrusion of the flexor tendons from the pulley system. The PIP joint could be reconstructed. (*B*) A second toe transfer was performed 48 hours after the accident. (*C, D*) The result at 1 year. No other surgery has been performed, although aesthetic refinements have been scheduled. (Copyright © 2015, Francisco del Piñal, MD.)

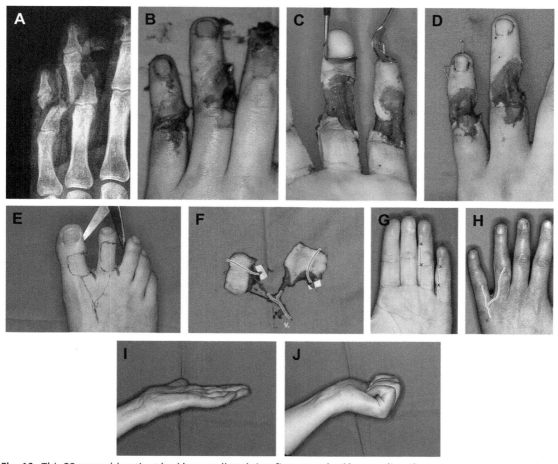

**Fig. 16.** This 22-year-old patient had her small and ring finger crushed by a sealing device, sustaining a combined thermal and crush injury. Because of the marginal blood supply to the digits, she was referred for treatment 48 hours after injury (*A, B*). The only inflow was through a small dorsal bridge shown here after debridement (*C, D*). Definitive fixation and re-establishment of the flow were performed in one stage using 2 digital flow-through free flaps (*E–H*). (*I, J*) Although her postoperative range of motion at the PIP was normal, to improve the active motion at the distal interphalangeal joint, tenolysis was performed. This eventually required the placement of a rod for rupture of the flexor digitorum profundus tendon of the small finger. The final results after all the procedures are shown. (Copyright © 2015, Francisco del Piñal, MD.)

does not yield a good functional result, at least in the senior author's experience. In fact, such replanted fingers ultimately become a burden to the rest of the hand. Second, no matter how long a second toe may be, it is still much shorter than a finger and moves poorly when transplanted to the hand. Therefore, the best indication for a single replant[20] (or a toe)[21] is when the amputation is distal to the PIP joint. When more than one finger has been amputated, the goal of the surgical intervention is to achieve anything close to the so-called acceptable hand. An acceptable hand has been defined as 1 with 3 fingers of near normal length, with near normal PIP joint motion, with good sensibility, with a functioning thumb. The term "acceptable hand" is so named because it is acceptable in both aesthetics and function (**Fig. 17**). By using toe transfers, lengthening procedures, finger transpositions, and so forth, the surgeon can change a badly damaged hand into an acceptable one (**Fig. 18**).[18,19,21]

## MANAGEMENT OF LATE PRESENTING CASES

Here, the topic of late reconstruction will be lightly touched upon. It should be understood, however, that late reconstruction corresponds to the largest patient group in the senior author's practice. Late and very late referrals are unfortunately very common. To varying degrees, they all share

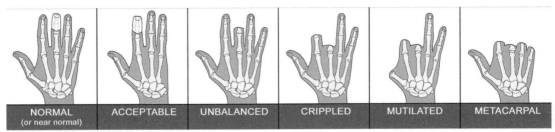

**Fig. 17.** Classification of finger injuries. In this sketch, the normal hand is roughly analogous to an unbalanced hand that has been improved with a second toe transfer. The acceptable hand is a crippled hand that is status post a toe transfer for the index finger and ray amputation of the middle finger. (*Adapted from* del Piñal F. The indications for toe transfer after "minor" finger injuries. J Hand Surg Br 2004;29:120–9; and del Piñal F, Herrero F, García-Bernal FJ, et al. Minimizing impairment in laborers with finger losses distal to the proximal interphalangeal joint by second toe transfer. Plast Reconstr Surg 2003;112:1000–11. Copyright © 2015, Francisco del Piñal, MD.)

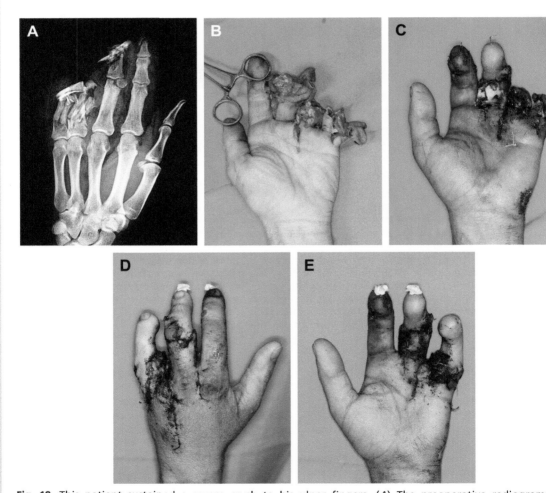

**Fig. 18.** This patient sustained a severe crush to his ulnar fingers. (*A*) The preoperative radiograms demonstrate longitudinal fractures from a crush. The fracture in the PIP joint of the middle finger was stabilized. (*B*) The pulleys are disrupted and the flexor tendons herniated. (*C*) Two days later, a second toe was transferred to the top of the base of the middle phalanx of the middle finger. (*D, E*) A week later (9 days after the injury), the contralateral second toe was transferred to the proximal phalanx of the small finger with a concomitant fourth ray amputation. The pictures shown are 16 days after the injury with all reconstructions done. (Copyright © 2015, Francisco del Piñal, MD.)

the following characteristics: marginal vascular supply to the hand, poor soft tissue coverage, deep infection, malaligned and nonunited bones, and a disabling lack of motion, that is, a frozen hand sometimes in association with deep infection. If there is still something of use distally, then a reconstructive effort is warranted, but the result is never going to be as satisfactory as that expected with the reconstruction of an acute injury. The patient should be warned that in severe cases an assisting hand is the goal...; sometimes much more can be achieved, but this not always appreciated.

The "solution" is to think in reverse: redebride, refix, revascularize, and recover. Toes and joints are liberally transferred to the injured hand in order to most closely approximate the "acceptable hand" (**Fig. 19**).[18,19,21] A consistent finding in

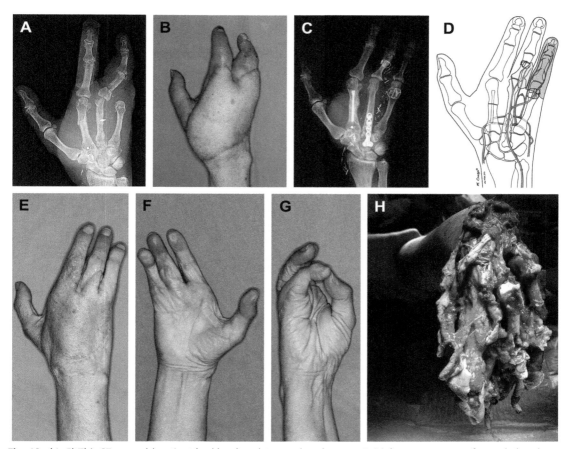

**Fig. 19.** (*A, B*) This 67-year-old patient had her hand trapped under a car. Initial surgery was performed elsewhere. Briefly, an anterolateral thigh flap was used for soft tissue coverage, together with transposition of the ring finger onto the third MP joint. The small finger was secondarily amputated. Furthermore, 7 additional surgical debridements for clearing deep infection were carried out over a 4-month period. Recommendation for amputation at the level of the distal forearm prompted the patient to seek a second opinion. The thumb had some motion, but the index and ring fingers had only sensibility preserved. The middle metacarpal and MP joint were found destroyed on the radiograms, with infection likely the cause. (*C, D*) The reconstruction was planned in 2 stages. At the first operation, the ulnar aspect of the ALT flap was thinned and the third metacarpal and MP joints, which were sequestrated, were radically debrided. The second metatarsal and the corresponding metatarsophalangeal joint and the contralateral second toe were transplanted. In the second operation, some extensor tendons were reconstructed, and the radial part of the flap was thinned. No other surgery has been performed. (*E–G*) An aesthetically pleasing and basic functioning hand was achieved, thereby justifying the surgical effort. Interestingly, neither the patient nor her husband (himself a doctor, who caused the accident) was happy with the final outcome. It should also be stated that a series of ill-advised surgeries were performed during her initial care course. However, one has to admit that in some cases the nature of the original injury can overwhelm even an expert surgeon and the care initially provided was quite good (picture supplied by the original surgeon) (*H*). (Copyright © 2015, Francisco del Piñal, MD.)

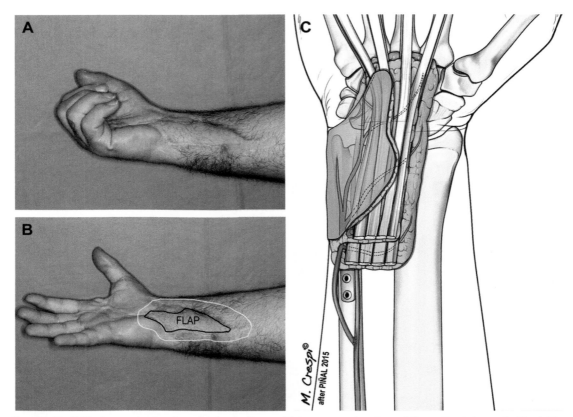

**Fig. 20.** (*A, B*) Flexion and extension obtained after multistage reconstruction of the patient shown in **Fig. 1.** The authors treated the malunion, excised scar tissue, and replace it with a well-vascularized free lateral arm flap, including an adipofascial extension (*yellow*) to encircle the flexor tendons, thus providing a better gliding environment. (*C*) Artistic rendering of the flap transfer. (Copyright © 2015, Francisco del Piñal, MD.)

these cases is the lack of a gliding environment for tendons and joints. The authors have had encouraging results by transferring vascularized adipofascial flaps (**Fig. 20**).[14] In summary, the reconstructive effort can be enormous, and the results are never going to be as good as when these injuries are managed acutely, but still there is room to achieve acceptable function.

## SUMMARY

Crush injuries rate among the most feared injuries for hand surgeons. Stiffness, deep infection, chronic pain, and late amputation are frequent outcomes. In the authors' experience, radical debridement of devitalized tissues, rigid fixation, and widespread usage of microsurgery to achieve rapid healing have dramatically altered the outcomes for this type of injury. In this work, the authors illustrate how adipofascial free flaps, along with free bone forming flaps, allow the surgeon to provide the ideal environment for healing. Toe transfers can dramatically improve function in digital defects.

## REFERENCES

1. Del Piñal F. Editorial: I have a dream... reflex sympathetic dystrophy (RSD or complex regional pain syndrome—CRPS I) does not exist. J Hand Surg Eur 2013;38:595–7.
2. Del Piñal F, García-Bernal FJ, Delgado J. Is posttraumatic first web contracture avoidable? Prophylactic guidelines and treatment-oriented classification. Plast Reconstr Surg 2004;113:1855–60.
3. Weinzweig N, Starker I, Sharzer LA, et al. Revisitation of the vascular anatomy of the lumbrical and interosseous muscles. Plast Reconstr Surg 1997;99:785–90.
4. Del Piñal F, Herrero F, Jado E, et al. Acute hand compartment syndromes after closed crush: a reappraisal. Plast Reconstr Surg 2002;110:1232–9.
5. Herzberg G, Comtet JJ, Linscheid RL, et al. Perilunate dislocations and fracture-dislocations: a multicenter study. J Hand Surg Am 1993;18:768–79.
6. Del Piñal F, Pisani D, García-Bernal FJ, et al. Massive hand crush: the role of a free muscle flap to obliterate the dead space and to clear deep infection. J Hand Surg Br 2006;31:588–92.

7. del Piñal F, Moraleda E, Rúas JS, et al. Minimally invasive fixation of fractures of the phalanges and metacarpals with intramedullary cannulated headless compression screws. J Hand Surg Am 2015; 40:692–700.

8. del Piñal F, García-Bernal FJ, Delgado J, et al. Overcoming soft-tissue deficiency in toe-to-hand transfer using a dorsalis pedis fasciosubcutaneous toe free flap: Surgical technique. J Hand Surg Am 2005;30: 111–9.

9. Sakai K, Doi K, Kawai S. Free vascularized thin corticoperiosteal graft. Plast Reconstr Surg 1991;87: 290–8.

10. Iorio ML, Masden DL, Higgins JP. Cutaneous angiosome territory of the medial femoral condyle osteocutaneous flap. J Hand Surg Am 2012;37:1033–41.

11. Garcia-Elias M, Dobyns JH, Cooney WP 3rd, et al. Traumatic axial dislocations of the carpus. J Hand Surg Am 1989;14:446–57.

12. Shuck J, Masden DL. Options for revascularization: artery versus vein: technical considerations. Hand Clin 2015;31:85–92.

13. del Piñal F, Herrero F. Extensor digitorum brevis free flap: anatomic study and further clinical applications. Plast Reconstr Surg 2000;105: 1347–56.

14. del Piñal F, Moraleda E, de Piero GH, et al. Outcomes of free adipofascial flaps combined with tenolysis in scarred beds. J Hand Surg Am 2014; 39:269–79.

15. Reagan DS, Grundberg AB, Reagan JM. Digital artery damage associated with closed crush injuries. J Hand Surg Br 2002;27:374–7.

16. del Piñal F, García-Bernal FJ, Delgado J, et al. Vascularized bone blocks from the toe phalanx to solve complex intercalated defects in the fingers. J Hand Surg Am 2006;31:1075–82.

17. del Piñal F, García-Bernal FJ, Regalado J, et al. The tibial second toe vascularized neurocutaneous free flap for major digital nerve defects. J Hand Surg Am 2007;32:209–17.

18. del Piñal F. The indications for toe transfer after "minor" finger injuries. J Hand Surg Br 2004;29: 120–9.

19. del Piñal F. Severe mutilating injuries to the hand: guidelines for organizing the chaos. J Plast Reconstr Aesthet Surg 2007;60:816–27.

20. May JW Jr, Toth BA, Gardner M. Digital replantation distal to the proximal interphalangeal joint. J Hand Surg Am 1982;7:161–6.

21. del Piñal F, Herrero F, García-Bernal FJ, et al. Minimizing impairment in laborers with finger losses distal to the proximal interphalangeal joint by second toe transfer. Plast Reconstr Surg 2003;112: 1000–11.

# Medial Femoral Trochlea Osteochondral Flap
## Applications for Scaphoid and Lunate Reconstruction

James P. Higgins, MD[a],*, Heinz K. Bürger, MD[b]

## KEYWORDS

- Osteochondral flap • Medial femoral trochlea • Medial femoral condyle
- Descending geniculate artery • Scaphoid nonunion • Vascularized bone • Kienböck disease

## KEY POINTS

- Vascularized osteochondral flaps are a new technique described for the reconstruction of challenging articular defects of the carpus.
- The medial femoral trochlea (MFT) osteochondral flap is supplied by the descending geniculate artery (DGA). This osteochondral flap has shown promise in the treatment of recalcitrant scaphoid proximal pole nonunions and advanced avascular necrosis of the lunate.
- The anatomy, surgical technique, and results are discussed, with clinical cases provided.

## INTRODUCTION

The DGA has become a versatile pedicle in reconstructive microsurgery. The DGA vessels supply the corticoperiosteal or corticocancellous medial femoral condyle (MFC) flap used in cases of nonunion of long bones, tubular bones of the hand, carpal and tarsal bones, and the craniofacial skeleton. In addition to providing bone from the apex of the condyle, the vessel branches have demonstrated the capability of providing cutaneous,[1] osteocutaneous,[2–4] or osteotendinous combinations[5] and even served as a useful recipient vessel in extremity reconstruction.[6]

The vascular distribution of this pedicle also includes periosteal vessels supplying the cartilage-bearing trochlea of the medial patellofemoral joint. The utility of harvesting this convex cartilaginous surface as a vascularized flap was described in a case report of scaphoid reconstruction of a recalcitrant proximal pole nonunion in 2008.[7] Cadaveric studies have described the pertinent vascular arcade supplying this bone and cartilage,[8,9] and an anatomic study elucidated the similarities between the convex curvature of the MFT and the proximal convex surfaces of the scaphoid, lunate, and capitate.[8] The authors have used this segment of bone and cartilage as a free osteochondral flap for various articular defects.[10] The most common applications have been reconstruction of recalcitrant scaphoid proximal pole nonunions[11,12] and advanced avascular necrosis of the lunate (Kienböck disease).[13]

## ANATOMY

The MFT flap shares the same vascular source vessel as the MFC corticoperiosteal flap. Both are supplied by periosteal vessels that are intimately adherent to the medial aspect of the distal

The authors have nothing to disclose.
[a] Curtis National Hand Center, MedStar Union Memorial Hospital, 3333 North Calvert Street, Baltimore, MD 21218, USA; [b] Privat Hospital Maria Hilf, Radetzkystrasse 35, Klagenfurt 9020, Austria
* Corresponding author.
*E-mail address:* anne.mattson@medstar.net

femur. This filigree of vessels represents the terminal branches of the DGA. The DGA originates from the superficial femoral artery (SFA) within the adductor hiatus of the distal thigh and travels distally. At the level of the adductor insertion on the medial condyle, the DGA divides into smaller caliber longitudinal and transverse periosteal branches. The longitudinal branch is used to harvest the MFC corticoperiosteal flap. The transverse branch courses anteriorly to the region of the cartilage-bearing medial trochlea. The convex osteochondral segment of the proximal-most aspect of trochlea is harvested as the MFT flap for articular reconstruction (**Fig. 1**).

## FLAP DESIGN

The osteochondral segment typically harvested for scaphoid and lunate reconstruction is approximately 2 cm × 1 cm × 1 cm, with the longest dimension measuring from proximal to distal. The segment is harvested from the proximal margin of the cartilage-bearing convex trochlea. This segment normally articulates with the medial patella and does not articulate with the tibia. The

flap carries cartilage on one surface only (**Fig. 2**). This is positioned during inset to articulate with the scaphoid fossa or lunate fossa of the radius (to recreate the greater curvature of the scaphoid or lunate, respectively).

The osteochondral segment is harvested in continuity with the transverse periosteal branch of the DGA. The DGA is harvested proximally to gain pedicle length and caliber as it approaches its origin from the SFA in the adductor canal. The maximal length of the pedicle is approximately 13 cm with an arterial caliber of approximately 1.5 mm at its takeoff from the SFA.

## HARVEST TECHNIQUE

When used for small articular defects, the MFT is usually harvested without a skin island to avoid excess bulk. The following description is the technique of harvest without skin. The authors have described the skin harvest on the DGA pedicle previously.[2]

An incision is created starting at the adductor hiatus, moving distally and anteriorly to the midpoint between the medial border of the

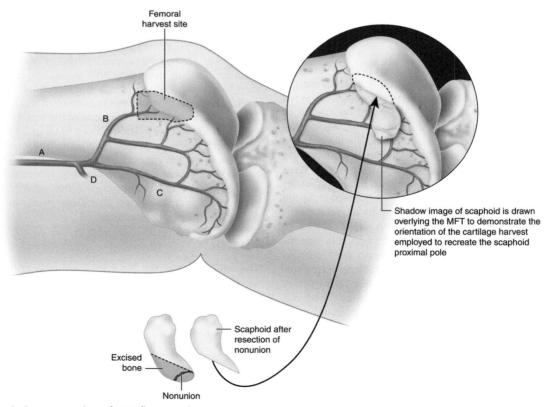

**Fig. 1.** Representation of MFT flap vascular pedicle. A, DGA. B, transverse branch. C, longitudinal branch. D, SGA. Area of desired osteochondral harvest shaded in green. Inset demonstrates orientation of harvested segment as it relates to area of scaphoid reconstruction. (Copyright 2013, The Curtis National Hand Center.)

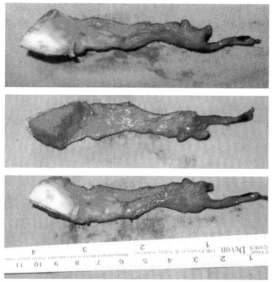

**Fig. 2.** Typical size and appearance of harvested MFT osteochondral flap. Note that the flap provides convex cartilage on one surface only. (*Top*: oblique view; *Middle*: posterior view; *Bottom*: anterior view.)

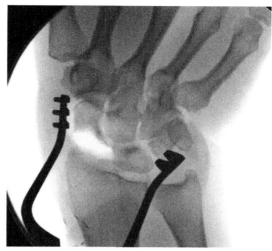

**Fig. 4.** Radiographic image of intraoperative scaphoid after generous resection of proximal pole nonunion. Note that the resection is performed beyond the proximal pole nonunion to accommodate a large flap segment and place the osteosynthesis site at the more favorable waist region of the scaphoid.

patella and the MFC. This skin incision is continued to the subfascial plane as the vastus medialis muscle is retracted anteriorly. The DGA can then be identified as the medial column of the femur is exposed. The DGA may be dissected as proximally as its origin from the SFA in the adductor canal. Branches coursing anteriorly to the vastus medialis and posteriorly to the medial thigh skin may be ligated. The skin branches (which include the saphenous artery) provide options for skin paddle harvest if desired.

Ligation and elevation of the pedicle from proximal to distal facilitate subsequent bone harvest. As the pedicle elevation reaches the region of the adductor tendon insertion, the vessels become intimately invested in the periosteum of the medial condyle. Three large branches are encountered: the transverse branch, the longitudinal branch, and the superomedial geniculate artery (SGA).

The SGA courses deep into the popliteal fossa in the retrocondylar sulcus of the femur. In approximately 10% of patients the DGA may be absent and the SGA may serve as the pedicle, requiring

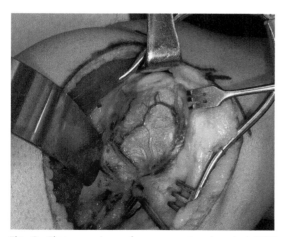

**Fig. 3.** Close-up view of convex osteochondral MFT and surrounding dense network of periosteal vessels. Distal leg is to the right; proximal leg is to the left.

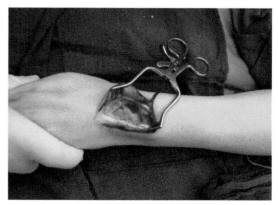

**Fig. 5.** Intraoperative view of completed scaphoid resection from dorsal approach. Note the volar wrist extrinsic ligament visible in the depth of the resection. Hand is to the left. The radial aspect of the wrist is shown in the top of the image.

dissection of this vessel from its origin off the popliteal artery.

The longitudinal branch serves as the pedicle for the (non–cartilage-bearing) MFC flap and is ligated when harvesting the MFT.

The transverse branch typically traverses the metaphyseal region and densely supplies the periosteum surrounding the MFT both on its medial aspect and proximal aspect (**Fig. 3**). This branch is preserved and elevated with its attachments to the trochlea. As the dissection approaches the trochlea, it is performed subperiosteally to protect the small vessels.

The width, length, and depth required is measured and the flap is then harvested using a saw and/or osteotomes. The most difficult maneuver is the sagittal cut because the patella remains in anatomic position during harvest. The authors find it most efficient to create the coronal and axial osteotomies with a power saw first. Knee extension then permits passage of a small curved osteotome directed from proximal to distal to carefully achieve the sagittal resection.

The joint capsule is closed, a drain is placed in the subcutaneous plane, and the skin is closed. No immobilization is required. Patients are permitted to ambulate immediately after surgery. It is common for a patient to have some discomfort with ambulation that resolves over 2 months to 4 months.

## FLAP INSET
### Wrist Exposure

Whether the MFT procedure is applied to scaphoid nonunion or a Kienböck case, the wrist exposure is performed at the outset of the operation to insure that the quality of the radius platform is adequate

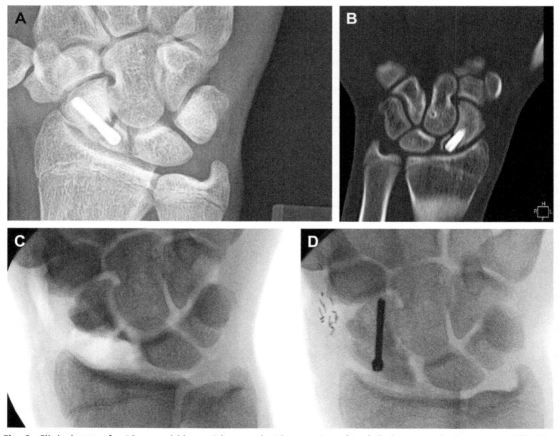

**Fig. 6.** Clinical case of a 16-year-old boy with a scaphoid nonunion after failed open reduction internal fixation via dorsal approach. (*A*) Preoperative anteroposterior radiograph. (*B*) Preoperative CT coronal image demonstrating the small size of the remaining proximal pole nonunited fragment. (*C*) Intraoperative fluoroscopic anteroposterior radiograph after resection of proximal scaphoid to level of scaphoid waist. Note the preserved concave cartilage shell of the scaphoid acetabulum. This is preserved to articulate with the capitate. (*D*) Anteroposterior radiograph 4 months after surgery demonstrating scaphoid union with excellent restoration of scaphoid morphology.

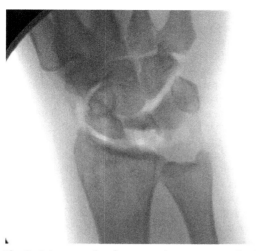

to pursue carpal reconstruction. The exploration also enables the surgeons to determine the dimensions of the osteochondral segment needed.

The wrist may be approached via either a volar or dorsal approach according to surgeon preference. For scaphoid reconstruction, the recipient vessel is either the volar branch of the radial artery (end-to-end) if volar approach is selected or the dorsal branch of the radial artery (end-to-side) if dorsal approach is selected. In cases of lunate reconstruction, the dorsal approach provides better visualization and ease of reconstruction.

### Preparation of the Carpus/Flap Fixation

The MFT flap provides a single convex cartilage-bearing surface that serves as the proximal-facing greater curvature of the newly reconstructed scaphoid or lunate. It therefore articulates with the native scaphoid or lunate fossa of the radius platform. The flap does not provide

**Fig. 7.** Intraoperative fluoroscopic anteroposterior image of lunate after resection of avascular and collapsed proximal segment. Note the preservation of the concave distal cartilage for articulation with the capitate.

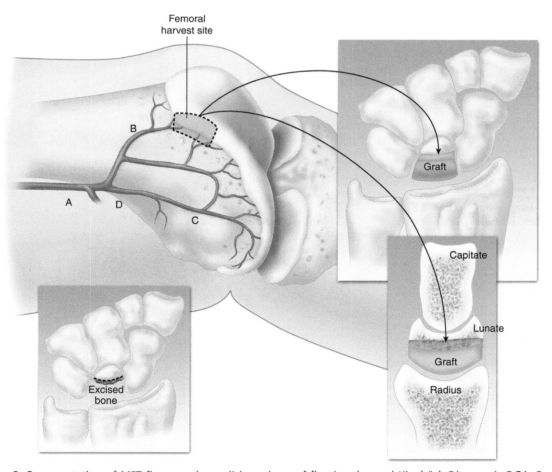

**Fig. 8.** Representation of MFT flap vascular pedicle and use of flap in advanced Kienböck Disease. A, DGA. B, transverse branch. C, longitudinal branch. D, SGA. Area of desired osteochondral harvest shaded in green. Inset demonstrates orientation of harvested segment as it relates to area of lunate reconstruction. (Copyright 2012, The Curtis National Hand Center.)

concave cartilage for recreation of the acetabulum of the scaphoid or the lunate. Thus these surfaces need to be preserved from the native carpus.

In the setting of scaphoid proximal pole nonunion, the nonunion site is resected generously while preserving the thin wafer of convex cartilage that articulates with the capitate (**Fig. 4**). With the wrist in flexion, the surgeon then generously resects further distally beyond the nonunion site to the midportion of the scaphoid (**Fig. 5**). This resection enables the surgeon to convert the difficult proximal pole nonunion into a waist level osteosynthesis. The segment of MFT is then carefully fashioned into a tightly fit reduction with the remaining distal scaphoid. Generous resection of the scaphoid to the level of the waist also enables the surgeon to harvest and inset a large osteochondral segment. The larger-sized segment facilitates

preservation of the periosteal vascular attachments and ease of screw fixation.

Cannulated screw fixation is directed through the cartilage surface of the flap across the waist-level osteosynthesis site and into the distal pole. This screw is often directed in a more longitudinal orientation than conventional scaphoid screw placement to achieve a good interface with the distal pole bone fragment and avoid the pathway of the previously failed screw fixation (**Fig. 6**).

In cases of advanced Kienböck disease, the lunate is subtotally resected (**Fig. 7**). Its diseased and collapsed proximal portion can be excavated with a scalpel and rongeur while carefully preserving the distal cartilage surface of the native lunate (**Fig. 8**). As in scaphoid reconstruction, the midcarpal joint need not be exposed. This maintains both the valuable linkage of the proximal row interosseous ligaments and the

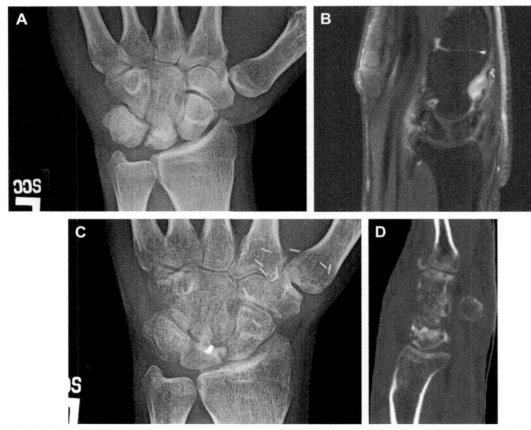

**Fig. 9.** A clinical case of a 28-year-old man with advanced Kienböck disease. (*A*) Preoperative anterioposterior radiograph demonstrating loss of carpal height. (*B*) Preoperative MRI sagittal image demonstrating coronal split of distal capitate cartilage surface. (*C*) Postoperative anterioposterior radiograph demonstrating restoration of carpal height, lunate morphology and vascularity. (*D*) Postoperative CT sagittal image demonstrating healing of reconstructed lunate with anatomic realignment of midcarpal concave surface of lunate.

concave cartilage surface effacing the midcarpal joint. If a significant coronal split with displacement exists, interosseous wire or fiber-wire coaptation of these segments may be performed to provide complete cartilage coverage of the midcarpal surface (**Fig. 9**). If there is no coronal split or the split is nondisplaced, a variety of fixation techniques may be planned (**Fig. 10**). The authors have used buried Kirschner wire fixation across the lunotriquetral joint and scapholunate joints, respectively (affixing the osteochondral flap), miniscrew fixation between larger segments of the native distal lunate into the flap, or complete absence of fixation with dependence on a tightly fashioned flap and the defect.

After careful measurement and sizing of the graft, the surgeon finds a satisfying and tight congruency between the flap and the evacuated lunate fossa.

## Flap Orientation

In the postoperative period, patients experience knee discomfort for 2 months to 4 months. They alter their gait for comfort. As in the setting of any knee surgery or injury, it is likely that they rely on their contralateral arm for assistance in ambulation, climbing stairs, or getting in or out of bed. For that reason, the authors most commonly harvest the ipsilateral MFT for scaphoid or lunate reconstruction.

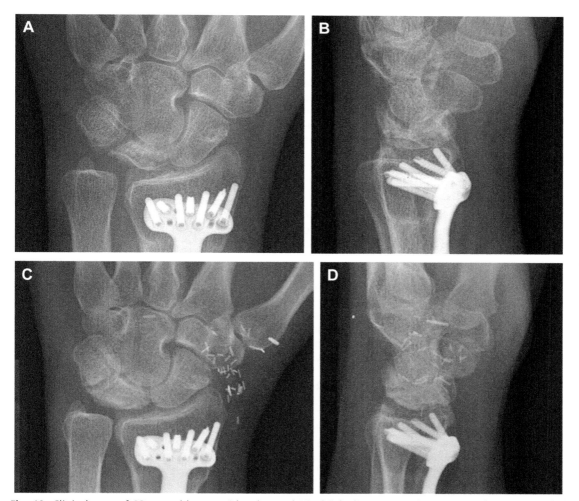

**Fig. 10.** Clinical case of 23-year-old man with advanced Kienböck disease. Despite attempted previous radial shortening osteotomy, the patient suffered from recurrent pain and evidence of further collapse. Preoperative (A) anteroposterior and (B) lateral radiograph demonstrating lunate collapse. Restoration of carpal height and lunate morphology are demonstrated on (C) anteroposterior (D) lateral radiographs 13 months after MFT reconstruction.

The volar or dorsal approach alters the orientation of the osteochondral segment during inset. In the most commonly used dorsal wrist approach, the flap dimensions when harvested from the ipsilateral knee correspond to the carpus as follows:

1. The proximal-to-distal harvest is measured to recreate the radial-to-ulnar dimensions of the scaphoid/lunate in the wrist.
2. The proximal trochlea is positioned radially; the distal trochlea is positioned ulnarly.
3. The anterior-to-posterior harvest is measured to recreate the proximal-to-distal dimension of the scaphoid/lunate in the wrist.
4. The anterior convex cartilage-bearing segment faces proximally in the wrist; the posterior cancellous surface of the harvested MFT faces distally in the wrist.
5. The medial-to-lateral harvest in the knee is measured to recreate the volar-to-dorsal dimensions of the scaphoid/lunate in the wrist.
6. The medial periosteum-bearing surface of the MFT is facing dorsally in the wrist to drape the vessels distally and gently draped into the snuffbox for anastomosis; the lateral cancellous bone surface of the harvested MFT faces volarly in the wrist.

## CLINICAL RESULTS

Two clinical series have been reported on the use of this flap. In 2013, Bürger and colleagues[11] reported on 16 patients who underwent MFT transfer for proximal pole scaphoid nonunion with an average of 14 months' follow-up (minimum 6 months). Fracture union was confirmed by CT scan in 15 of 16 patients; 12 of 16 patients reported complete pain relief whereas 4 of 16 reported improvement without complete pain relief. Preoperative and postoperative range of motion was similar.

In 2014, Bürger and colleagues[13] also reported on 16 cases of osteochondral MFT flap transfers for lunate reconstruction for advanced Kienböck disease with mean follow-up of 19 months (minimum 12 months). Healing was confirmed in 15 of 16 reconstructed lunates. Lichtman staging remained unchanged in 10 patients, improved in 4 patients, and worsened in 2 patients. All but 1 patient experienced improvement in wrist pain (12 of 16 patients with complete relief; 3 of 16 patients with incomplete relief). Wrist motion at follow-up averaged 50° extension and 38° flexion, similar to preoperative measurements. Average

grip strength at follow-up was 85% of the contralateral side.

## SUMMARY

The MFT flap provides vascularized osteochondral bone for reconstruction of small convex articular defects. Promising early clinical reports suggest that it may provide a novel solution to articular problems requiring replacement of damaged cartilage surfaces. Further research is under way to explore several areas requiring investigation, including donor site morbidity, long-term radiographic and clinical prevention of arthritis, and the importance of subchondral perfusion of vascularized cartilage survival within an intrasynovial environment. The expansion of this donor site for other clinical indications is also under way.

## REFERENCES

1. Acland RD, Schusterman M, Godina M, et al. The saphenous neurovascular free flap. Plast Reconstr Surg 1981;67:763–74.
2. Iorio ML, Masden DL, Higgins JP. Cutaneous angiosome territory of the medial femoral condyle osteocutaneous flap. J Hand Surg Am 2012;37:1033–41.
3. Pelzer M, Reichenberger M, Germann G. Osteo-periosteal-cutaneous flaps of the medial femoral condyle: a valuable modification for selected clinical situations. J Reconstr Microsurg 2010;26:291–4.
4. Martin D, Bitonti-Grillo C, De Biscop J, et al. Mandibular reconstruction using a free vascularised osteocutaneous flap from the internal condyle of the femur. Br J Plast Surg 1991;44:397–402.
5. Huang D, Wang HW, Xu DC, et al. An anatomic and clinical study of the adductor magnus tendon-descending genicular artery bone flap. Clin Anat 2011;24:77–83.
6. Higgins JP. Descending geniculate artery: the ideal recipient vessel for free tissue transfer coverage of below-the-knee amputation wounds. J Reconstr Microsurg 2011;27:525–9.
7. Kalicke T, Burger H, Muller EJ. A new vascularized cartilague-bone-graft for scaphoid nonunion with avascular necrosis of the proximal pole. Description of a new type of surgical procedure. Unfallchirurg 2008;111:201–5.
8. Hugon S, Koninckx A, Barbier O. Vascularized osteochondral graft from the medial femoral trochlea: anatomical study and clinical perspectives. Surg Radiol Anat 2010;32:817–25.

9. Iorio ML, Masden DL, Higgins JP. The limits of medial femoral condyle corticoperiosteal flaps. J Hand Surg Am 2011;36:1592–6.

10. Higgins JP, Bürger HK. Osteochondral flaps from the distal femur: expanding applications, harvest sites, and indications. J Reconstr Microsurg 2014; 30:483–90.

11. Bürger HK, Windhofer C, Gaggl AJ, et al. Vascularized medial femoral trochlea osteocartilaginous flap reconstruction of proximal pole scaphoid non-unions. J Hand Surg Am 2013;38:690–700.

12. Higgins JP, Bürger HK. Proximal scaphoid arthroplasty using the medial femoral trochlea flap. J Wrist Surg 2013;2:228–33.

13. Bürger HK, Windhofer C, Gaggl AJ, et al. Vascularized medial femoral trochlea osteochondral flap reconstruction of advanced Kienböck disease. J Hand Surg Am 2014;39:1313–22.

# Vascularized Small-Bone Transfers for Fracture Nonunion and Bony Defects

 CrossMark

Ai Dong Deng, MD[a], Marco Innocenti, MD[b],
Rohit Arora, MD[c], Markus Gabl, MD[c], Jin Bo Tang, MD[a],*

## KEYWORDS

- Vascularized bone grafting • Fracture nonunion • Scaphoid • Lunate • Kienbock disease
- Medial femoral condyle • Pedicled distal radial grafting • Osteoperiosteal or corticoperiosteal flaps

## KEY POINTS

- Vascularized small-bone grafting is an efficient and often necessary surgical approach for nonunion or necrosis of several bones in particular sites of the body, including scaphoid, lunate, distal ulna, and clavicle.
- The medial femoral condyle is an excellent graft source that can be used in treating scaphoid, ulna, clavicle, or lower-extremity bone defects, including nonunion.
- Vascularized bone grafting to the small bones, particularly involving reconstruction of damaged cartilage surfaces, should enhance subchondral vascular supply and help prevent cartilage regeneration.
- Pedicle distal radial bone grafting is still a viable option as a technically easier way to treat scaphoid nonunion or revascularization of Kienböck disease.
- Vascularized osteoperiosteal and corticoperiosteal flaps are useful for treating nonunion of long bones.

## INTRODUCTION

Vascularized bone grafting has frequently been used in reconstruction of long-bone defects, because vascular supply to the graft will ensure better healing to the defect size. Vascularized bone grafting for small-bone defects or nonunion is necessary only in some special clinical conditions, such as nonunion of scaphoid fractures, or defects in small bones such as clavicles, radius or ulna, facial bones, and tarsal bones in the foot.[1–5]

The sources of such bone grafts vary. Typically, vascularized iliac bone grafting has been used as a free transfer to many parts of the body, and pedicled bone chips taken from the distal radius have been used in the hand and wrist.[1,2,6,7] The medial femoral condyle (MFC) has emerged more recently as one of the most versatile donor sites in the treatment of challenging bone reconstruction. This graft donor site, described by Sakai and colleagues[8] in 1991, has recently gained popularity thanks to the work of Burger, Higgins, and others.[9–13] The current application of small-bone grafting in 3 units in 3 countries, China, Italy, and Austria, are summarized in later discussion. The indications and applications of small-bone grafting in the 3 units are summarized in **Table 1**.

The authors have nothing to disclose.
[a] Department of Hand Surgery, Affiliated Hospital of Nantong University, 20 West Temple Road, Nantong 226001, Jiangsu, China; [b] Plastic Surgery, University of Florence Careggi University Hospital, CTO, Largo Palagi 150139, Florence, Italy; [c] Department of Trauma Surgery and Sports Medicine, Medical University Innsbruck, Anichstrasse 35, A-6020, Innsbruck, Austria
* Corresponding author.
*E-mail address:* jinbotang@yahoo.com

Clin Plastic Surg 44 (2017) 267–285
http://dx.doi.org/10.1016/j.cps.2016.11.005

**Table 1**
**The current application of vascularized small-bone grafting in 3 units in China, Italy, and Austria**

|  | Nantong, China | Florence, Italy | Innsbruck, Austria |
|---|---|---|---|
| Free MFC graft | Scaphoid<br>Ulna<br>Clavicle<br>Lunate (advanced Kienböck) | Scaphoid<br>Ulna<br>Clavicle<br>Navicular bone | Scaphoid<br>Tibia<br>Metacarpal<br>— |
| Free iliac<br>bone graft | —<br>— | —<br>— | Scaphoid<br>Lunate (advanced Kienböck) |
| Distal radial<br>graft[a] | Scaphoid<br>Lunate (Kienbock) | —<br>— | —<br>— |

[a] A graft based on a pedicle of the 1,2 or 2,3 intercompartmental arteries (ICSRAs) for nonunion of the scaphoid or the fourth and fifth ICSRA for Kienbock disease.

## MEDIAL FEMORAL CONDYLE AS A GRAFT DONOR IN RECONSTRUCTION OF SMALL-BONE DEFECTS

Originally described as a periosteal or corticoperiosteal flap based on the descending genicular artery (DGA), this flap has evolved into a more structural graft including a variable amount of cancellous bone and finally into an osteochondral graft, including a small amount of the articular cartilage of the MFC.[9,10] From a structural point of view, this graft belongs to the family of flat bone flaps, such as the scapula and, more importantly, the iliac crest, and is therefore indicated in reconstructions of small defects that for some reason require vascularized bone.

Maxillofacial surgery and hand surgery are the 2 main fields of application of the procedure to a variety of conditions; nonunions, tumors, and infections are the most common abnormalities that benefit from an MFC graft. This flap provides a very well-vascularized bone block and a thick periosteum that may be significantly larger than the bone flap in order to overlap the junction with the host bone, improving the blood supply and the ability to heal. In addition, in the case of intraoral location of the flap, the periosteum is quickly colonized by the neighboring mucosa, providing optimal and fast integration with the surrounding tissues.

In the upper limbs, recalcitrant nonunion of the forearm bones and clavicle, scaphoid nonunion, necrosis of the proximal pole of the scaphoid, and Kienböck disease have been the pathologic conditions most frequently treated by an MFC graft. More recently, this graft has been successfully used in metacarpal and phalangeal reconstruction as well as tarsal reconstruction.

An MFC graft is actually a very versatile graft. In addition, the donor site morbidity is inconspicuous,[14] and the harvesting technique is relatively straightforward.

### Surgical Anatomy and Harvesting Technique

The surgical anatomy and the harvesting technique have been described in detail by several authors, who progressively refined the anatomic knowledge of the region and added many technical details to the procedure.

This flap is based on the DGA system. The DGA rises from the superficial femoral artery and runs distally, deep and posterior to the vastus medialis muscle. Usually it bifurcates 0.7 cm distal to its origin in 2 branches: the saphenous artery, which supplies the skin of the medial aspect of the knee, and a terminal, periosteal branch that supplies a rich periosteal network on the medial condyle. In this typical vascular configuration, the pedicle of a medial condyle flap may be up to 8 cm long. However, in about 30% of cases, the periosteal branch of the DGA is extremely small or even absent.[15] In those circumstances, the superior medial genicular artery, a short vessel that arises directly from the popliteal artery, is the main contributor to the periosteal network and the pedicle of such a flap.

The patient is placed supine with hips extrarotated and abducted, and the knee flexed at 80°. A sterile tourniquet is suggested but not mandatory. A longitudinal incision is placed over the projection of the posterior margin of the vastus medialis muscle and extended over the MFC. The DGA may be visualized close to the femur and to the posteromedial aspect of the vastus medialis muscle. After dedicating some branches to the muscle and its tendon, the artery supplies a rich periosteal plexus on the MFC together with the superior medial genicular artery (**Fig. 1**). The flap may be tailored in a variety of forms according to the specific need of the recipient area. It may be constituted only of periosteum and a thin layer of cortex, but it can be also a vascularized corticocancellous bone graft if a block of cancellous

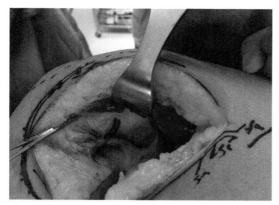

**Fig. 1.** The DGA and the periosteal vascular network on the MFC.

bone is included in the harvest. Finally, it may be an osteochondral graft when a small portion of cartilage is harvested (**Fig. 2**). The donor site morbidity is negligible, and according to Higgins and colleagues,[16,17] a graft up to 7 cm long may be safely harvested.

## Applications to Different Sites of the Body

Applications of this flap to different parts of the body are illustrated in later discussion through a few cases in Plastic Surgery, University of Florence Careggi University Hospital, Florence, Italy.

### Reconstruction of defects in ulna

A 45-year-old man suffered an open fracture of the radius and ulna of the left forearm. A nonunion of the ulna fracture was initially treated by conventional corticocancellous bone graft from the iliac crest. The graft united with the proximal stump of the recipient bone, but a nonunion recurred distally (**Fig. 3**A). An MFC corticoperiosteal flap was harvested from the contralateral knee, based on the DGA. Some parallel slots were made by saw on the inner surface of the graft (**Fig. 3**B) in order to make it foldable (**Fig. 3**C) and wrap it around the site of nonunion. The plate was stable and therefore left in place. There was radiologic evidence of successful union 3 months after surgery (**Fig. 3**D).

### Clavicle reconstruction

A 52-year-old woman suffered an unstable nonunion after conservative treatment of a fracture of the left clavicle. Two attempts at reconstruction by means of autologous corticocancellous bone from the iliac crest failed over the following 3 years. When the patient was referred to the authors, radiographs showed atrophic nonunion of the clavicle. Movement at the glenohumeral joint was limited and painful. A reconstruction by means of corticocancellous MFC was performed, and a new locking compression plate was used to stabilize the graft (**Fig. 4**A). The vascular pedicle was anastomosed to the thoracoacromial artery and

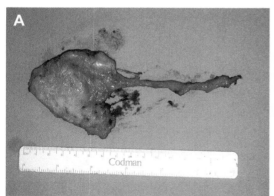

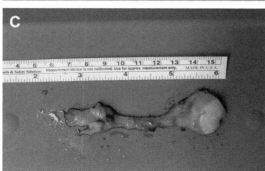

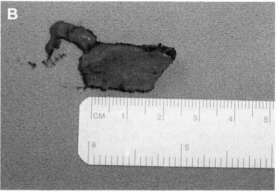

**Fig. 2.** (*A*) MFC may be harvested including periosteum and a thin layer of cortex only (*A*), or as a bone block including cancellous bone (*B*). The osteochondral graft includes a small portion of cartilage (*C*).

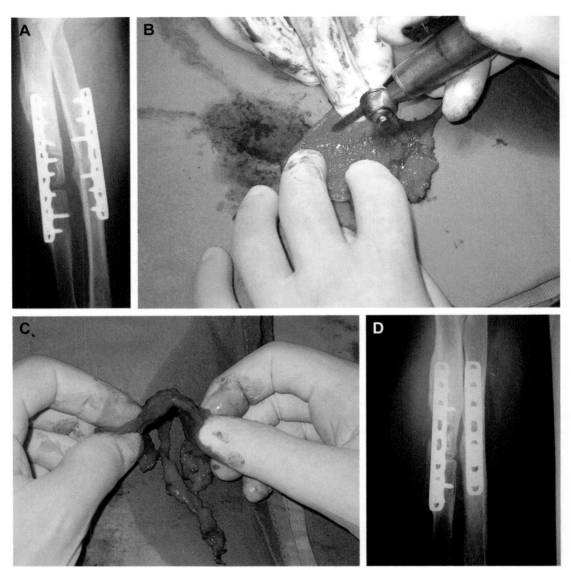

**Fig. 3.** (*A*) Atrophic nonunion at the distal junction of a conventional corticocancellous bone graft in the ulna. (*B*) Parallel slots were made by saw on the inner surface of the graft in order to interrupt the cortex. (*C*) Subsequently, the flap was wrapped around the bone defect. (*D*) Bone healing 3 months postoperatively.

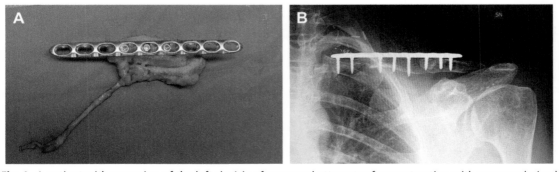

**Fig. 4.** A patient with nonunion of the left clavicle after several attempts of reconstruction with nonvascularized bone graft. (*A*) Preplating of the MFC with a locking compression plate. (*B*) Bone healing at 4 months.

vein. At 4 month follow-up, the patient was pain free and had recovered functional range of motion (ROM) at the affected shoulder. Radiographs showed union of the graft on both sides 6 months after surgery (**Fig. 4**B).

### Navicular bone reconstruction

A 63-year-old man underwent multiple attempts at reconstruction of the navicular bone of the right foot after traumatic loss of the bone. The last one was an implant of a synthetic spacer, which totally failed in providing stability to the mid foot (**Fig. 5**A). The patient was not able to load on the foot and needed crutches to walk. After removal of the spacer (**Fig. 5**B) and aggressive debridement of the defect, the authors used a free medial condyle flap to achieve a stable fusion of the mid foot. The graft was harvested as a bone block with a redundant periosteal flap and tailored according to a wax template corresponding to the tridimensional defect (**Fig. 5**C). The oversize periosteal flap was able to overlap the junction with the tarsal bones and the graft stabilized with a single screw (**Fig. 5**D). An end-to-end anastomosis was performed with the anterior tibial artery. Full and pain-free weight-bearing was possible 3 months after surgery.

### *Practical Tips and Comments on the Medial Femoral Condyle Transfer*

The MFC probably represents the most useful innovation in vascularized bone grafts. Over its direct competitor, the iliac crest, MFC has shown several advantages in clinical practice, including the low morbidity at the donor site and easy dissection and possibility to customize the graft according to the defect. However, a drawback of the procedure is some anatomic variability of the pedicle, because in about 30% of cases the feeding pedicle is the superior medial genicular artery, which is quite short.

Current indications for MFC grafting are "difficult" small defects that need vascularized bone such as nonunions of the clavicle or the bones of forearm, hand, and foot and situations in maxillofacial surgery that depend on the ability of the thick periosteum to be colonized by the oral mucosa. Finally, the osteochondral version of the flap has opened up new perspectives in the reconstruction of the proximal pole of scaphoid and lunate.

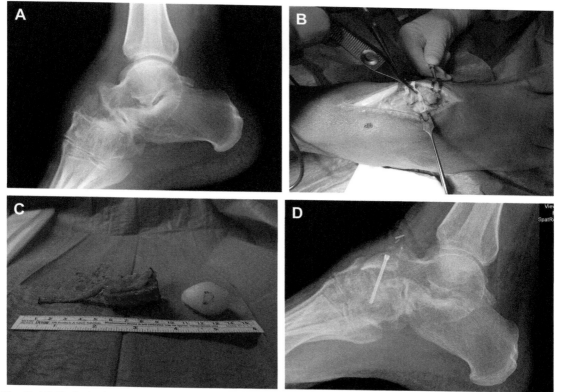

**Fig. 5.** (*A*) Navicular bone loss. (*B*) The removal of a synthetic spacer previously implanted after traumatic navicular bone loss. (*C*) The MFC is tailored according to a 3-dimensional template of the defect. (*D*) The bone healing at 3 months.

## FREE VASCULARIZED BONE GRAFTS FOR CHALLENGING INDICATIONS
### *Vascularized Iliac Bone Grafting: Kienböck Disease*

In the treatment of advanced Kienböck disease (ie, Lichtman stage 3), the authors reconstruct the fractured lunate by a free vascularized iliac bone graft and external fixation. The details of the surgical procedure used at the Medical University Innsbruck in Austria were described in a previous report.[18]

Because poor vascularity is a cause of avascular necrosis in Kienböck disease and bony

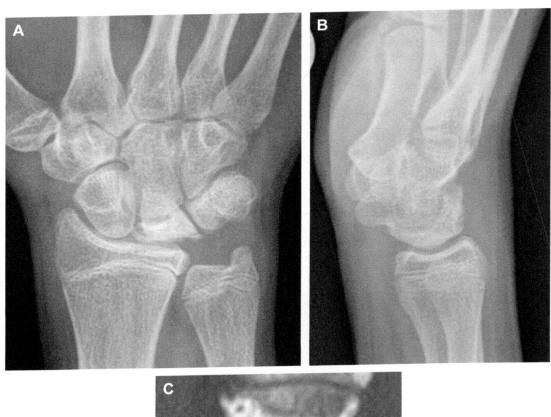

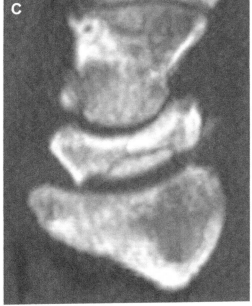

**Fig. 6.** (*A, B*) Collapse of the lunate with loss of lunate height. (*C*) CT scan confirmed his diagnosis of stage 3B Kienböck disease.

impairment occurs in stage 3 disease, lunate revascularization and vascularized bone transfer are reasonable. The authors consider the biomechanical properties of the iliac bone graft to be superior to those of the distal radius. Schnitzler and colleagues[19] demonstrated that the dense cancellous structure of the iliac crest graft is mechanically superior to other donor sites. Bone volume and bone turnover of the distal radius are lower; trabeculae are thinner, and the cortices are only half as thick as the iliac crest.[19]

An external fixator prevents direct load bearing of the lunate and protects the graft until osseointegration is achieved. Because revascularization leads to increased osteoclastic activity, which weakens the bone during the early postoperative period,[20] the authors use an external fixator for 8 weeks after surgery to neutralize compression forces that might displace the graft and be detrimental during incorporation. In their described procedure, the dense-structured cancellous bone with its strong cortical bone from the iliac crest is placed on the palmar aspect of the lunate, where the maximal axial load is applied.[21]

The authors illustrate their surgical methods in a 17-year-old boy. He presented with pain at the dorsal wrist and collapse of the lunate with loss of lunate height (**Fig. 6**A). Computed tomographic (CT) scan confirmed his diagnosis of stage 3B Kienböck disease (**Fig. 6**B). Intraoperatively, a volar approach to the lunate was used (**Fig. 7**A). Note the dorsal external fixator already applied. The core lunate and the necrotic bone were debrided, leaving the cartilage shell of the lunate. A vascularized tricortical iliac bone graft based on the deep circumflex iliac artery was harvested (**Fig. 7**B). The graft was shaped to fit into the lunate (**Fig. 7**C) and fixed with a Kirschner wire, and the pedicle was end-to-side anastomosed to the ulnar artery. An external fixator was used for 8 weeks. Eleven years later, radiographs showed the reconstructed lunate height had been maintained with only minor arthritic changes in the lunate facet (**Fig. 8**).

## Vascularized Medial Femoral Condyle Osteochondral Bone Graft: Scaphoid Proximal Pole Necrosis

This method has been used by many surgeons. The authors share similar views and illustrate the method in a case with scaphoid pole necrosis from Medical University Innsbruck.

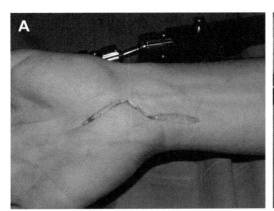

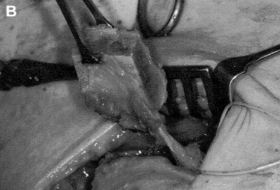

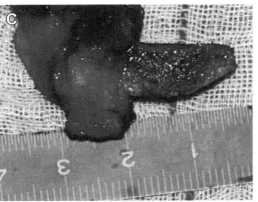

**Fig. 7.** (*A*) A volar approach to the lunate was used. (*B*) A vascularized tricortical iliac bone graft based on the deep circumflex iliac artery was harvested. (*C*) The graft was shaped to fit into the lunate, ready to be inserted and fixation with a Kirschner wire. An external fixator was then used for 8 weeks.

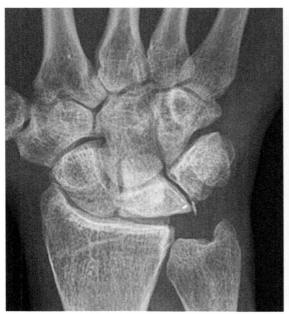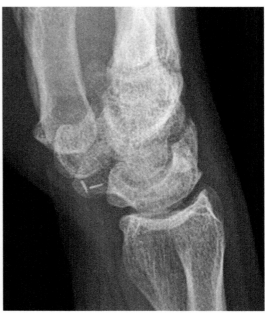

**Fig. 8.** Eleven years later, radiographs show the reconstructed lunate height had been maintained with only minor arthritic changes in the lunate facet in posteroanterior and lateral views.

A 29-year-old male farmer presented with pain in his right wrist after initial trauma, a fall during work on his outstretched right hand, 8 years previously. Radiograph showed proximal pole nonunion (**Fig. 9**). The ROM of the wrist was extension 55° and flexion was 45°. CT scan showed fragmented proximal pole of the scaphoid (see **Fig. 9**). Wrist arthroscopy was performed to clarify the cartilage condition of the scaphoid facet. The proximal pole was fragmented, and the scaphoid facet showed no degenerative changes (see **Fig. 9**). The authors decided to resect the proximal pole and to replace it with an MFC graft. An osteochondral bone graft was shaped to fit into the defect created from resection of the proximal scaphoid (see **Fig. 9**). The convex surface of the graft faced the scaphoid facet of the distal joint surface of the radius. The graft was fixed using a volar locking plate (see **Fig. 9**), and the pedicle was connected with an end-to-side anastomosis to the radial artery. Postoperative radiographs of the knee show the donor site defect filled with bone substitute (**Fig. 10**). A 14-month follow-up radiograph shows an incorporated bone graft with no signs of scapholunate instability (see **Fig. 10**). The periosteum of the graft probably enhances formation of a stable tissue layer, because it covers the scapholunate ligamentous complex. At follow-up, wrist extension was 55° and flexion was 50°. He noted pain of scale 2 after manual work.

### Vascularized Medial Femoral Condyle Corticoperiosteal Flap: Metacarpal Head Nonunion

Sakai and colleagues[8] described free vascularized thin, corticoperiosteal flaps based on the articular branch of the DGA in the treatment of nonunions of the humerus, ulna, and metacarpals. The authors take a similar surgical approach and illustrate it in a case here.

A 31-year-old man presented with an intra-articular fracture of the fourth metacarpal head (**Fig. 11**). CT showed a volarly displaced head fragment that was fixed with a cannulated headless screw from a dorsal approach. Postoperative radiographs confirmed anatomic reconstruction with stable fixation (see **Fig. 11**). Six months later, the screw was removed in another institution because its dorsal prominence was causing extensor synovitis.

Eight months after the initial surgery, the patient was referred to the authors with pain of scale 4, loss of flexion of 40°, and extension lag of 10°. Radiographs showed a collapsed and necrotic metacarpal head (see **Fig. 11**). Possible options, including joint fusion, prosthetic replacement, arthroplasty, or osteochondral graft, were discussed with the patient, and the decision was made to replace the necrotic head with an osteochondral graft, that is, an MFC graft. Intraoperatively, the necrotic fragment was resected, preserving the radial and ulnar collateral ligaments (see **Fig. 11**). An osteochondral bone graft was shaped to fit into the defect created from

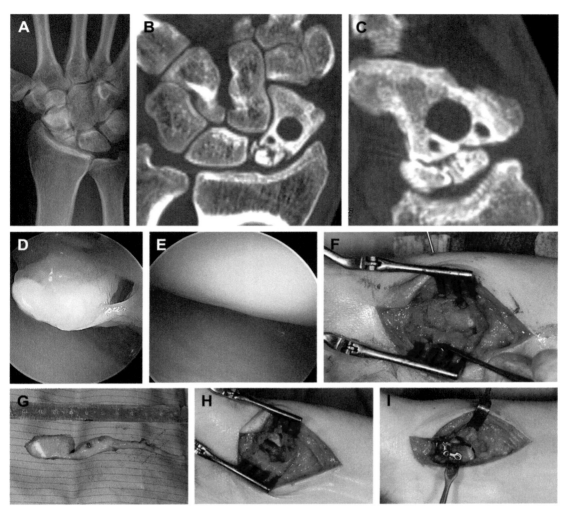

**Fig. 9.** Proximal pole nonunion of the scaphoid of a 29-year-old male farmer. (*A, B*) Plain radiographs and (*C*) CT scan shows fragmented proximal pole of the scaphoid. (*D*). Wrist arthroscopy shows fragmentation of the proximal pole. (*E*) The scaphoid facet had no degenerative changes. (*F*) An MFC graft was harvested. (*G*) The graft was shaped to fit into the defect in the proximal scaphoid. (*H*) The convex surface of the graft faced the scaphoid facet of the distal radial articular surface. (*I*) The graft was fixed using a volar locking plate.

resection (see **Fig. 11**). The convex surface of the graft faced the base of the proximal phalanx. The graft was fixed using screws, and the pedicle was anastomosed end to end to the second metacarpal artery. Radiographs taken 24 months after surgery showed a united graft with no signs of instability (**Fig. 12**). The ROM of the metacarpophalangeal joint was flexion 70° and no extension lag. The patient reported no pain.

### Free Vascularized Osteoperiosteal Graft with Corticoperiosteum of a Medial Femoral Condyle: Tibial Nonunion

An extension of the existing MFC graft is to include more periosteal components, making it more suitable in treating nonunion of the tibia. The authors illustrate the surgical methods using a case from the Medical University Innsbruck.

A 29-year-old man presented with symptomatic longstanding nonunion of the distal tibia after plate fixation. Six months after primary surgery, the plate fixation failed, making full weight-bearing impossible for the patient (**Fig. 13**). CT scan showed atrophic nonunion with bony defect of 3 cm (see **Fig. 13**). Intraoperatively, the nonunion was debrided; the broken plate was removed, and an intramedullary nail was inserted (see **Fig. 13**). A free vascularized osteoperiosteal with some amount of corticoperiosteal graft from the MFC was harvested (see **Fig. 13**) and fixed into the bony defect using 2 screws. Radiographs

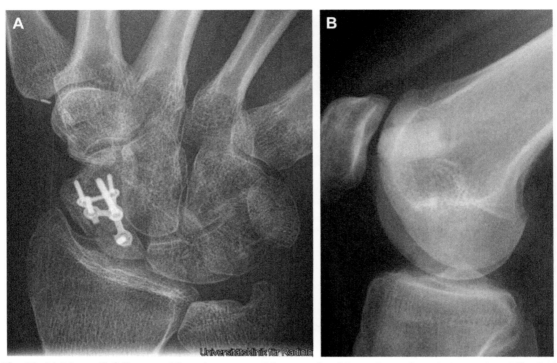

**Fig. 10.** At 14-month follow-up, (*A*) an incorporated bone graft with no signs of scapholunate instability in a plain radiograph; (*B*) the donor site defect in the knee area had been filled with bone substitute.

taken at final follow-up (at 26 months) confirmed bone union (**Fig. 14**), and the patient was capable of full weight-bearing and returned to his previous work level.

## Consideration of Indications, Variations in Graft Designs, and Practical Tips

In cases where the authors need an osteochondral bone graft to replace necrotic cartilage with collapsed subchondral bone, they use the free vascularized osteochondral bone flap (ie, MFC) based on the DGA. In advanced Kienböck disease, where strong cortical bone is needed to restore the collapsed lunate height, the authors use the tricortical free iliac bone graft based on the deep circumflex iliac artery with an additional external fixator. In cases of long-bone nonunion with minor bone defect (<3 cm), they use an osteo-periosteal or corticoperiosteal free MFC graft in addition to rigid bone fixation.

Based on clinical series in Innsbruck, following the goals of stability and viability, using a free vascularized bone graft from the iliac crest enabled a mean recovery to 98° of wrist flexion-extension arc and to 45° of wrist deviation arc. Assessment of radiological results in their patients showed an average Ståhl index of 0.4 and an average carpal height index of 0.54 at final follow-up.

Radiologically, the initial restoration of the carpal height could be maintained for an average of 13 years in the collapsed lunate stage 3A and 3B. Free vascularized bone graft from the iliac crest has been found to be strong enough to carry the applied loads for a long period of time. It has also been proven beneficial to tailor the graft adequately, especially to the long sagittal diameter of the lunate.[22]

In cases where bone replacement is prolonged, subchondral bone collapse and complete resorption of cartilage may occur.[23] In cases like avascular necrosis of the proximal pole of the scaphoid after fracture nonunion, Kienböck disease, or bone defects after tumor resection, the recipient bone has biologically unfavorable characteristics. These considerations support the choice of a vascularized osteochondral autograft with a reliable vascular and bone integration, leading to biomechanically stable graft incorporation.[24]

## VASCULARIZED BONE GRAFTS FOR BONE NONUNION OR NECROSIS IN THE HAND
### Variations and Preferences in Donor Sites

In the Affiliated Hospital of Nantong University, China, 10 surgeons on the authors' team have different preferences in treating scaphoid

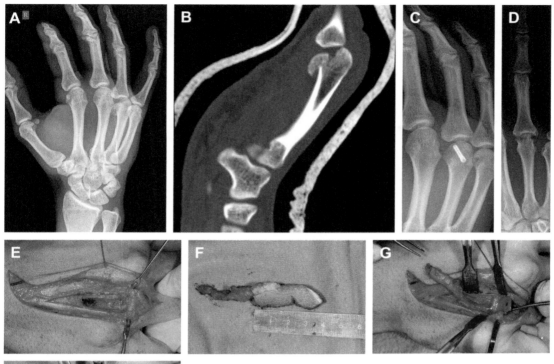

Fig. 11. An intra-articular fracture of the fourth metacarpal head of a 31-year-old man. (A) A preoperative plain radiograph shows the fourth metacarpal head fracture. (B) CT shows a volarly displaced head fragment. (C) Screw fixation and removal of the screw in another institution 6 months after screw fixation. (D) Eight months after the initial surgery, radiographs show a collapsed and necrotic metacarpal head. (E) An osteochondral MFC graft was decided. Intraoperatively the necrotic fragment was resected, preserving the radial and ulnar collateral ligaments. (F) The graft was shaped to fit into the defect created from resection. (G, H) The convex surface of the graft faced the base of the proximal phalanx. The graft was fixed using screws.

nonunion or necrosis: 2 use the MFC, and the other 8 use the distal radial bone based on the 1,2 or 2,3 intercompartment supraretinacular arteries (1,2 ICSRA and 2,3 ICSRA); none use nonvascularized graft or vascularized iliac bone grafts. In addition, some perform decompression and distal radial bone graft based on the fourth and fifth extensor compartment arteries in early-stage Kienböck disease.

Two practical reasons account for variations in deciding donor sites among surgeons in this unit: First, the 10 attending surgeons have different preferences or experience levels in individual graft techniques. Some tend to use those that they have been using for many years. Second, easy harvest of donor tissue in the same surgical field of the recipient hand and wrist represents advantages in deciding their surgical options. The authors illustrate the methods currently in use in this unit through 5 cases:

1. *Free vascularized MFC grafting for scaphoid nonunion:* In a 58-year-old man presenting with pain of the left wrist with radiographic diagnosis of nonunion of the left scaphoid waist fracture (**Fig. 15**).
2. *1,2 ICSRA-based pedicled distal radial bone grafting for scaphoid nonunion:* In a 33-year-old man presenting with pain of the left wrist with radiographic diagnosis of nonunion of the left scaphoid wrist fracture (**Fig. 16**).
3. *Free vascularized MFC grafting for advanced Kienböck disease:* In a 42-year-old man presenting with Lichtman stage 3 Kienböck disease of the right wrist (**Fig. 17**).
4. *Decompression and pedicled bone grafting (fourth and fifth intercompartmental artery pedicled distal radial graft) for early-stage Kienböck disease:* In a 46-year-old woman and another 47-year-old woman with right wrist pain diagnosed as stage 1 Kienböck disease (**Fig. 18**).

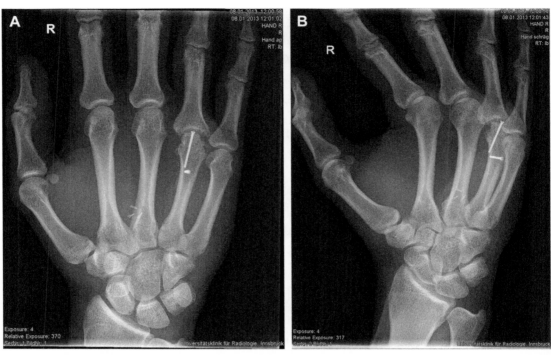

**Fig. 12.** Radiographs taken 24 months after surgery show a healed graft with no signs of instability. (*A*) Posteroanterior view. (*B*) Lateral view.

## Considerations and Practical Tips

The authors believe that 1,2 ICSRA- or 2,3 ICSRA-based pedicled distal radial grafts remain viable options in treating nonunion of the scaphoid fracture, although recent reports suggest that the MFC may be an even better graft source. They recommend that either pedicled or free vascularized bone grafting should be used in nonunion of the scaphoid. This approach does not mean that nonvascularized bone grafting does not lead to healing in some cases, rather vascularized bone grafts, particularly those based on a pedicled bone graft, represent an easy and efficient way to correct the nonunion. Some have moved to the use of an MFC, and the outcomes have been very good.

For Kienböck disease, the authors' team members have widely varying views on the need for vascularized bone grafting in the early stages of this disease. Only 2 team members perform such grafts for early-stage Kienböck disease. The authors feel that the revascularization of the lunate after such surgeries could be the result of decompression after a part of the bone is taken from the center of the lunate, rather than bringing in blood supply, because a decompression procedure alone can be efficient. In addition, early-stage Kienböck

disease may heal spontaneously or with simple splinting. Therefore, the authors maintain that the bone chip taken from the lunate should be not exceed one-fourth of the size of the lunate, and the need for this surgery should be fully explained to patients before surgery. It should not be routine for early-stage Kienböck disease.

For advanced Kienböck disease, the authors consider the MFC an excellent donor site if a part of cartilage is included in the graft. Future reports should compare the outcomes of the different graft sources for advanced Kienböck disease.

## FUTURE CHALLENGES

Vascularized bone grafts have been proven effective in promoting the healing of chronic nonunions, restoring vascularity to osteonecrotic bone, and reconstituting segmental bone defects resulting from trauma, infection, or tumor resection. Nonvascularized osteochondral grafts, known as mosaic transfers, have been used successfully in many indications. Although nonvascularized grafts have limited osteogenic capacity and require creeping substitution of the graft bone, vascularized grafts preserve viable osteocytes and blood

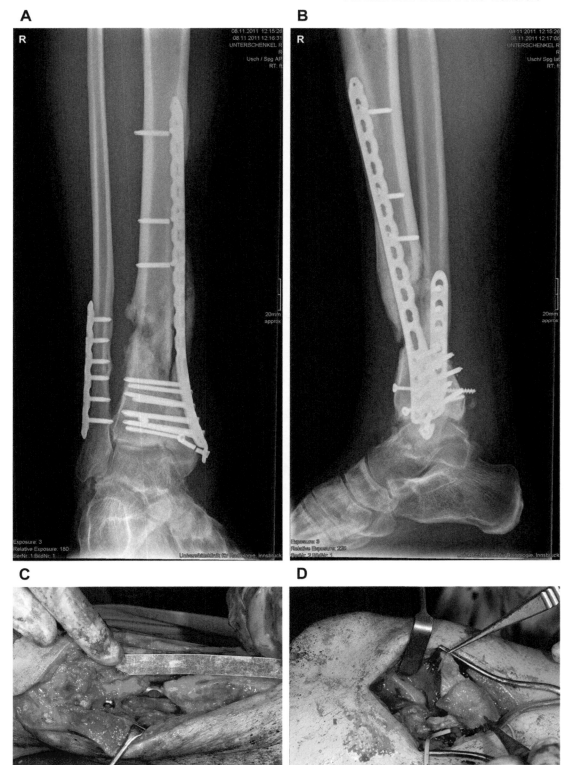

**Fig. 13.** Nonunion of the distal tibia after plate fixation in a 29-year-old man. (*A*) Six months after plate fixation, nonunion of the tibia was found in radiographs. (*A*) Posteroanterior view. (*B*) Lateral view. (*C*) Intraoperatively, the nonunion was debrided; the broken plate removed, and an intramedullary nail was inserted. (*D*) A free vascularized osteoperiosteal with some amount of corticoperiosteal graft from the MFC was harvested and fixed into the bony defect using 2 screws.

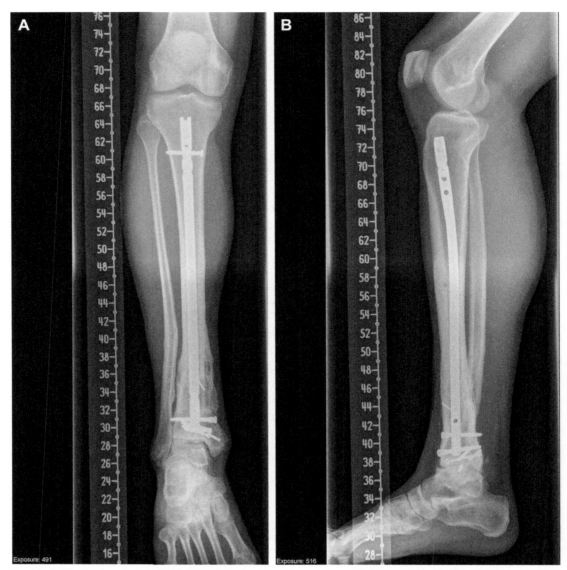

**Fig. 14.** Radiographs taken at final follow-up at 26 months confirmed bone union. (*A*) Posteroanterior view. (*B*) Lateral view.

supply, resulting in faster incorporation and healing.

## Osteochondral Defects of the Joints

Osteochondral lesions of convex joint surfaces, resulting from trauma, infection, aseptic necrosis, or tumor resection, are challenging for the surgeon.[3,4,25–29] Total replacement and joint fusion might not always be possible, and for some patients, are also not acceptable options.[1,2,29–32] In the wrist, limited bone fusions and bone resection can be considered, but are always associated with substantial loss of ROM. In selected cases,

osteochondral replacement of nonunions and bone defects may preserve the involved joints and active motion.

## Nonunion or Necrosis of Small Bones in the Hand

In the hand and wrist, recalcitrant nonunion of the joint surfaces in the carpal bones, the metacarpals, and phalanges often present with small and poor-quality segments after multiple previous surgical fixation attempts or in the case of aseptic necrosis. In these circumstances, a nonvascularized graft is inadequate because of the absence of blood

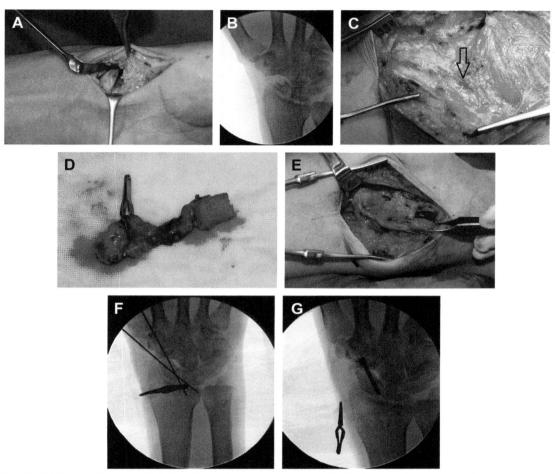

**Fig. 15.** A 58-year-old man with left wrist scaphoid non-union. (*A, B*) The bony defect was seen in the operating table and with mini-C arm X-ray machine during surgery. (*C*) The course of the DGA and the site (indicated with an *arrow*) where it courses deep to nourish the MFC to be harvested. (*D*) The MFC has been harvested, ready to be transferred to the scaphoid. (*E, F*) Temporary K-wire fixations and final headless screw fixation. The scaphoid healed, and the patient remained asymptomatic at 2 years follow-up.

supply or poor quality of joint cartilage. A vascularized osteochondral flap of a contour similar to the convex joint surface is a better way to reconstruct the necrotic and diminutive joint surface.[33,34]

Viability of chondrocytes is a concern with osteochondral grafts, because 50% of nourishment to these cells comes from the subchondral vascular network.[35] The vascularized MFC is a valuable graft source when including a part of the cartilage surface—making an osteochondral flap.

## Nonunion of Long Bones in the Lower Extremities

Reconstruction of segmental long-bone defects in the lower extremities has been reported in the literature, with the free fibular graft the most popular and reliable technique. Treatment of recalcitrant fracture nonunions with minor bony defect (<3 cm) can be successfully treated with a free vascularized osteoperiosteal or corticoperiosteal MFC graft.[36] Corticoperiosteal flaps were found to be more efficient in bone production than periosteal flaps.[37] This difference has been attributed to better preservation of the deepest layer of the periosteum (so-called cambium layer) thought to be responsible for most of the osteogenetic activity of the periosteum.[34] The combination of rigid fracture fixation and the osteogenetic capacity of the corticoperiosteal flap may produce good results in difficult nonunions without major bone defects.

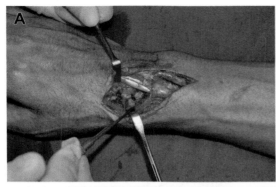

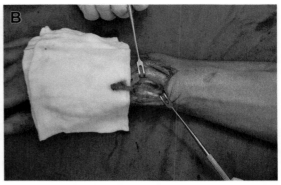

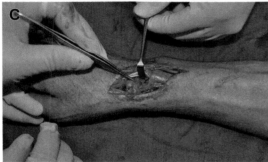

**Fig. 16.** A 33-year-old man with left scaphoid waist fracture and nonunion. (*A*) Bony defect in the scaphoid with nonunion. (*B*) Harvesting the 1,2 ICSRA-based distal radial graft. (*B*) After the graft was transferred to the defect site of the scaphoid.

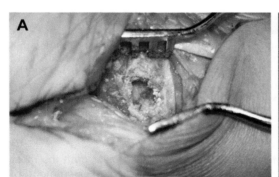

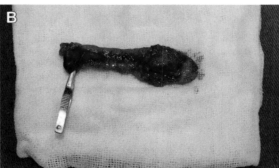

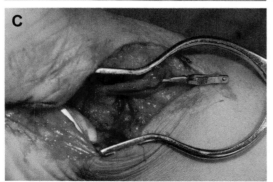

**Fig. 17.** A 42-year-old man with advanced Kienbock disease. (*A*) A bone defect was created through taking the necrotic bone in the lunate. (*B*) The MFC graft was taken. (*C*) The graft was placed to the defect site of the lunate.

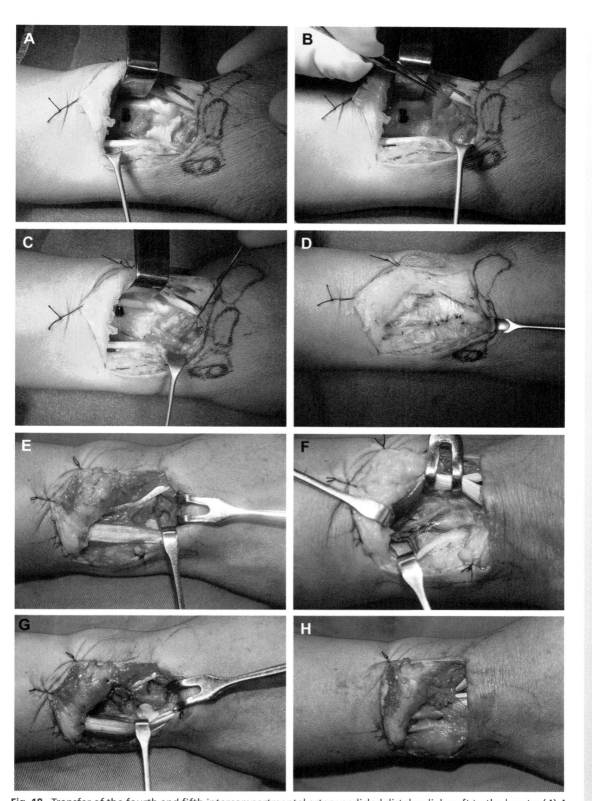

**Fig. 18.** Transfer of the fourth and fifth intercompartmental artery pedicled distal radial graft to the lunate. (*A*) A 46-year-old woman, with early-stage Kienbock disease in the right hand. Through a dorsal approach, decompression of the lunate was decompressed through drilling a round hole (1 cm) in the center of the lunate. A bone was taken from the distal radius. (*B*) Rotating the bone chip based on the vascular pedicle. Note the preservation of at site of attachment of the vascular pedicle. (*C*) Transfer of the bone to the lunate. (*D*) Closure of the carpal joint capsule. (*E–H*) A similar decompression and pedicled bone transfer to the lunate of the right hand of a 47-year-old woman. The 2 patients remained asymptomatic at follow-up 3 years later.

## SUMMARY

Vascularized small bone grafting is an efficient and useful surgical option for nonunion or necrosis of several particular anatomic sites. In particular, the MFC is an excellent graft source and can be used in treating scaphoid nonunion, ulnar, clavicle, or lower-extremity bone defects, including nonunion. The authors believe that vascularized bone grafting to the small bones, particularly those including cartilage surfaces, is important for subchondral vascular supply and in preventing regeneration of the joint surface. Pedicle distal radial bone grafting is still a viable option, representing a technically more feasible way to treat scaphoid nonunion or revascularization after Kienböck disease. The osteoperiosteal or corticoperiosteal flap is useful for nonunion of a long bone.

## REFERENCES

1. Ferguson DO, Shanbhag V, Hedley H, et al. Scaphoid fracture non-union: a systematic review of surgical treatment using bone graft. J Hand Surg Eur Vol 2016;41:492–500.
2. Pinder RM, Brkljac M, Rix L, et al. Treatment of scaphoid nonunion: a systematic review of the existing evidence. J Hand Surg Am 2015;40:1797–805.e3.
3. Elgammal A, Lukas B. Vascularized medial femoral condyle graft for management of scaphoid nonunion. J Hand Surg Eur Vol 2015;40:848–54.
4. Kamrani RS, Farhoud A, Nabian MH, et al. Vascularized posterior interosseous pedicled bone grafting for infected forearm nonunion. J Hand Surg Eur Vol 2016;41:441–7.
5. Brandtner C, Hachleitner J, Buerger H, et al. Combination of microvascular medial femoral condyle and iliac crest flap for hemi-midface reconstruction. Int J Oral Maxillofac Surg 2015;44:692–6.
6. Hirche C, Heffinger C, Xiong L, et al. The 1,2-intercompartmental supraretinacular artery vascularized bone graft for scaphoid nonunion: management and clinical outcome. J Hand Surg Am 2014;39:423–9.
7. Payatakes A, Sotereanos DG. Pedicled vascularized bone grafts for scaphoid and lunate reconstruction. J Am Acad Orthop Surg 2009;17:744–55.
8. Sakai K, Doi K, Kawai S. Free vascularized thin corticoperiosteal graft. Plast Reconstr Surg 1991;87:290–8.
9. Bürger HK, Windhofer C, Gaggl AJ, et al. Vascularized medial femoral trochlea osteochondral flap reconstruction of advanced Kienböck disease. J Hand Surg Am 2014;39:1313–22.
10. Higgins JP, Burger HK. Proximal scaphoid arthroplasty using the medial femoral trochlea flap. J Wrist Surg 2013;2:228–33.
11. Hamada Y, Hibino N, Kobayashi A. Expanding the utility of modified vascularized femoral periosteal bone-flaps: an analysis of its form and a comparison with a conventional-bone-graft. J Clin Orthop Trauma 2014;5:6–17.
12. Del Pinal F, Innocenti M. Evolving concepts in the management of the bone gap in the upper limb. Long and small defects. J Plast Reconstr Aesthet Surg 2007;60:776–92.
13. Houdek MT, Wagner ER, Wyles CC, et al. New options for vascularized bone reconstruction in the upper extremity. Semin Plast Surg 2015;29:20–9.
14. Rao SS, Sexton CC, Higgins JP. Medial femoral condyle flap donor-site morbidity: a radiographic assessment. Plast Reconstr Surg 2013;131:357e–62e.
15. García-Pumarino R, Franco JM. Anatomical variability of descending genicular artery. Ann Plast Surg 2014;73:607–11.
16. Katz RD, Parks BG, Higgins JP. The axial stability of the femur after harvest of the medial femoral condyle corticocancellous flap: a biomechanical study of composite femur models. Microsurgery 2012;32:213–8.
17. Endara MR, Brown BJ, Shuck J, et al. Torsional stability of the femur after harvest of the medial femoral condyle corticocancellous flap. J Reconstr Microsurg 2015;31:364–8.
18. Gabl M, Lutz M, Reinhart C, et al. Stage 3 Kienbock's disease: reconstruction of the fractured lunate using a free vascularized iliac bone graft and external fixation. J Hand Surg Br 2002;27:369–73.
19. Schnitzler CM, Biddulph SL, Mesquita JM, et al. Bone structure and turnover in the distal radius and iliac crest: a histomorphometric study. J Bone Miner Res 1996;11:1761–8.
20. Aspenberg P, Wang JS, Jonsson K, et al. Experimental osteonecrosis of the lunate. Revascularization may cause collapse. J Hand Surg Br 1994;19:565–9.
21. Iwasaki N, Minami A, Miyazawa T, et al. Force distribution through the wrist joint in patients with different stages of Kienbock's disease: using computed tomography osteoabsorptiometry. J Hand Surg Am 2000;25:870–6.
22. Arora R, Lutz M, Deml C, et al. Long-term subjective and radiological outcome after reconstruction of Kienböck's disease stage 3 treated by a free vascularized iliac bone graft. J Hand Surg Am 2008;33:175–81.
23. Malinin T, Ouellette EA. Articular cartilage nutrition is mediated by subchondral bone: a long- term autograft study in baboons. Osteoarthritis Cartilage 2000;8:483–91.
24. Tanaka Y, Omokawa S, Fujii T, et al. Vascularized bone graft from the medial calcaneus for treatment

of large osteochondral lesions of the medial talus. Foot Ankle Int 2006;27:1143–7.

25. Haefeli M, Schaefer DJ, Schumacher R, et al. Titanium template for scaphoid reconstruction. J Hand Surg Eur Vol 2015;40:526–33.

26. Citlak A, Akgun U, Bulut T, et al. Partial capitate shortening for Kienböck's disease. J Hand Surg Eur Vol 2015;40:957–60.

27. Peters SJ, Degreef I, De Smet L. Avascular necrosis of the capitate: report of six cases and review of the literature. J Hand Surg Eur Vol 2015;40:520–5.

28. Liodaki E, Xing SG, Mailaender P, et al. Management of difficult intra-articular fractures or fracture dislocations of the proximal interphalangeal joint. J Hand Surg Eur Vol 2015;40:16–23.

29. Frueh FS, Calcagni M, Lindenblatt N. The hemi-hamate autograft arthroplasty in proximal interphalangeal joint reconstruction: a systematic review. J Hand Surg Eur Vol 2015;40:24–32.

30. Yeoh D, Tourret L. Total wrist arthroplasty: a systematic review of the evidence from the last 5 years. J Hand Surg Eur Vol 2015;40:458–68.

31. Mattila S, Waris E. Unfavourable short-term outcomes of a poly-L/D-lactide scaffold for thumb trapeziometacarpal arthroplasty. J Hand Surg Eur Vol 2016;41:328–34.

32. Saltzman BM, Frank JM, Slikker W, et al. Clinical outcomes of proximal row carpectomy versus four-corner arthrodesis for post-traumatic wrist arthropathy: a systematic review. J Hand Surg Eur Vol 2015;40:450–7.

33. Dodds SD, Halim A. Scaphoid plate fixation and volar carpal artery vascularized bone graft for recalcitrant scaphoid nonunions. J Hand Surg Am 2016; 41:e191–8.

34. Adani R, Tarallo L, Caccese AF, et al. Microsurgical soft tissue and bone transfers in complex hand trauma. Clin Plast Surg 2014;41:361–83.

35. Huntley JS, Bush PG, McBirnie JM, et al. Chondrocyte death associated with human femoral osteochondral harvest as performed for mosaicplasty. J Bone Joint Surg Am 2005;87:351–60.

36. Cavadas PC, Landın L. Treatment of recalcitrant distal tibial nonunion using the descending genicular corticoperiosteal free flap. J Trauma 2008;64:144–50.

37. Camilli JA, Penteado CV. Bone formation by vascularized periosteal and osteoperiosteal grafts. an experimental study in rats. Arch Orthop Trauma Surg 1994;114:18–24.

# Compound or Specially Designed Flaps in the Lower Extremities

Bruno Battiston, MD[a],*, Davide Ciclamini, MD[a],
Jin Bo Tang, MD[b],*

## KEYWORDS

- Perforator flap • Propeller flap • Combined transfer • Osteoperiosteal flaps • Soft tissue defects
- Leg and foot

## KEY POINTS

- Novel and combined tissue transfers from the lower extremity provide new tools to combat soft tissue defects of the hand, foot, and ankle, or fracture nonunion.
- Flaps can be designed for special purposes, such as providing a gliding bed for a grafted or repaired tendon or for thumb or finger reconstruction.
- A variety of propeller flaps can cover soft tissue defects of the leg and foot.
- In repairing severe bone and soft tissue defects of the lower extremity, combined approaches, including external fixators, one-stage vascularized bone grafting, and skin or muscle flap coverage of the traumatized leg and foot, have become popular.

## INTRODUCTION

The history of plastic surgery has been marked by the creation and subsequent evolution of flaps. Cutaneous flaps have undergone evolution during the past few decades. Ger[1] demonstrated the importance of muscle alone as a flap, and Taylor and colleagues[2,3] introduced osseous flaps in the form of vascularized iliac crest and fibula flaps. In a recent meta-analysis of lower limb reconstruction, Bekara and colleagues[4] report that the 5 most commonly used flaps were latissimus dorsi (accounting for 26% of all free vascularized flap transfers in lower extremities), anterolateral thigh (20%), rectus abdominis (9%), gracilis (8%), and serratus anterior (6%). These flaps were categorized as muscular (58%), fasciocutaneous (42%), or fascial (1%). These flaps are still the workhorses in reconstruction of the lower limb and are the most common flaps in clinical practice.

Beyond the introduction of new flaps, there has been a continuous push toward optimization of reconstructive techniques, both in terms of minimization of donor-site defects or morbidity and in refinements of the reconstructed site and function. In the last 3 decades, the advent of perforator flaps, described by Koshima and Soeda in 1989[5] and by Allen and Treece in 1994,[6] was a major technical advancement in reconstructive surgery. Since then, some new flaps have been described and many existing flaps have been improved, whereas donor-site morbidity decreased gradually with the muscle-sparing approach of perforator flaps. The community of reconstructive surgeons, moving away from the concept of the "reconstructive ladder," gradually embraced the "reconstructive elevator" concept[7] armed with many new advanced tools.

The authors have nothing to disclose.
[a] U.O.C. Traumatology, Hand Surgery, Microsurgery, A.S.O. Città della Salute e della Scienza, CTO - Hospital, Via Gianfranco Zuretti, 29, 10126 Torino, Italy; [b] Department of Hand Surgery, The Hand Surgery Research Center, Affiliated Hospital of Nantong University, 20 West Temple Road, Nantong 226001, Jiangsu, China
* Corresponding author.
*E-mail addresses:* bruno.battiston@virgilio.it; jinbotang@yahoo.com

Clin Plastic Surg 44 (2017) 287–297
http://dx.doi.org/10.1016/j.cps.2016.11.006

This article reviews the most used or recently proposed flaps, focusing especially on the European experience, with the acknowledgment that flap surgery is subject to experimentation by and imagination of surgeons, which are a starting point, to be completed over the years for each innovative flap.

## FROM FREE PERFORATOR FLAPS TO PEDICLED FLAPS BASED ON PERFORANT VESSELS

Today, perforator flaps are universally considered the final frontier of flap harvesting, because they allow sparing of the muscle, taking just the skin and a subcutaneous tissue layer as a flap. The term "perforator flap" was first used by Koshima and Soeda in 1989 to describe flaps supported by "perforator vessels,"[5] which they defined as small vascular branches going from a main vessel to the skin and "perforating" all the structures (muscle, fascia, and so forth) before distributing to dermal and subdermal vascular networks to support the cutaneous layer. These small branches may also become the only circulatory source of the flap or even a receiving vessel for free flaps, which requires special skills (ie, supermicrosurgery).[7]

Despite the Gent consensus on perforator flaps,[8] the definition of perforator flaps is still subject to debate. Nevertheless, the authors generally agree with the Gent terminology, which defines the flap by the name of the underlying nutrient vessel, even though many of the most commonly used perforator flaps are referred to by their "popular" name, such as an anterolateral thigh flap (ALT). Perforator flaps are an important part of daily clinical practice, and the ALT flap is actually the most frequently used free perforator flap, because it is capable of covering a great variety of loss of substance.

Several surgeons have used the concepts of perforator flaps in limb reconstructive surgery to harvest local flaps supported by small perforating branches.[9] Their experience especially underscores 2 aspects of the technique: first, the difficulty of pedicle dissection, demanding high microsurgical skills; and second, the absence of microvascular anastomosis, simplifying the procedure. They refer to these reconstructions as microsurgical nonmicrovascular procedures. One main advantage of such approaches may be the use of local resources to reconstruct lost tissue with the "like-to-like" concept. Experience with these local flaps led to the use of a skin island supplied with blood through a perforator pedicle that may be rotated through at least 90°

to 180°: the propeller flap.[10] Besides having a more reliable vascular pedicle than traditional flaps, propeller flaps allow for great freedom in design and for wide mobilization, extending the possibility of reconstructing difficult wounds with local tissues and minimal donor-site morbidity.[10] Understanding the possibilities of this surgical technique, several surgeons have begun to use perforating branches to harvest non–well-defined and described flaps in a "freestyle" manner.

In the authors' experience, perforator propeller flaps used in a freestyle manner can be used with positive results in the upper and lower limb for the treatment of traumatic loss of substance, as well as after tumor excisions or burns, and in other conditions (Fig. 1). In selected cases, even complex defects may be treated with propeller flaps harvested as composite flaps. In 2009, the authors reported a successful case of reconstruction of the dorsal aspect of the index finger with extensor tendon loss by means of a composite propeller flap rotated 180° and based on the dorsal metacarpal artery; this included the extensor proprius indicis tendon to restore the continuity of the extensor common tendon of the index finger.[11]

## PEDICLED CUTANEOUS FLAPS BASED ON PERFORANT VESSELS (PERFORATOR FREESTYLE FLAPS): BENEFITS AND RISKS

A vigorous debate has arisen around freestyle pedicled perforator flaps and propeller flaps, in particular around their safety in clinical practice. Propeller flaps are an appealing option for coverage of a large range of defects, because besides having a more reliable vascular pedicle than traditional flaps, they allow for greater freedom in design and for wider mobilization, extending the possibility of reconstructing difficult wounds with deep tissue defects with local tissues and minimal donor-site morbidity.[12]

Despite the widespread use of free perforator flaps, pedicled perforator flaps and propeller perforator flaps seem not to be as widely used, probably because of the danger of vascular complications caused by transfer of a flap attached only by its vascular pedicle, which is prone to shearing, kinking, and trauma. Bekara and colleagues[4] concluded from their meta-analysis that free and pedicled propeller flaps have similar risks of failure and development of complications. Although partial necrosis is more serious in a pedicled propeller flap than in a free flap, these flap types afford similar levels of coverage success (coverage failure: free flap

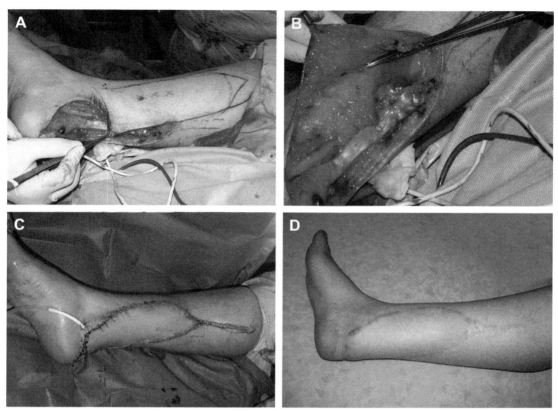

**Fig. 1.** (*A*) Loss of substance at lower leg and Achilles region after tumor resection. The Achilles tendon has been reconstructed with an allograft, and a local perforator propeller flap based on a branch from the posterior tibial artery is prepared. (*B*) The small perforating vessel is identified and dissected. (*C*) The reconstruction at the end of the operation. (*D*) Final result 1 year later.

5% vs pedicled-propeller flaps 3%). D'Arpa and colleagues[13] reported complete survival of 79 (93%) of 85 freestyle pedicled perforator flap transfers. Six flaps (7%) had vascular complications that were managed with venous supercharging (2 cases), derotation (1 case), conservative management (2 cases), or secondary skin grafting (1 case). In a case series of 34 patients with moderate loss of substance of torso and extremities, Gunnarsson and colleagues[14] reported that reconstructive goals were achieved in all cases without any total flap loss or major complications. Minor complications occurred in 7 (21%) of 34 cases, consisting of venous congestion leading to distal tip necrosis or epidermolysis. Although there was partial flap loss in 4 cases, necrosis never affected more than 10% of the total flap size.[14] The European debate around freestyle perforator and propeller flaps continues, but there is no concrete evidence that these flaps pose substantially greater risk than the traditional free flap.

## PEDICLED BONE FLAPS

Local vascularized bone grafts are a good choice for the reconstruction of bone and soft tissue loss in both lower and upper extremities. The use of vascularized bone grafts from the distal radius for scaphoid nonunions or Kienbock disease is well established.[15] What is new is the use of small vascular grafts for special types of reconstructions. A reverse-flow second dorsal metacarpal artery (SDMA) bone flap was successfully used for reconstruction of distal finger phalanx bony loss, with the vascularized bone flap mobilized on its reverse SDMA pedicle and pivoted at the level of the distal anastomoses between the palmar and dorsal metacarpal arteries.[16] A free corticocancellous bone graft from the distal radius and nail bed reconstruction with a homodigital dorsal reverse adipofascial flap based on an exteriorized pedicle were also successfully used in a case of hand distal phalanx loss.[17]

## OSTEOPERIOSTEAL FLAPS

The periosteum of the medial femoral condyle and supracondylar region can be harvested as a free flap with or without cancellous bone.[18–21] This flap provides a thin and pliable sheet of osteogenic tissue that can be transferred to sites of problematic fracture nonunions. It is usually harvested as a free flap for the reconstruction of bone defects and recalcitrant nonunion of long and short bones, including clavicle, humerus, radius, ulna, metacarpal, femur, tibia, phalanx, carpal and tarsal bones, orbit, maxilla, mandible, and skull, and in many applications other than limb reconstruction.

Quite recently the indications of this flap were broadened by including some cartilage with the osteoperiosteal graft. In fact, the medial femoral trochlea (MFT) provides a source of convex osteocartilaginous vascularized bone that has been demonstrated to have a contour similar to the proximal scaphoid. Thus, the MFT graft may be used for the treatment of very proximal scaphoid nonunions: the proximal scaphoid pole is completely resected and reconstructed by means of a portion of vascularized medial femoral condyle and trochlea with its cartilaginous stock, which is anastomosed to the palmar branch of the radial artery (**Fig. 2**). Higgins and Burger[19] published an excellent series on this flap demonstrating a high rate of union, acceptable range of wrist motion, and significant pain relief.

In addition, many new applications are created. For upper limbs, the medial femoral condyle flap has been successfully used in a nonunion of the proximal phalanx of the dominant thumb. The MFC flap has also been shaped into a "neophalanx" for phalangeal reconstruction.[22]

The MFT flap has been also harvested to restore distal bone stock in septic terminal digital bone loss. The flap has proven very useful in restoring pulp pinch function, because it is capable of resisting resorption, nonunion, and reactivation of infection.[23]

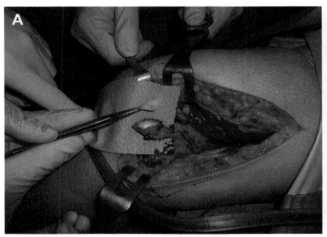
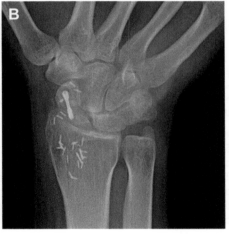
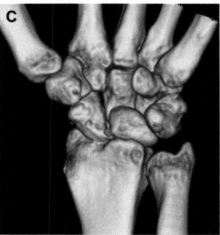

**Fig. 2.** (A) Harvesting of the osteochondral graft from the medial femoral condyle with its vascular pedicle for a scaphoid nonunion. It is cut precisely to the shape of the scaphoid proximal pole. (B) Three-month postoperative radiograph shows bone union. (C) CT shows healing of the fracture.

## FILLET FLAPS

Amputated non-replantable tissues offer an invaluable source of composite flaps (either free or pedicled) or grafts that readily can be used to restore some important structures and functions.

In treating a severe limb trauma or performing replantation, surgeons should immediately reconstruct all important structures, when possible. In the absence of extensive contamination, any amputated part should be considered a source of graft material: simple or composite, vascularized or not.[24] Moreover, in a multilimb accident, all "spare parts" from the foot are useful for hand reconstruction.

New applications of this concept frequently appear, even in nonemergency settings, for example, utilization of skin from deformed and useless fingers to cover defects in the hand, as published half a century ago.[25]

## GLIDING FLAPS

Transfer of vascularized tissues into an exhausted bed is a common practice in treatment of recalcitrant nonunions, radiotherapy wounds, or scarred nerves. This concept has been recently underscored by some European experiences in extending the indications to failed tenolysis or to any situation in which the bed was expected to be inadequate, providing gliding surfaces to delicate functional structures.[26]

## UNIQUE DESIGNS OF FLAPS

Flaps can be designed based on vascular supplies to fit the needs of the recipient site. The authors use a "3-leaf flap" designed by Yajun Xu and colleagues[27] as an example to illustrate how varied flap designs can improve specific tissue repairs. The 3-leaf flap consists of 3 flaps from the dorsal foot based on the tibial anterior artery and its 2 branches on the dorsal foot, transferred to cover multiple soft tissue defects in the hand in 50 patients since 1996 by Xu and colleagues. The flap design and vascular supply are shown in **Fig. 3**. In order to avoid flap necrosis, none of the flaps (leaves) should

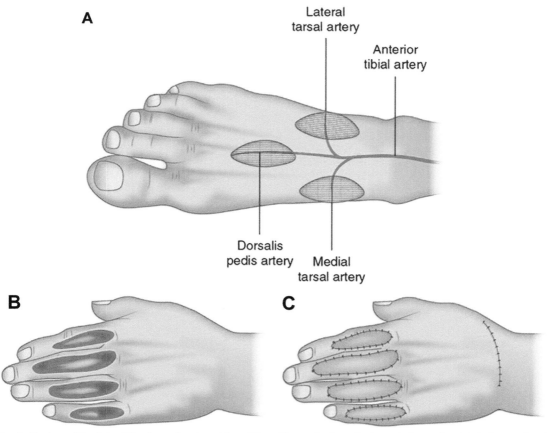

**Fig. 3.** Design of the 3-leaf flap from the dorsal foot (A) and its use in the soft tissue defects of multiple fingers (B, C).

exceed 6 × 1 cm. One 3-leaf flap needs only one set of an artery and a vein to be connected to recipient vessels. One such 3-leaf flap from each foot can be used to cover a hand with degloving injury of 3 fingers in a hand (**Fig. 4**). When 2 such flaps are needed to repair one hand, 2 sets of arteries and veins are connected to vessels in the recipient hand. The first method is that the artery and vein of the dorsal 3-leaf flap are connected to the radial artery and cephalic vein, and the artery and vein of the palmar flap are connected to the common digital artery and cephalic vein through a V-shaped vein graft. The second method is to place 2 sets of vascular anastomoses on the dorsum of the hand: the 2 arteries are connected to 2 ends of the transected radial artery. The 2 veins are connected to veins of the dorsal hand. The sensory nerve in the foot can be sutured to common digital nerves if possible, which offers the possibility of sensory recovery in fingers. The key point is that each leaf should be small enough to avoid flap necrosis; the width of each leaf should not usually exceed 1 cm. If both volar and dorsal aspects of multiple fingers are lost, 2 sets of such flaps should be harvested to cover the defect. In literature, surgeons have recommended various combinations of flaps or bone transfers for thumb or finger reconstruction.[28–31]

## INDEPENDENT OR COMBINED USE OF PROPELLER FLAPS FOR FOOT AND ANKLE REPAIR

Several propeller flaps or skin flaps nourished by vessels supplying the cutaneous nerves can be harvested for tissue repair of the legs and ankles, independently or in combination. In a review of their use of 142 pedicled propeller perforator flaps in leg and ankle repairs, Xu and colleagues found partial necrosis in 6 flaps (for which skin grafts were later necessary) and venous congestion in 8 flaps (it was necessary to remove skin sutures to decompress the pedicle sites). These complications are 2 major complications after flap transfer. The rich experience of this team in the use of perforator flaps is also detailed later in the section on flap designs.

Two combinations are possible: (1) *For dorsal foot repair*: A flap based on nutrient vessels of the superficial fibular nerve and a flap based on a perforator of the fibular artery above the ankle or a perforator of the anterior tibial artery anterior to the ankle. (2) *For ankle and dorsolateral foot repair*: A flap based on sural nerve nutrient vessels with a flap based on a perforator of the posterior tibial artery. Some of these flaps are described later and are presented in **Figs. 5** and **6**.

### An Anterolateral Leg Flap Based on Nutrient Vessels of the Superficial Fibular Nerve

An anterolateral leg flap based on nutrient vessels of the superficial fibular nerve is used for dorsal foot coverage. The flap pivot point is 3 to 5 cm above the intersection point of the middle and lateral one-third of a line between the medial and lateral malleoli of the ankle. The central axis of this flap is the line connecting the fibular head with the rotation point of the flap. The upper margin can extend to three-fourths of the lower leg, which is the entry point of the perforator and can be detected with Doppler signal. The flap can go up to the borderline of lateral and posterior aspects of the leg and anteriorly up to the tibia. The vascular pedicle should be longer (eg, 2 cm longer) than needed to leave room for rotation and extended use.

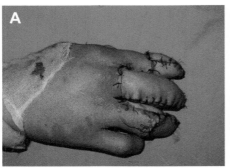
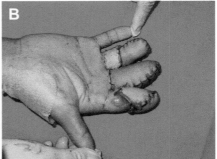

**Fig. 4.** Multiple finger degloving injury repaired with 2 sets of the 3-leaf flap. (*A*) Dorsal view after transfer. (*B*) Palmar view after transfer. (*Courtesy of* Yajun Xu, MD, Jiangsu, China.)

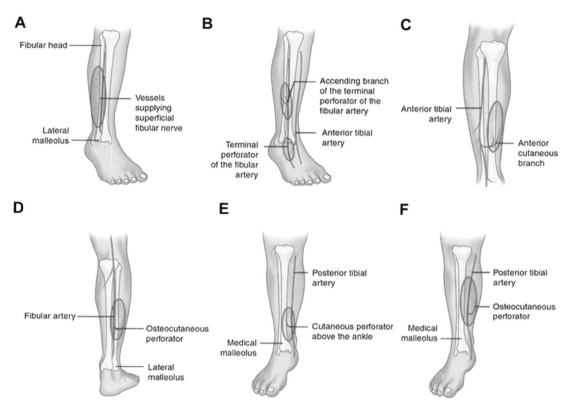

**Fig. 5.** Various propeller perforator flaps in the leg can be used for leg, ankle, or foot soft tissue repairs. (*A*) An anterolateral leg flap based on nutrient vessels of the superficial fibular nerve. (*B*) An anterolateral leg flap based on anterior or lateral perforator of the terminal branch of the fibular artery. (*C*) An anterolateral leg flap based on the perforator of the anterior tibial artery above the ankle. (*D*) A posterior leg flap based on the lateral perforator of the fibular artery above the ankle. (*E*) A posterior leg flap based on a perforator of the posterior tibial artery. (*F*) A posterior leg flap based on a perforator of the posterior tibial artery at the lower one-third leg.

## An Anterolateral Leg Flap Based on Anterior or Lateral Perforator of the Terminal Branch of the Fibular Artery

The pivot point is 3 to 4 cm above the lateral condyle of the ankle. If the terminal branch of the fibular artery is ligated, then the flap rotation point can be at the tip of the lateral malleolus of the ankle. Therefore, the rotation point can vary over a large range (5 cm). The axis of the flap is from the fibular head to the anterior border of the lateral malleolus. The flap's upper margin should be within the midpoint between the fibular head and the lateral malleolus, anteriorly but not over the tibial ridge and posteriorly or over the posterior border of the fibula. An anterolateral leg flap based on the perforator of the anterior tibial artery above the ankle, with a pivot point 2 to 4 cm above the ankle (ie, entry point of the cutaneous artery). This flap can be harvested with a width 3 to 5 cm over the anterolateral aspect of the lower leg.

## A Posterior Leg Flap Based on the Lateral Perforator of the Fibular Artery Above the Ankle

A posterior leg flap based on the lateral perforator of the fibular artery above the ankle, with a pivot point intersecting the middle and lower one-third from the fibular head to the lateral malleolus, is just posterior to the fibula. This flap can be harvested from the anterior border of the fibula to the midline of the posterior leg, with its upper limit the neck of the fibula. A posterior leg flap is based on the perforator of the posterior tibial artery, with the pivot point 2 to 4 cm above the midpoint between the medial border of the Achilles tendon and the medial malleolus. The flap upper margin should not extend beyond 10 cm below the knee. The posterior border is up to the posterior midline of the leg. A posterior leg flap based on a perforator of the posterior tibial artery at the lower one-third of the leg, with the pivot point 5

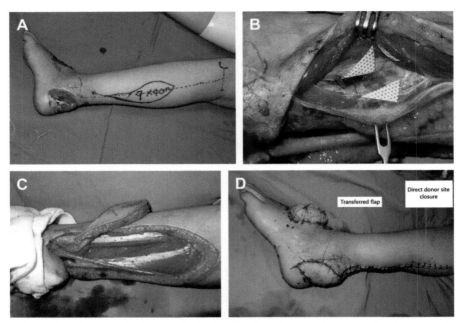

**Fig. 6.** A soft tissue defect repaired with a posterior leg flap based on the lateral perforator of the fibular artery above the ankle. (*A*) Flap margin. (*B*) The perforators were dissected. (*C*) Flap ready to rotate. (*D*) Flap coverage in the ankle and direct donor site closure. (*Courtesy of* Yajun Xu, MD, Jiangsu, China.)

to 6 cm above the medial malleolus of the ankle, with upper border up to 10 cm below the knee, can be used for repair of the medial aspect of the heel.

## NEW COMPLEX APPROACHES WITH FLAPS

Microsurgical free flaps are now used in almost all surgical fields. In orthopedics, for example, simultaneous treatment of fractures and associated soft tissue injuries is so widespread as to constitute a new "orthoplastic approach" for extremity trauma.[32,33] Microsurgical flaps, especially in a composite setting, may treat severe combined tissue losses in one step. However, microsurgical techniques are not alternatives to the traditional reconstructive methods familiar in the literature. In the lower limb, the authors have learned to use free vascularized fibular grafts supported by circular external fixation, depending on the amount of bone loss and the condition of the concomitant soft tissues. In this way, they combine biological and mechanical support to obtain good results in the treatment of such severe injuries (**Fig. 7**). This approach allows the patient early postoperative weight-bearing on the injured leg, because the frame protects the graft. As the load increases throughout treatment, the initial stiff coupling of the frame wires to the bone becomes more and more elastic, causing the "automatic

dynamization" of the external frame. Therefore, the fibular graft becomes more and more stressed and, in accordance with Wolff's laws, becomes hypertrophic. In some cases, the Ilizarov system allows for contemporary length discrepancy correction through distraction at the interface tibia-fibular graft.

Reconstruction of combined bone and soft tissue defects involves more than a simple decision of the techniques to be adopted: it is also a question of timing. In traumatic cases, if the lesion is clean or sufficiently debrided, the authors may consider an "all-in-one" reconstruction by means of bone grafts, osteosynthesis, and coverage flaps. If the general condition of the patient is critical and/or the lesion is highly contaminated, a reconstruction in 2 or more stages is suggested, especially in traumatic instances.[34] Nonetheless, some surgeons suggest immediate composite free flaps even in complex traumatic cases.[35]

In free flap transfer, some "tricks" may facilitate surgery. Brunelli and colleagues[36] reported the outcomes of a series of microsurgical fingertip reconstructions with partial toe transfers in which the vascular pedicle was exteriorized and subsequently excised after the transfer had become established. The aim of this technique was to provide better aesthetic and functional outcomes.

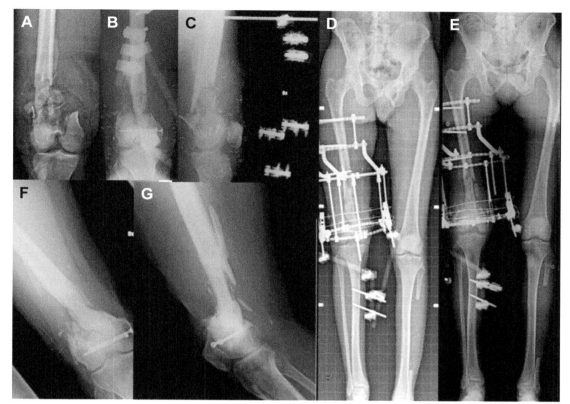

**Fig. 7.** Initial treatment according to damage-control concepts with temporary external fixation (*A–C*). Twenty days after the first operation, a biological support is added, covering the large bone defect by means of a peroneal vascularized graft stabilized with an Ilizarov apparatus (*D, E*). (*F, G*) The final result 10 months after the first treatment with complete bone integration and hypertrophy of the fibula.

Some advances come not through the description of new flaps or ideas but instead through the use of new imaging techniques or new devices. Digital technology allows one not only to improve the planning of reconstructions but also to create "3D" models that may serve in device construction (preformed plates) and better functional restoration. 3D models are helpful in complex reconstructions of 3-dimensional defects (as in oncologic resections), especially in the craniofacial setting.[37]

## SUMMARY

Novel and combined tissue transfers from the lower extremity offer new tools to address some of the most difficult problems, such as scaphoid nonunion of the scaphoid and soft tissue defects of the hand, foot, and ankle. Flaps can be harvested and designed for special purposes, such as providing a gliding bed for a grafted or repaired tendon and for thumb or finger reconstruction. A variety of propeller flaps can be harvested to cover soft tissue defects in the leg and foot. In repairing severe bone and soft tissue defects of the lower extremity, combined approaches are often necessary, including use of external fixators, one-stage vascularized bone grafting, and skin or muscle flap coverage of the traumatized leg and foot.

## REFERENCES

1. Ger R. The technique of muscle transposition in the operative treatment of traumatic and ulcerative lesions of the leg. J Trauma 1971;11: 502–10.
2. Taylor GI, Townsend P, Corlett R. Superiority of the deep circumflex iliac vessels as the supply for free groin flaps. Clinical work. Plast Reconstr Surg 1979;64:745–59.
3. Taylor GI, Miller GD, Ham FJ. The free vascularized bone graft: a clinical extension of microvascular techniques. Plast Reconstr Surg 1975;55: 533–44.

4. Bekara F, Herlin C, Somda S, et al. Free versus perforator-pedicled propeller flaps in lower extremity reconstruction: what is the safest coverage? A meta-analysis. Microsurgery 2016. [Epub ahead of print].

5. Koshima I, Soeda S. Inferior epigastric artery skin flaps without rectus abdominis muscle. Br J Plast Surg 1989;42:645–8.

6. Allen RJ, Treece P. Deep inferior epigastric perforator flap for breast reconstruction. Ann Plast Surg 1994;32:32–8.

7. Masia J, Olivares L, Koshima I, et al. Barcelona consensus on supermicrosurgery. J Reconstr Microsurg 2014;30:53–8.

8. Blondeel PN, Van Landuyt KH, Monstrey SJ, et al. The "Gent" consensus on perforator flap terminology: preliminary definitions. Plast Reconstr Surg 2003;112:1378–83.

9. Georgescu AV, Matei I, Ardelean F, et al. Microsurgical nonmicrovascular flaps in forearm and hand reconstruction. Microsurgery 2007;27: 384–94.

10. Teo TC. The propeller flap concept. Clin Plast Surg 2010;37:615–26.

11. Gottlieb LJ, Krieger LM. From the reconstructive ladder to the reconstructive elevator. Plast Reconstr Surg 1994;93:1503–4.

12. Battiston B, Artiaco S, Antonini A, et al. Dorsal metacarpal artery perforator-based propeller flap for complex defect of the dorsal aspect in the index finger. J Hand Surg Eur Vol 2009;34: 807–9.

13. D'Arpa S, Cordova A, Pignatti M, et al. Freestyle pedicled perforator flaps: safety, prevention of complications, and management based on 85 consecutive cases. Plast Reconstr Surg 2011;128: 892–906.

14. Gunnarsson GL, Jackson IT, Westvik TS, et al. The freestyle pedicle perforator flap: a new favorite for the reconstruction of moderate-sized defects of the torso and extremities. Eur J Plast Surg 2015; 38:31–6.

15. Mathoulin C, Haerle M, Vandeputte G. Vascularized bone grafts in carpal bone reconstruction. Ann Chir Plast Esthet 2005;50:43–8.

16. Katz TL, Hunter-Smith DJ, Matthew Rozen W. Reverse second dorsal metacarpal artery vascularized bone flap for index distal bone loss: a case report. Microsurgery 2016;36:250–3.

17. Müller NA, Calcagni M, Giesen T. Treatment of painful nonunion of the distal phalanx in the finger with bone graft and dorsal reverse adipofascial flap based on an exteriorized pedicle. Tech Hand Up Extrem Surg 2015;19:115–9.

18. Sakai K, Doi K, Kawai S. Free vascularized thin corticoperiosteal graft. Plast Reconstr Surg 1991;87: 290–8.

19. Higgins JP, Burger HK. Proximal scaphoid arthroplasty using the medial femoral trochlea flap. J Wrist Surg 2013;2:228–33.

20. Ferguson DO, Shanbhag V, Hedley H, et al. Scaphoid fracture non-union: a systematic review of surgical treatment using bone graft. J Hand Surg Eur Vol 2016;41:492–500.

21. Elgammal A, Lukas B. Vascularized medial femoral condyle graft for management of scaphoid nonunion. J Hand Surg Eur Vol 2015;40:848–54.

22. Ruston JC, Amin K, Darhouse N, et al. The vascularized medial femoral corticoperiosteal flap for thumb reconstruction. Plast Reconstr Surg Glob Open 2015;3:e492.

23. Henry M. Free vascularized medial femoral condyle structural flaps for septic terminal digital bone loss. J Hand Microsurg 2015;7:306–13.

24. Tos P, Ciclamini D, Titolo P, et al. Bank tissue concepts in microsurgical reconstruction of mangled hands. In: Battiston B, Georgescu AV, Soucacos PN, editors. Frontiers in microsurgery of the upper extremity. Athens (Greece): Konstantaras Medical Publications; 2016. p. 181–5.

25. Cave EF, Rowe CR. Utilization of skin from deformed and useless fingers to cover defects in the hand. Ann Surg 1947;125:126.

26. del Piñal F, Moraleda E, de Piero GH, et al. Outcomes of free adipofascial flaps combined with tenolysis in scarred beds. J Hand Surg Am 2014;39: 269–79.

27. Xu YJ, Shou KS, Zhang QR. Clinical application of the trifoliated flap from the dorsal foot. Chin J Microsurg 2003;26:14–6.

28. Wang H, Chen C, Li J, et al. Modified first dorsal metacarpal artery island flap for sensory reconstruction of thumb pulp defects. J Hand Surg Eur Vol 2016;41:177–84.

29. Zhang G, Ju J, Li L, et al. Combined two foot flaps with iliac bone graft for reconstruction of the thumb. J Hand Surg Eur Vol 2016;41: 745–52.

30. Wang ZT, Sun WH. Cosmetic reconstruction of the digits in the hand by composite tissue grafting. Clin Plast Surg 2014;41:407–27.

31. Tang JB, Elliot D, Adani R, et al. Repair and reconstruction of thumb and finger tip injuries: a global view. Clin Plast Surg 2014;41:325–59.

32. Battiston B, Antonini A, Tos P, et al. Microvascular reconstructions of traumatic-combined tissue loss at foot and ankle level. Microsurgery 2011;31: 212–7.

33. Battiston B, Santoro D, Lo Baido R, et al. Treatment of acute bone defects in severe lower limb trauma. J Orthop Traumatol, in press.

34. Battiston B, Vasario G, Ciclamini D, et al. Reconstruction of traumatic losses of substance at the elbow. Injury 2014;45:437–43.

35. Cavadas PC, Thione A. Complex upper extremity macro-replantation. In: Battiston B, Georgescu AV, Soucacos PN, editors. Frontiers in microsurgery of the upper extremity. Athens (Greece): Konstantaras Medical Publications; 2016. p. 161–6.

36. Brunelli F, Spalvieri C, Rocchi L, et al. Reconstruction of the distal finger with partial second toe transfers by means of an exteriorised pedicle. J Hand Surg Eur Vol 2008;33:457–61.

37. Succo G, Berrone M, Battiston B, et al. Step-by-step surgical technique for mandibular reconstruction with fibular free flap: application of digital technology in virtual surgical planning. Eur Arch Otorhinolaryngol 2015;272:1491–501.

# Complex Microsurgical Reconstruction After Tumor Resection in the Trunk and Extremities

Omar N. Hussain, MD, M. Diya Sabbagh, MD,
Brian T. Carlsen, MD*

## KEYWORDS

- Microsurgery • Extremities • Sarcoma • Flap • Limb salvage surgery • Trunk

## KEY POINTS

- Soft tissue tumors of the trunk and extremities represent a challenge because of the paucity of soft tissue and the relative close proximity with critical structures.
- A multidisciplinary team approach should be adopted, especially for the trunk and lower extremity.
- Every attempt should be made to preserve a limb. When amputation is inevitable, the remaining limb must be optimized to maintain function or to improve prosthesis control.
- Several flaps can be used to cover soft tissue defects in the trunk and extremity. Biological and synthetic materials can add to the wide variety of options in the armamentarium of the reconstructive surgeon.

## GENERAL CONSIDERATIONS IN ONCOLOGIC RECONSTRUCTION

Thorough evaluation of the patients' health status, functional demands, location, and extent of the tumor as well as the tissue loss expected with tumor ablation procedures must be done before attempting any course of treatment. A multidisciplinary team approach also helps the reconstructive surgeon in selecting the appropriate flap for the defect and minimizing donor site defects, especially for trunk and lower extremity reconstruction.[1] Accurate assessment of the defect, meticulous dissection of the recipient site, precise microvascular anastomoses, and proper flap insets are essential factors for an optimal outcome. The timing of the reconstruction depends on the surgeon's preference and the patients' medical status, but it is preferable to do the reconstruction immediately after tumor resection. This approach decreases the number of operations and minimizes contamination of deep tissues and structures.[2–4]

Reconstruction in patients with cancer is unique, as adjuvant chemotherapy and radiation therapy can affect wound healing and flap survival; neoadjuvant radiation therapy usually creates a zone of injury that extends beyond the margins of resection. Furthermore, patients with cancer are well known to be hypercoagulable and, therefore, have a higher risk for venous thromboembolism. Chemotherapy, radiation, and immobilization further increase the risk of thromboembolic events in this special patient population. All of these factors make oncologic reconstruction more challenging and necessitates careful planning and individualization of treatment plans.[2,5–9]

## GOALS OF RECONSTRUCTION IN THE TRUNK

The primary goals of chest wall reconstruction are stabilization of thoracic skeletal defects that may

The authors have nothing to disclose.
Division of Plastic and Reconstructive Surgery, Mayo Clinic, 200 First Street, Rochester, MN 55905, USA
* Corresponding author.
E-mail address: Carlsen.Brian@mayo.edu

Clin Plastic Surg 44 (2017) 299–311
http://dx.doi.org/10.1016/j.cps.2016.11.008
0094-1298/17/© 2017 Elsevier Inc. All rights reserved.

plasticsurgery.theclinics.com

alter respiratory mechanics, obliteration of intra-thoracic dead space, protection of vital intrathoracic structures and suture lines, and soft tissue coverage of extrathoracic defects.[10] Other considerations include avoiding lung herniation, counteracting substantial shrinking of the thorax, leading to thoracoplastylike effect, preventing entrapment of the scapula in posterior resections, protecting mediastinal organs against external impact, and maintaining a good cosmetic chest contour.[11] Additional challenges exist when reconstructing the lower extremities. These challenges include restoring painless function be it ambulation in regard to the lower extremity or fine dexterity and hand function in regard to the upper extremity. The slower rate of nerve regeneration and the higher incidence of flap failure and wound complications add to the complexity of extremity reconstruction.[2,3,5,12,13]

## FREE TISSUE TRANSFER FOR TRUNK RECONSTRUCTION

Chest wall tumors account for most indications for chest wall reconstruction in large retrospective series, which include primary lung cancer, primary chest wall tumors, contiguous breast cancer, and metastases.[14–18] The most common benign chest wall tumors are osteochondromas, chondromas, fibrous dysplasia, and desmoid tumors. The most common primary malignancies are soft tissue sarcoma, chondrosarcoma, and Ewing sarcoma.[18] Wide local excision is the mainstay of treatment. High-grade malignancies and desmoid tumors typically require 4-cm margins of normal tissue, whereas low-grade malignancies are typically resected with 1- to 2-cm margins. Bony involvement for many lesions necessitates resection of the entire rib or sternum with resection margin guidelines of one normal rib above and below the level of involvement.[18–20] The excision of tumors with a wide margin of normal tissue leads to large defects that routinely require complex reconstruction of the chest wall and soft tissue coverage.[14–17] Chest wall reconstruction after tumor resection should be approached in a systematic fashion. Depending on the type of tumor, extent of resection, and history of radiation, reconstructive options include primary closure, skin grafts, local flaps, pedicled muscular, musculocutaneous flaps, and free flaps.

The chest wall is divided into the anterior, lateral, and posterior regions. Prosthetic skeletal reconstruction is typically reserved for anterior chest wall defects greater than 5 cm or involving 3 or more contiguous ribs because of the increased chance of paradoxic chest wall motion.[18,21] Posterior chest wall defects can tolerate up to a 10-cm diameter resection because of support from the scapula unless the defect extends beyond the fourth rib where entrapment of the scapula can occur during movement of the arm.[15] However, the reconstructive plan must be tailored to each individual patient. Patients with borderline pulmonary function may require reconstruction for smaller defect to avoid postoperative insufficiency, and others with rigid chest walls from radiation or adhesions may tolerate larger defects without affecting pulmonary function.[22] Synthetic options for skeletal support include polytetrafluoroethylene, polypropylene, Vicryl, mesh-methyl methacrylate sandwich, methyl methacrylate neo-ribs, osteosynthesis systems, and dedicated sternal prostheses.[11,15] Biological options include autogenous tensor fascia latae, rib grafts, bovine pericardium, or acellular dermal matrix.[14,21,23]

Intrathoracic infection from ongoing airway or esophageal leak is a life-threatening condition often attributed to the presence of a persistent pleural space and continuing empyema.[24,25] Intrathoracic muscle transposition can augment the closure of the leak with well-vascularized tissue and prevent recurrence and the long-term sequelae of ongoing infection.[25] This transposition can be performed with pedicled pectoralis major, serratus anterior, latissimus dorsi, and omentum flaps.[17,26–29] In complex cases after multiple operations, local muscles are often no longer available for reconstruction because of transection or previous attempts at reconstruction. Intrathoracic free tissue transfer has been shown to provide an abundance of well-vascularized tissue with the versatility of accessing the entire intrathoracic cavity and reducing morbidity by covering the fistula repair and obliterating the pleural dead space in a single operation.[27–29]

Extrathoracic soft tissue coverage should be anticipated preoperatively and requires a combined effort between the extirpative surgeon and the reconstructive surgeon for coverage of prosthetic devices, maintenance of intrathoracic integrity, and restoration of aesthetic contours while improving survival and minimizing donor site morbidity.[10,11,14–18,20–23] Anticipation of further resections for recurrence is necessary to maximize the use of local flaps while preserving options for future reconstruction, and a variety of reconstructive algorithms have been described.[17,29–32]

Recurrence is common after resection of soft tissue sarcoma in the chest, with 23% of patients experiencing a recurrence and 38% of those presenting as a local recurrence an average of 11.6 months after resection.[33] The only factor improving survival after surgical resection of high-grade soft tissue sarcomas is wide negative margins in primary, recurrent, and metastatic lesions.[34] The workhorse flaps of thoracic reconstruction are the pectoralis major, latissimus dorsi, and vertical rectus abdominis muscle (VRAM) or transverse rectus abdominis muscle (TRAM) flaps.[10] Local options are limited when local muscles are invaded by tumor or have previously been sacrificed. Irradiated local muscle has also been shown to have an increase in complications when compared with nonirradiated muscle transposition for soft tissue coverage even leading to complete flap loss.[26] In these cases of compromised local options, microsurgical augmentation of superiorly based rectus abdominis flaps with supercharged inferior epigastric vessels or free flap reconstruction can provide well-vascularized soft tissue coverage from outside the zone of injury[17,29] (Fig. 1).

Recipient vessels for anterior chest reconstruction are most commonly the internal mammary and thoracodorsal arteries.[17,27–31] If these vessels have been included in the resection, the proximal transected stumps can be used end to end for arterial inflow. Other options include the lateral thoracic, subclavian, thoracoacromial, external carotid, and transverse cervical arteries.[17,30,31] Posterior chest wall reconstruction is most commonly performed with the thoracodorsal artery as the recipient vessel.[17,27–31] The circumflex scapular or a regional intercostal artery can also be used. The venous comitantes for the arteries are most commonly used for recipient veins. Other options include transposition of the external jugular and the cephalic veins.

Complex microsurgical reconstruction after tumor resection in the trunk reduces the morbidity of prolonged hospital stays, multiple operations for debridement, and open wounds in patients in whom local flap reconstruction is not feasible.[25,27–32] Three microsurgical methods are generally used in chest wall reconstruction. Microvascular augmentation of blood flow in pedicled flaps via supercharging/turbocharging, free flap reconstruction of complex intrathoracic defects, and free flap reconstruction of extrathoracic soft tissue defects.[17,24,25,27–31,35]

Large central chest wall defects can be challenging when local flaps are not possible because of resection or vascular compromise. Pedicled VRAM/TRAM flaps serve well in this setting because they provide the volume to obliterate dead space and provide very large skin paddles.[10,16,17,29,31,32] In patients with abdominal scars from prior abdominal operations, microvascular augmentation with supercharging/turbocharging of the inferior epigastric vessels and

even using bilateral inferior epigastric vessels as a bipedicled flap has been shown to improve perfusion.[17,29] It is worth noting that vascular insufficiency can be identified before ligation of vessels by placing clamps on the inferior epigastric artery and vein and observing the flap. When performing pedicled VRAM/TRAM flaps in patients with history of internal mammary artery radiation or abdominal scars, microsurgical augmentation of inferior epigastric vessels can salvage flaps showing vascular insufficiency or enable transposition of a larger, well-perfused musculocutaneous bipedicled flap. In these circumstances, abandoning attempts of relying on these vessels for pedicle flap perfusion may be ill advised and free tissue transfer should be considered.

Complications after pneumonectomy or partial pneumonectomy can result in chronic empyema and bronchopleural fistula requiring multiple thoracotomies, drainage, and attempts at repair.

## OUTCOMES FOR TRUNK RECONSTRUCTION

Buttressing airway and esophageal leak and pleural space obliteration improve patient outcomes.[23,35] Arnold and Pairolero[24] reported a 73% success rate in 100 consecutive cases when performing open drainage with fistula repair, buttressing the repair with intrathoracic muscle transposition, and obliterating the pleural space.[23,35] Another study by Chen and colleagues[25] reported a 100% success rate in treatment of bronchopleural fistulae and chronic empyema with one-stage free latissimus dorsi and serratus anterior muscle flaps in 5 patients with 4 to 7 prior thoracotomies.[26] Similarly, Hammond, and colleagues[27] reported an 80% success in treating 5 patients with bronchopleural fistulae and empyema with free rectus abdominis and latissimus dorsi flaps. In addition, 2 patients with complex intrathoracic wounds were successfully treated with free omentum flap and latissimus dorsi flap coverage. Finally, Walsh and colleagues[28] reported 100% resolution using free flaps in the treatment of empyema and bronchopleural fistula in 6 patients. In patients with bronchopleural fistulae and chronic empyema and no local options, free flaps can reliably provide the necessary volume of well-vascularized muscle to buttress fistula repair and obliterate dead space in a single stage.

Free flap extrathoracic reconstruction is infrequent but indicated when local muscles have previously been excised, irradiated, transected, or used in prior reconstruction attempts. Cordeiro and colleagues[29] identified 2 groups that benefitted from free flaps over a 10-year experience of 192

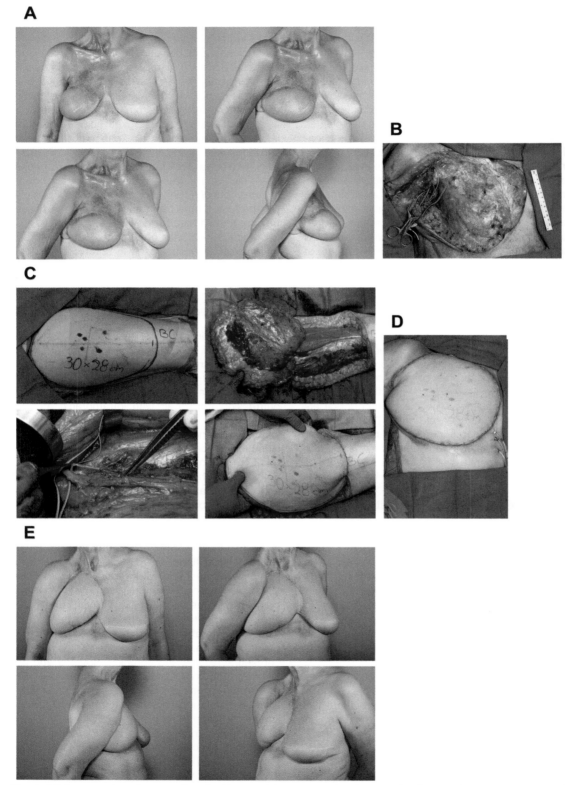

**Fig. 1.** (*A*) Preoperative photographs of a 69-year-old woman with a history of right-sided breast cancer treated with a mastectomy, lymphadenectomy, and radiation therapy for positive nodes. Five years later, she developed a

chest wall reconstructions with 20 free flaps, including 13 unilateral rectus abdominis musculocutaneous flaps, one bilateral rectus abdominis muscle flap, 2 contralateral latissimus dorsi flaps, and 4 forearm filet flaps. The first group were best reconstructed with free rectus abdominis musculocutaneous flaps for large central defects with transected internal mammary vessels and sacrificed latissimus dorsi muscles from prior posterolateral thoracotomies. The second group is best served with forearm filet flap reconstruction of the shoulder when oncologically safe after forequarter amputations (**Fig. 2**).

Free tissue transfer provides the benefit of distant nonirradiated tissue with the versatility of flap selection and choice of recipient vessel location allowing unrestricted extrathoracic soft tissue coverage in patients with no local options. The ability to use various flaps can allow the reconstructive team to simultaneously raise the flap while the extirpative surgeon is resecting the chest wall tumor reducing operative time and need for position changes. The reconstructive surgeon who is able to use these microsurgical techniques can provide reliable well-vascularized coverage in the most complex chest wounds. It is important to adhere to the basic principles of chest wall reconstruction and use the simplest, reliable option of intrathoracic or extrathoracic soft tissue coverage. Complete reconstruction in a single stage at time of resection should be the goal in order to shorten the duration of hospitalization and recovery in patients who often have already had a prolonged course.

# MICROSURGICAL EXTREMITY RECONSTRUCTION
## Soft Tissue Tumors of the Extremities

Extremities are complex structures, and tumors can arise from any of the several tissue types that comprise them. Fortunately, most upper extremity tumors are benign, the most common ones being ganglion cysts, enchondromas, and lipomas. Malignant tumors are fairly uncommon and account for less than 3% of upper extremity tumors. Sarcomas represent most upper extremity

malignancies, with 15% of soft tissue sarcomas occurring in the upper extremity; most of these tumors are located proximal to the wrist.[36,37] Soft tissue sarcomas, however, occur more frequently in the lower extremities in comparison with the upper extremities with a 3:1 ratio.[38] With the exception of nerve sheath tumors, all musculoskeletal tumors have a mesodermal cell origin; therefore, benign and malignant tumors present similarly. Malignant tumors can be misdiagnosed as lipoma, ganglion cyst, or even infection in some cases, which highlights the importance of always maintaining a high index of suspicion.[3,7,38,39]

## Amputation Versus Limb Salvage

Once a malignant lesion in an extremity has been identified, the treatment plan usually involves radical resection or wide excision of the malignant mass. In the extremities, *radical resection* often means amputation, either above or below the elbow or knee. Historically, amputation of the involved extremity was the mainstay of treatment of soft tissue sarcomas because local excision resulted in high rates of recurrence.[3,5,40–44]

Reconstructive surgeons who participate in the management of soft tissue defects following tumor resection are often confronted with the dilemma of whether to attempt to salvage a limb or proceed with amputation. The decision to attempt heroic measures to save the limb or to amputate generally depends on the location of the tumor, degree of invasion, number of compartments involved with the inherent loss of function, and the soft tissue defect that is expected to result from tumor resection. Moreover, if limb-preserving surgery would result in significant loss of function and morbidity, it should not be attempted and radical resection with amputation should be taken into consideration.[1,2,4,5,12,13] When the decision to proceed with amputation has been made, the residual limb should be optimized for an eventual prosthesis fitting. Every attempt should be made to provide adequate bony length below a joint to allow for the attachment of the prosthesis sleeve. In case of below-knee amputation, a 14-cm residual limb length is required to allow for weight

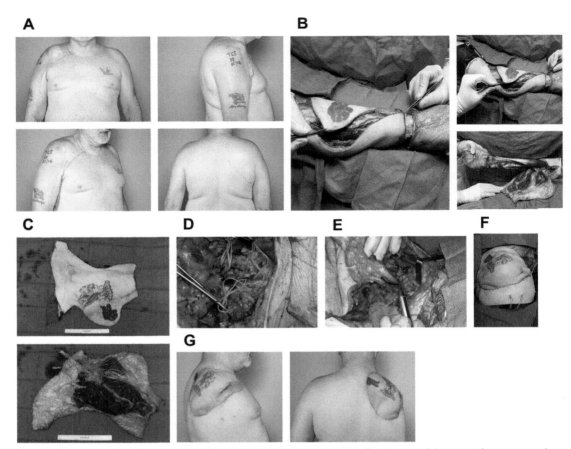

**Fig. 2.** (*A*) Preoperative photographs with planned resection margins of a 60-year-old man with recurrent chondrosarcoma of the right shoulder requiring forequarter amputation with planned fillet free flap reconstruction. (*B*) Harvest of right forearm fillet flap including volar deep and superficial musculature, basilic vein, median and ulnar nerves, and brachial artery. (*C*) The fillet flap. (*D*) Recipient vessels (*red vessel loops*: internal jugular vein; *blue vessel loops*: stump of subclavian artery). (*E*) Median nerve coaptation to upper trunk of brachial plexus for neuroma protection and potential prosthetic control. Basilic vein end-to-side anastomosis with Cook-Swartz Doppler probe in view. (*F*) Flap inset. (*G*) Three months postoperative follow-up.

bearing with a prosthetic limb and to minimize energy expenditure with ambulation.[3–5,8,43,45,46]

Residual limb coverage goals vary between upper and lower extremities. In both the upper and lower extremities, a primary objective is to provide adequate coverage and padding of bony prominences without excess or redundant soft tissue. The lower extremity residual limb, on the other hand, will be used for ambulation and weight bearing; thus, careful selection of flaps should be done to minimize late complications. Despite the numerous advances in prosthetics, the currently available prostheses still fall short in restoring form, function, and sensation, especially in regard to the upper extremity. Therefore, every attempt should be made to preserve the limb.[8,47,48] When amputation is inevitable, the principle of spare parts should be used when the soon-to-be

amputated limb can be used for reconstruction of large defects, obliterate dead space, and provide coverage for the residual limb (see **Fig. 2**). This practice allows for prosthesis fitting and faster return of functionality. It is possible to harvest the flap before amputation, which significantly reduces ischemia time.[49,50]

Advancements in microsurgery and the increased efficacy of the available chemoradiation therapies have made limb salvage operations the gold standard in treating soft tissue tumors. Wide tumor resection, often referred to as an en bloc resection, is the removal of the mass together with at least a 2- to 3-cm surrounding margin of normal tissue.[51] The hand and foot represent a challenge because they are composed of multiple compartments with little soft tissue in each compartment and specialized, glabrous skin for weight bearing and grasp. Moreover, important structures exist in close proximity; the delicate biomechanical balance that is necessary to produce a fine movement requires multiple structures to work in concert. Wide margin excision disrupts this balance because of loss of tendons, muscles, nerves, and bone, which eventually results in severe functional impairment. This unique set of challenges makes the role of the reconstructive microsurgeon more important; a successful reconstruction is not just measured by adequate wound coverage and padding of bony prominences but also by preservation of function, sensation, and cosmesis.

In the lower extremity, several studies have found no difference in the functional outcome between patients who were treated with amputation versus those in whom limb salvage surgeries were done.[12] Soltanian and colleagues[8] found that outcomes depend more on patient socioeconomic status and resources rather than on the initial treatment plan. The knee plays a critically important role in ambulation, and every attempt to salvage the knee should be made to improve the patients' ability to ambulate independently.

## TARGETED MUSCLE REINNERVATION

Whether the treatment approach is to perform a radical resection or wide local excision, the principles of targeted muscle reinnervation can help with future neuroma pain and improve prosthetic control. Neuromas can be a source of chronic pain and prevent use of a prosthesis. Souza and colleagues have shown that giving the transected nerve a distal target and a vascularized scaffold on which axons can regenerate is associated with less neuroma formation[52] (see **Fig. 2**). In another study, they also showed that targeted muscle repair gives patients with upper extremity amputation more motor control and, therefore, better function with prosthesis.[52,53] Targeted muscle reinnervation technique provides better outcomes than just transecting the damaged nerve or burying it. Moreover, it effectively restores the continuity of the peripheral nervous system and encourages nerve regeneration.[54–56]

## GOALS OF EXTREMITY RECONSTRUCTION

When considering extremity reconstruction, function is the primary consideration. For the lower extremity, this means the soft tissue must be robust, stable (resistant to further breakdown), tolerate dependence, fit well into a shoe, and tolerate weight bearing if on the weight-bearing end of the limb. Similar priorities can apply to an amputated limb in that the limb must fit well (not too bulky) into the prosthetic and tolerate weight bearing and shear forces. Function is also critically important for upper extremity reconstruction, but the priorities differ. In the upper limb, preserve joint mobility such that the hand can be positioned in space and its grip, pinch, and grasp functions maintained or restored. For both the upper and lower limbs, the coverage must be stable to tolerate these functions and pain free. Finally, aesthetics are important as both extremities are often exposed to the outside world.

## MICROSURGICAL RECONSTRUCTION OF EXTREMITIES

More so than the trunk and proximal limbs, the distal extremities have very limited local soft tissue to provide a stable bed for a skin graft or to enable local pedicle flap coverage. In these areas, free tissue transfer is often necessary for limb salvage. Multiple studies have shown that free tissue transfer reconstruction is associated with more favorable outcomes.[39,41,57] Among the benefits of using free flaps is avoidance of sacrificing tissue in an extremity that was already compromised by tumor resection; there is also usually no need to sacrifice a major vessel of the extremity, as can be the case for pedicled flaps. To avoid interruption of distal extremity circulation, end-to-side arterial anastomoses should be performed whenever possible. An exception is when the recipient vessels were transected during the tumor resection, in which case, vascular reconstruction or a flow-through flap should be considered. Free flaps also provide a large volume of vascularized tissue and help in establishing a stable wound bed that can withstand radiation therapy if need be following surgical resection. Moreover, using healthy, well-vascularized tissue that has not been exposed to radiation (if given preoperatively) can optimize healing and reduce the risk of infection. Finally, use of free tissue transfer provides greater flexibility in obtaining surgical margins that greatly influences recurrence and survival rates.[6,41,57,58]

Muscle free flaps with skin graft coverage are particularly useful in extremity reconstruction because of their propensity to atrophy with improved shape and contour in comparison with fasciocutaneous flaps. In addition, they tend to become more adherent to the deep structures and skeleton and are, therefore, less mobile. These features, in the authors' opinion, make these flaps preferable for the weight bearing lower extremity and palm of the hand where tissue glide can be very problematic. The flap atrophy also improves the contour on the other surfaces of the foot allowing for improved aesthetics and shoe wear. Muscle flaps are often the only appropriate option for overweight and obese patients, the incidence of which continues to grow worldwide. Although they can be useful in reconstructing defects over joints, their deep surface tends to become more adherent than fasciocutaneous flaps and may compromise joint motion. Another disadvantage is their decreased capacity for elevation and reinset if future operations are or become necessary.

Fasciocutaneous flaps, on the other hand, can offer their own set of advantages. The skin is thicker and has a less-scarred appearance. Their thickness and composition provide a friction-free surface for the underlying tendons and joints making them ideal flaps for joint coverage and tendon glide, such as the elbow, knee, ankle, and dorsal surface of the hand and foot.[1,59,60] In addition, fasciocutaneous flaps better facilitate secondary procedures, such as bone grafting and tendon transfer. However, one must carefully consider the thickness of such flaps at their donor site. A simple way to do this is simply to pinch the skin and subcutaneous tissue. If the tissue is too thick for the anticipated recipient site, debulking with suction or excisional lipectomy can be an option in the future. However, in many areas on the extremity the subcutaneous fat layer is so thin that a perfect match with a fasciocutaneous flap may not be possible.

## FREE TISSUE TRANSFER FOR UPPER EXTREMITY RECONSTRUCTION

Upper extremity reconstruction should focus on restoring function first and foremost. During tumor resection, adjacent nerves and vessels may be resected and appropriate reconstruction should be attempted. Nerve, tendon, and bone grafting may be done immediately or delayed based on the individual case. Ideally, reconstruction should be attempted early to allow for a faster return to premorbid condition. When nerve grafting is needed, autologous graft is preferred. Tendon transfers or functional muscle transfer should be considered when tumor resection results in loss of a functional compartment or when motor nerves are not expected to regenerate. Tendons can be harvested from the great toe extensors or the contralateral palmaris longus. Transfer of an innervated segment of gracilis muscle with neural anastomosis to the anterior or posterior interosseous motor nerves can improve finger and wrist flexion and extension. The gracilis and rectus femoris muscle are good options to restore elbow flexion.[1,59–63]

When reconstructing soft tissue defects, an assortment of free flaps may be used depending on the location and size of the defect. The latissimus dorsi flap is considered one of the workhorse flaps in upper extremity reconstruction. It can be harvested with or without a skin paddle and is usually used to cover large defects and for obliteration of dead spaces. It can be combined with the serratus muscle or the scapular/parascapular flap to increase the flap size and can also be used to cover smaller defects by harvesting a hemi-latissimus flap, which is made possible by the predictable branching of the thoracodorsal artery into 2 distinct descending and transverse branches. The rectus abdominis flap is a reliable flap that can be used to cover medium to large complex defects in the upper extremity. This flap can be oriented vertically, transversely, or obliquely; intramuscular dissection can be done to increase the pedicle length. The gracilis flap can be used to cover small- to medium-sized defects and can be used for functional reconstruction of the forearm defects where flexion and extension of the wrist or digits is lost following tumor resection.[51,58,59]

The radial forearm fasciocutaneous flap is one of the workhorse flaps in hand reconstruction. It is thin and proves to be useful in covering defects that require minimal bulk. The anterolateral thigh (ALT) flap provides a large, thin skin paddle with minimal donor site morbidity. It is based on the descending branch of the lateral femoral circumflex artery with a perforator that can almost always be found midpoint of a line extending from the anterior superior iliac spine and the superolateral aspect of the patella. Harvesting the lateral femoral cutaneous nerve allows for a sensate flap. A portion of the vastus lateralis muscle can also be incorporated for dead space obliteration. A lateral arm flap is thin, which makes it ideal for reconstructing defects of the hand and distal forearm. It has multiple perforators, which allow using the harvested flap in multiple segments. Moreover, a segment of the vascularized humerus bone, triceps tendon, and the lower lateral cutaneous nerve, which can provide a sensate reconstruction, can be harvested with the flap.[1,39,61–64]

## FREE TISSUE TRANSFER FOR LOWER EXTREMITY RECONSTRUCTION

Lower extremity reconstruction should be approached in a systematic fashion based on the location and size of the defect. Flap selection is an important consideration and depends on many different factors. As a general rule, fasciocutaneous flaps are preferred overlying joints and where tendon glide is critical, such as the knee, ankle, and dorsum of the foot. However, wound size and body habitus may make fasciocutaneous flaps inadequate or inappropriate even in these locations. In addition, fasciocutaneous flaps are ideal when future operations are planned, such as bone grafting and tendon transfer, as they are better able to tolerate re-elevation and inset. A drawback of fasciocutaneous flaps, however, is their lack of atrophy and challenge to replicate the thin soft tissues of the knee, distal leg, and foot even after aggressive debulking (**Fig. 3**). Muscle flaps with skin graft, on the other hand, undergo extensive atrophy and for this reason often have the best results in regard to shape and contour. They also tend to be more adherent to the deep tissues providing a more stable soft tissue platform for ambulation for reconstruction of the weight-bearing limb or foot (**Fig. 4**). Disadvantages of muscle flap and skin graft include the scarred appearance, lack of motion/gliding over joints and tendons, and their lack of tolerance for re-elevation and inset if future operations are required.

In the proximal lower extremity, there is relatively abundant musculature that can allow for a stable bed for skin graft or pedicle flap coverage from the abdomen in the form of a TRAM or VRAM flap or from the neighboring thigh in the form of an ALT or anteromedial thigh flap. However, in some situations free tissue transfer can be necessary because of the extent of resection and poor quality of the surrounding tissues damaged by radiation or repeated operations. In these circumstances, large flaps are indicated. The TRAM flap can provide the size and bulk necessary to fill the void while providing healthy skin coverage. For larger defects, obese individuals, and/or those without any pannus for a TRAM flap, a latissimus dorsi muscle flap and skin graft may be most appropriate.

Reconstruction of defects around the knee can be particularly challenging. There is a paucity of soft tissue; the skin is very thin, yet it allows extreme flexion and a wide range of motion. A pedicle gastrocnemius muscle flap can be used for many defects. However, for tumor reconstruction, this is often less desirable for several potential reasons: its limited size to cover an extensive resection, resection of its pedicle in the resection, and radiation injury. The anterior surface of the knee presents unique challenges. The native skin and soft tissue is specialized to allow for full knee extension without tissue buckling and full flexion without contracture. Reconstructing this specialized soft tissue that will allow for this wide range of motion in a similar manner is quite difficult. Adding to the complexity is the paucity of nearby recipient vessels.[43,65–68]

Recipient vessels choice varies based on the location of the defect and the available vasculature following tumor resection. Common recipient vessels include the popliteal artery, the superficial femoral artery, anterior tibial artery, and the

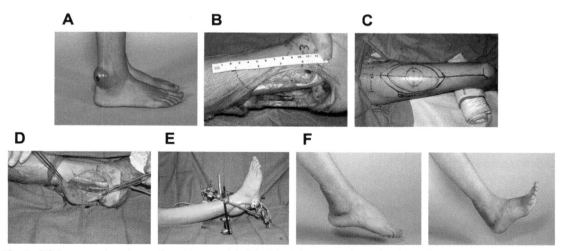

**Fig. 3.** (*A*) Preoperative views of an 11-year-old girl with right posterolateral ankle soft tissue sarcoma including most of the Achilles tendon and peroneal tendon sheath. (*B*) Intraoperative photographs of resection bed. (*C*) Markings for right ALT flap with template of wound. Tensor fascia lata is marked as well and will be subsequently used in functional reconstruction of the Achilles tendon. (*D*) Flap inset with the tensor fascia lata positioned against the Achilles tendon for functional reconstruction. (*E*) Postoperative photograph with the flap in place. The external fixator was used in this case as a kickstand to protect the flap and keep the ankle in dorsiflexion. (*F*) Two-year follow-up after liposuction and debulking of the flap.

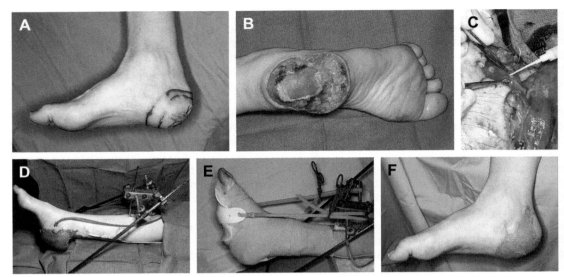

**Fig. 4.** (*A*) Preoperative appearance of a 60-year-old woman with recurrent verrucous carcinoma. (*B*) Image shown following tumor resection with exposure of the residual calcaneus and tendons. The posterior tibial artery was resected and the tibial nerve divided. (*C*) The tibial nerve was coapted to the obturator nerve for neuroma control and in hopes to improve protective sensation of the flap. (*D*) Protection of the flap is facilitated with an external fixator that also allows for a compressive wrap and footplate splint (*E*). (*F*) The flap proved resilient to weight bearing and atrophied nicely for an aesthetic contour that allows for easy shoe wear without the need for orthotics.

descending branch of the lateral circumflex femoral artery. Venous anastomoses are performed to the venae comitantes or to the greater saphenous vein. The best choice for recipient vessels is debatable and should be individualized to patients; recipient vessel choice should be made based on vessel size match, vessel availability, and the location where vascular anastomosis will be performed while accounting for any zone of injury. For anterior knee wounds, the senior author often prefers the anterior tibial artery. Although it is distal to the wound, in tumor cases this is less of a concern than traumatic wounds and it allows for easier inset and patient positioning in the operating room. In addition, it is less prone to compression postoperatively. When all options have been exhausted, perforator-based flaps (supermicrosurgery) can be performed.[69–72]

For defects of the lower leg that are above the foot and ankle, muscle flaps with skin graft coverage are preferred because of their improved contour and shape. Free tissue transfer is indicated when local flaps are inadequate because of size, reach, or damage from radiation. Unlike the thigh, local soft tissue is scarce and may be compromised by radiation or vascular disease.[2,73–75]

Amputation is still considered the gold standard for ablation of tumors involving the foot. Tumor resection with clear margins often leaves little to be reconstructed. Moreover, the excellent rehabilitation and prosthetic options for below-the-knee amputations allow for a faster recovery and return to function.[2,76] However, exceptions exist and microsurgery offers a variety of options for reconstruction. The goals of reconstruction should be to allow weight bearing during ambulation and padding of bony prominences. Also, reconstruction should eventually allow the use of shoe wear or orthotic devices. Bulky flaps may be durable and protect bony prominence but are often insensate and may not accommodate shoe wear. The foot is often visible, and bulky flaps can also be unsightly. Similar to knee reconstruction, achieving all the goals of reconstruction in one operation is often difficult. Flap choice must be individualized based on each case's needs and desired outcomes.[77–81] The senior author usually prefers muscle and skin graft coverage of the foot because of its capacity to atrophy and improved stability for weight-bearing purposes (see **Fig. 4**). However, fasciocutaneous flaps around the ankle may be preferred to improve ankle motion and allow for Achilles tendon reconstruction (see **Fig. 3**). An external fixator can be used to elevate the lower extremity, especially in cases of ankle reconstruction whereby the flap may be located in a dependent area (see **Figs. 3** and **4**).[82] The fixator also allows for protection of the flap and easy monitoring in the postoperative period.

## SUMMARY

Microsurgical reconstruction is the gold standard of reconstruction following tumor resection. The reconstructive surgeon who is able to use these microsurgical techniques can provide reliable, well-vascularized coverage in the most complex chest and extremities defects. It is important to adhere to the basic principles of reconstruction and use the simplest, reliable option for soft tissue coverage. Complete reconstruction in a single stage at time of resection should be the goal in order to shorten the duration of hospitalization and recovery in patients who often have already had a prolonged course.

## ACKNOWLEDGMENTS

The authors are grateful for Dr Karim Bakri's, MD assistance in the case presented in **Fig. 2**.

## REFERENCES

1. Saint-Cyr M, Langstein HN. Reconstruction of the hand and upper extremity after tumor resection. J Surg Oncol 2006;94:490–503.
2. Zenn MR, Levin LS. Microvascular reconstruction of the lower extremity. Semin Surg Oncol 2000;19: 272–81.
3. Barner-Rasmussen I, Popov P, Böhling T, et al. Microvascular reconstruction after resection of soft tissue sarcoma of the leg. Br J Surg 2009;96:482–9.
4. Chang EI, Nguyen AT, Hughes JK, et al. Optimization of free-flap limb salvage and maximizing function and quality of life following oncologic resection: 12-year experience. Ann Surg Oncol 2016;23: 1036–43.
5. Engel H, Lin CH, Wei FC. Role of microsurgery in lower extremity reconstruction. Plast Reconstr Surg 2011;127:228S–38S.
6. Ferguson PC. Surgical considerations for management of distal extremity soft tissue sarcomas. Curr Opin Oncol 2005;17:366–9.
7. Kandel R, Coakley N, Werier J, et al. Surgical margins and handling of soft-tissue sarcoma in extremities: a clinical practice guideline. Curr Oncol 2013; 20:E247–54.
8. Soltanian H, Garcia RM, Hollenbeck ST. Current concepts in lower extremity reconstruction. Plast Reconstr Surg 2015;136:815e–29e.
9. Gomes M, Khorana AA. Risk assessment for thrombosis in cancer. Semin Thromb Hemost 2014;40: 319–24.
10. Bakri K, Mardini S, Evans KK, et al. Workhorse flaps in chest wall reconstruction: the pectoralis major, latissimus dorsi, and rectus abdominis flaps. Semin Plast Surg 2011;25:43–54.
11. Thomas PA, Brouchet L. Prosthetic reconstruction of the chest wall. Thorac Surg Clin 2010;20:551–8.
12. MacKenzie EJ, Bosse MJ. Factors influencing outcome following limb-threatening lower limb trauma: lessons learned from the Lower Extremity Assessment Project (LEAP). J Am Acad Orthop Surg 2006;14:S205–10.
13. Higgins TF, Klatt JB, Beals TC. Lower Extremity Assessment Project (LEAP)–the best available evidence on limb-threatening lower extremity trauma. Orthop Clin North Am 2010;41:233–9.
14. Arnold PG, Pairolero PC. Chest-wall reconstruction: an account of 500 consecutive patients. Plast Reconstr Surg 1996;98:804–10.
15. Deschamps C, Tirnaksiz BM, Darbandi R, et al. Early and long-term results of prosthetic chest wall reconstruction. J Thorac Cardiovasc Surg 1999; 117:588–91.
16. Mansour KA, Thourani VH, Losken A, et al. Chest wall resections and reconstruction: a 25-year experience. Ann Thorac Surg 2002;73:1720–5.
17. Chang RR, Mehrara BJ, Hu QY, et al. Reconstruction of complex oncologic chest wall defects: a 10-year experience. Ann Plast Surg 2004;52:471–9.
18. Shah AA, D'Amico TA. Primary chest wall tumors. J Am Coll Surg 2010;210:360–6.
19. Somers J, Faber LP. Chondroma and chondrosarcoma. Semin Thorac Cardiovasc Surg 1999;11: 270–7.
20. King RM, Pairolero PC, Trastek VF, et al. Primary chest wall tumors: factors affecting survival. Ann Thorac Surg 1986;41:597–601.
21. McCormack PM. Use of prosthetic materials in chest-wall reconstruction. Assets and liabilities. Surg Clin North Am 1989;69:965–76.
22. Sodha NR, Azoury SC, Sciortino C, et al. The use of acellular dermal matrices in chest wall reconstruction. Plast Reconstr Surg 2012;130:175S–82S.
23. Weyant MJ, Bains MS, Venkatraman E, et al. Results of chest wall resection and reconstruction with and without rigid prosthesis. Ann Thorac Surg 2006;81: 279–85.
24. Arnold PG, Pairolero PC. Intrathoracic muscle flaps. An account of their use in the management of 100 consecutive patients. Ann Surg 1990;211: 656–60.
25. Chen HC, Tang YB, Noordhoff MS, et al. Microvascular free muscle flaps for chronic empyema with bronchopleural fistula when the major local muscles have been divided–one-stage operation with primary wound closure. Ann Plast Surg 1990; 24:510–6.
26. Arnold PG, Lovich SF, Pairolero PC. Muscle flaps in irradiated wounds: an account of 100 consecutive cases. Plast Reconstr Surg 1994;93:324–7.
27. Hammond DC, Fisher J, Meland NB. Intrathoracic free flaps. Plast Reconstr Surg 1993;91:1259–64.

28. Walsh MD, Bruno AD, Onaitis MW, et al. The role of intrathoracic free flaps for chronic empyema. Ann Thorac Surg 2011;91:865–8.

29. Cordeiro PG, Santamaria E, Hidalgo D. The role of microsurgery in reconstruction of oncologic chest wall defects. Plast Reconstr Surg 2001;108: 1924–30.

30. Tukiainen E, Popov P, Asko-Seljavaara S. Microvascular reconstructions of full-thickness oncological chest wall defects. Ann Surg 2003;238:794–801.

31. Losken A, Thourani VH, Carlson GW, et al. A reconstructive algorithm for plastic surgery following extensive chest wall resection. Br J Plast Surg 2004;57:295–302.

32. Cohen M, Ramasastry SS. Reconstruction of complex chest wall defects. Am J Surg 1996;172:35–40.

33. McMillan RR, Sima CS, Moraco NH, et al. Recurrence patterns after resection of soft tissue sarcomas of the chest wall. Ann Thorac Surg 2013;96: 1223–8.

34. Perry RR, Venzon D, Roth JA, et al. Survival after surgical resection for high-grade chest wall sarcomas. Ann Thorac Surg 1990;49:363–8.

35. Arnold PG, Pairolero PC. Intrathoracic muscle flaps: a 10-year experience in the management of life-threatening infections. Plast Reconstr Surg 1989; 84:92–8.

36. Zyluk A, Mazur A. Statistical and histological analysis of tumors of the upper extremity. Obere Extremität 2015;10:252–7.

37. Ann-Marie Plate GS, Posner MA. Malignant tumors of the hand and wrist. J Am Acad Orthop Surg 2006;14:680–92.

38. Ring A, Kirchhoff P, Goertz O, et al. Reconstruction of soft-tissue defects at the foot and ankle after oncological resection. Front Surg 2016;3:15.

39. Lohman RF, Nabawi AS, Reece GP, et al. Soft tissue sarcoma of the upper extremity: a 5-year experience at two institutions emphasizing the role of soft tissue flap reconstruction. Cancer 2002;94:2256–64.

40. Murray PM. Soft tissue sarcoma of the upper extremity. Hand Clin 2004;20:325–33.

41. Ghert MA, Davis AM, Griffin AM, et al. The surgical and functional outcome of limb-salvage surgery with vascular reconstruction for soft tissue sarcoma of the extremity. Ann Surg Oncol 2005; 12:1102–10.

42. Groundland JS, Binitie O. Reconstruction after tumor resection in the growing child. Orthop Clin North Am 2016;47:265–81.

43. Han G, Bi WZ, Xu M, et al. Amputation versus limb-salvage surgery in patients with osteosarcoma: a meta-analysis. World J Surg 2016;40:2016–27.

44. Hwang JS, Mehta AD, Yoon RS, et al. From amputation to limb salvage reconstruction: evolution and role of the endoprosthesis in musculoskeletal oncology. J Orthop Traumatol 2014;15:81–6.

45. Chiang YC, Wei FC, Wang JW, et al. Reconstruction of below-knee stump using the salvaged foot fillet flap. Plast Reconstr Surg 1995;96:731–8.

46. Gallico GG 3rd, Ehrlichman RJ, Jupiter J, et al. Free flaps to preserve below-knee amputation stumps: long-term evaluation. Plast Reconstr Surg 1987;79: 871–8.

47. Fitzgibbons P, Medvedev G. Functional and clinical outcomes of upper extremity amputation. J Am Acad Orthop Surg 2015;23:751–60.

48. Waters RL, Perry J, Antonelli D, et al. Energy cost of walking of amputees: the influence of level of amputation. J Bone Joint Surg Am 1976;58:42–6.

49. Oliveira IC, Barbosa RF, Ferreira PC, et al. The use of forearm free fillet flap in traumatic upper extremity amputations. Microsurgery 2009;29:8–15.

50. Levin LS, Erdmann D, Germann G. The use of fillet flaps in upper extremity reconstruction. J Am Soc Surg Hand 2002;2:39–44.

51. Muramatsu K, Ihara K, Yoshida K, et al. Musculoskeletal sarcomas in the forearm and hand: standard treatment and microsurgical reconstruction for limb salvage. Anticancer Res 2013;33:4175–82.

52. Souza JM, Cheesborough JE, Ko JH, et al. Targeted muscle reinnervation: a novel approach to postamputation neuroma pain. Clin Orthop Relat Res 2014;472: 2984–90.

53. Cheesborough JE, Smith LH, Kuiken TA, et al. Targeted muscle reinnervation and advanced prosthetic arms. Semin Plast Surg 2015;29:62–72.

54. Kapelner T, Jiang N, Holobar A, et al. Motor unit characteristics after targeted muscle reinnervation. PLoS One 2016;11:e0149772.

55. Gart MS, Souza JM, Dumanian GA. Targeted muscle reinnervation in the upper extremity amputee: a technical roadmap. J Hand Surg Am 2015;40: 1877–88.

56. Carlsen BT, Prigge P, Peterson J. Upper extremity limb loss: functional restoration from prosthesis and targeted reinnervation to transplantation. J Hand Ther 2014;27:106–13.

57. Lopez JF, Hietanen KE, Kaartinen IS, et al. Primary flap reconstruction of tissue defects after sarcoma surgery enables curative treatment with acceptable functional results: a 7-year review. BMC Surg 2015; 15:71.

58. Kim JY, Subramanian V, Yousef A, et al. Upper extremity limb salvage with microvascular reconstruction in patients with advanced sarcoma. Plast Reconstr Surg 2004;114:400–8.

59. Chim H, Ng ZY, Carlsen BT, et al. Soft tissue coverage of the upper extremity: an overview. Hand Clin 2014;30:459–73.

60. Scheker LR, Ahmed O. Radical debridement, free flap coverage, and immediate reconstruction of the upper extremity. Hand Clin 2007;23:23–36.

61. Wang D, Levin LS. Composite tissue transfer in upper extremity trauma. Injury 2008;39:S90–6.
62. Schaverien MV, Hart AM. Free muscle flaps for reconstruction of upper limb defects. Hand Clin 2014;30:165–83.
63. Saint-Cyr M, Gupta A. Indications and selection of free flaps for soft tissue coverage of the upper extremity. Hand Clin 2007;23:37–48.
64. Sforzo CR, Scarborough MT, Wright TW. Bone-forming tumors of the upper extremity and Ewing's sarcoma. Hand Clin 2004;20:303–15.
65. Umezawa H, Sakuraba M, Miyamoto S, et al. Analysis of immediate vascular reconstruction for lower-limb salvage in patients with lower-limb bone and soft-tissue sarcoma. J Plast Reconstr Aesthet Surg 2013;66:608–16.
66. Li X, Zhang Y, Wan S, et al. A comparative study between limb-salvage and amputation for treating osteosarcoma. J Bone Oncol 2016;5:15–21.
67. Ong YS, Levin LS. Lower limb salvage in trauma. Plast Reconstr Surg 2010;125:582–8.
68. Reddy V, Stevenson TR. MOC-PS(SM) CME article: lower extremity reconstruction. Plast Reconstr Surg 2008;121:1–7.
69. Louer CR, Garcia RM, Earle SA, et al. Free flap reconstruction of the knee: an outcome study of 34 cases. Ann Plast Surg 2015;74:57–63.
70. Hong JP, Koshima I. Using perforators as recipient vessels (supermicrosurgery) for free flap reconstruction of the knee region. Ann Plast Surg 2010; 64:291–3.
71. Manoso MW, Boland PJ, Healey JH, et al. Limb salvage of infected knee reconstructions for cancer with staged revision and free tissue transfer. Ann Plast Surg 2006;56:532–5.
72. Weinberg H, Kenan S, Lewis MM, et al. The role of microvascular surgery in limb-sparing procedures for malignant tumors of the knee. Plast Reconstr Surg 1993;92:692–8.
73. Serletti JM, Deuber MA, Guidera PM, et al. Atherosclerosis of the lower extremity and free-tissue reconstruction for limb salvage. Plast Reconstr Surg 1995;96:1136–44.
74. Serafin D, Voci VE. Reconstruction of the lower extremity. Microsurgical composite tissue transplantation. Clin Plast Surg 1983;10:55–72.
75. Serafin D, Sabatier RE, Morris RL, et al. Reconstruction of the lower extremity with vascularized composite tissue: improved tissue survival and specific indications. Plast Reconstr Surg 1980;66:230–41.
76. Lange RH. Limb reconstruction versus amputation decision making in massive lower extremity trauma. Clin Orthop Relat Res 1989;243:92–9.
77. Karakousis CP, DeYoung C, Driscoll DL. Soft tissue sarcomas of the hand and foot: management and survival. Ann Surg Oncol 1998;5:238–40.
78. Medina MA 3rd, Salinas HM, Eberlin KR, et al. Modified free radial forearm fascia flap reconstruction of lower extremity and foot wounds: optimal contour and minimal donor-site morbidity. J Reconstr Microsurg 2014;30:515–22.
79. Sugg KB, Schaub TA, Concannon MJ, et al. The reverse superficial sural artery flap revisited for complex lower extremity and foot reconstruction. Plast Reconstr Surg Glob Open 2015;3:e519.
80. Korompilias AV, Lykissas MG, Vekris MD, et al. Microsurgery for lower extremity injuries. Injury 2008;39:S103–8.
81. Erdmann D, Sundin BM, Yasui K, et al. Microsurgical free flap transfer to amputation sites: indications and results. Ann Plast Surg 2002;48:167–72.
82. Ting BL, Abousayed MM, Holzer P, et al. External fixator kickstands for free soft tissue flap protection: case series and description of technique. Foot Ankle Int 2013;34:1695–700.

# Pediatric Microsurgery
## A Global Overview

Ali Izadpanah, MD[a], Steven L. Moran, MD[b],*

**KEYWORDS**

- Microsurgery • Pediatric • Free tissue transfer • Children

**KEY POINTS**

- Pediatric microsurgical procedures have successful outcomes similar to adult reconstructions.
- Free tissue transfer can provide immediate reconstruction of defects without the need for tissue expansion, skin grafting, or muscle sacrifice.
- Dedicated microsurgical centers should perform the bulk of these procedures given the small structures involved and ancillary pediatric expertise which may be required for adequate post-operative care.

## INTRODUCTION

Early in the evolution of pediatric microsurgery, Gilbert[1] thought that the small vessels in children could pose a technical limitation for free tissue transfer and suggested that a minimum vessel diameter of 0.7 mm was safe for microanastomoses. Vessels smaller than this were initially considered too small for reliable outcomes. As microsurgical expertise has improved, allowing for the safe transfer of smaller and more refined flaps, free tissue transfer has continued to gain popularity for the management of pediatric soft tissue and bony defects. Over the past 2 decades, pediatric microsurgery has been shown to be technically feasible and reliable.[2–7]

The major advantage of free tissue transfer in children is the ability to reconstruct defects in a single stage. Historically, soft tissue reconstruction in children has required the use of skin grafting, tissue expansion, or pedicled flaps; surgeons would typically follow *the reconstructive ladder* in choosing a surgical procedure. Split-thickness skin grafting and tissue expansion are techniques that can produce scarring and require several operative procedures or multiple dressing changes to achieve a healed wound. The use of local flaps or pedicled muscle flaps can add further injury and donor site morbidity to an already traumatized extremity. With the advent of free perforator flaps, such as the anterolateral thigh (ALT) flap and superficial circumflex iliac artery perforator (SCIP) flap, donor site morbidity is minimized and no muscle needs to be violated.[8] With present day technology, the authors advocate for using the "reconstructive elevator" and bypass more traditional techniques for the benefits of free tissue transfer in children, allowing for single-stage reconstruction and in many cases primary closure of the donor site. This article reviews the present state-of-the-art in pediatric microsurgery using a global perspective.

## CATEGORIES OF MICROSURGERY IN CHILDREN

Pediatric microsurgery is primarily performed for the reconstruction of congenital defects as well as following trauma and tumor extirpation. Most *elective* pediatric microsurgery is performed for the reconstruction of congenital facial deformities

The authors have nothing to disclose.

[a] Department of Orthopedic Surgery, Mayo Clinic, 200 First Street Southwest, Rochester, MN 55905, USA;
[b] Division of Plastic Surgery, Department of Surgery, Mayo Clinic, 200 First Street Southwest, Rochester, MN 55905, USA
* Corresponding author.
*E-mail address:* Moran.steven@mayo.edu

plasticsurgery.theclinics.com

and congenital hand anomalies. Traumatic defects and tumor reconstructions, while seen less frequently than in the adult population, can pose particular challenges; in these cases, the reconstructive surgeon must allow for ongoing growth and minimize donor site morbidity. Here, the authors provide an overview of the more frequently performed pediatric microvascular procedures within these major categories of congenital deformity, trauma, and tumor.

## Congenital Defects

### Facial asymmetry

Congenital facial anomalies requiring free tissue transfers include Romberg hemifacial atrophy, hemifacial microsomia, facial clefts, and Treacher Collins syndrome.[9–15] Many of these patients have some component of facial asymmetry due to a combination of soft tissue and bony hypoplasia. The use of local tissue for the treatment of these deformities is limited and can create further facial morbidity. Free nonvascularized fat or dermal grafts can have unpredictable absorption, and prosthetic implants run the risk of extrusion and infection over time. Adipofascial free flaps have been shown to be an effective alternative for these cases.[9] Shintomi and colleagues[16] used a de-epithelialized groin flap with dermis down for integration into the native fascia with the flap's fatty side against the facial skin for prevention of skin contracture.

Despite Shintomi's results, the most commonly used free flap for soft tissue augmentation after Romberg hemifacial atrophy is the scapular and parascapular flaps. These flaps, when combined with their local fascial extension, provide reliable thick tissue that can be safely contoured and secured to the underlying skeleton to avoid migration due to gravity.[9] These flaps provide a large amount of tissue, and the vascular pedicle is long, with a diameter of greater than 1 mm even in young children; however, the donor site is conspicuous and can hypertrophy.

In addition to scapular and parascapular flaps, the use of free omentum to improve facial asymmetry has also been described.[17] The omentum has large donor vessels, and the vascularized fatty tissue can be folded on itself, allowing flexibility in correcting deformities. The disadvantage of using this flap is the need for a laparotomy, the lack of structural support within the flap, and the potential for seroma formation. Laparoscopic omentum harvest makes this a more appealing option in adolescents, but not for infants and toddlers because the omentum is poorly developed in young children.

In Romberg syndrome, the timing of surgery is controversial, and many think that it should only be undertaken after the disease process is quiescent. In comparison, recent studies have shown benefits of the vascularized flap on the native tissue after transfer, even during times of active disease.[16,18] Earlier placement of free vascularized tissue in theory could necessitate further surgery following the completion of facial growth; however, the authors have found that for smaller contour defects remaining after free tissue transfer, free fat injections from the gluteal, abdominal, or inguinal regions can improve the cosmetic result while avoiding an extended secondary major surgical procedure.[19,20]

### Clefts

Another condition that may benefit from free tissue transfers is the residual wide cleft lip and palate, which have failed primary repair using the local tissue.[21,22] Futran and Haller[22] originally reported on the use of the free radial forearm flap for the correction of large residual fistulas with good outcomes. Further work by MacLeod and colleagues[23] also reported good results with the use of the free radial forearm flap with and without bone for large palatine defects.

### Facial reanimation

The history and nuances of free tissue transfer for facial paralysis are beyond the scope of this review; however, any surgeon embarking on the treatment of this condition needs to have a thorough understanding of the surgical techniques available to treat this heterogeneous condition. In chronic facial nerve palsies, the possibilities of functional return after nerve repair or decompression are minimal due to the deterioration of the motor end plates on the muscle. In such cases, the only option for active motion is the use of functional muscle transfers with either local pedicled flaps or free muscle. Many of the local transfers cannot produce synchronous involuntary facial expressions (particularly smile) to match the contralateral side. The free gracilis functional transfer has become the standard treatment to restore smile in cases of nerve absence or injury.[24–32]

The 2-staged technique, which classically consists of cross-facial nerve grafting followed by muscle transfer and neurotization, produces minimal donor site morbidity and can allow for synchronous restoration of smile. Recent reports have noted an 11% failure rate with this procedure due to flap complications and the unpredictability of nerve ingrowth from the contralateral side.[33] Bae and colleagues[27] explored the choice of motor nerves to neurotize the transplanted muscle for achieving synchronous and spontaneous function; their results demonstrated that the final outcomes in commissural movement after both cross-facial nerve grafting and neurotization of free functional gracilis using the masseter nerve were similar. In 2009, Terzis and Olivares[34] published Terzis' lifetime experience with the use of both pectoralis minor muscle and free gracilis in 32 children followed for 5 years or longer. The study noted improvement in smile in all children with the ability of the muscle to grow with the child and provide increasing function over time.

## Hand and Upper Limb Anomalies

Congenital hand deformities in children are common, with an incidence of 1.97 per 1000 live births.[35] Although most children with congenital anomalies do well with standard reconstructive procedures, there are 3 groups of children who can benefit from free tissue transfers: (1) children with absent digits; (2) children with radial hypoplasia; and (3) children with pseudoarthrosis of the forearm. Each group will be discussed in further detail.

The causes of congenital absent digits include adactyly, symbrachydactyly, transverse failure of formation, cleft hand, and congenital constriction ring syndrome (or amniotic band syndrome).[36,37] Great toe or second toe transfer is a means of improving hand function in these children.[38] The primary goal of reconstruction is to establish a useful thumb for opposition. If a thumb is already present, then reconstructive measures should focus on the creation of a stable post to which the child may oppose the thumb. If possible, the creation of a second finger can allow for the utilization of chuck pinch. In addition, a second finger will allow for stabilization of remaining fingers or hypoplastic digits during precision pinch (**Fig. 1**). A thumb and 2 fingers allow for power grasp, key pinch, and chuck grip and should be considered the goal for reconstruction of the adactylous or congenitally deficient hand.[39]

Jones and Kaplan[40] have described the indications for free toe transfer to the thumb as (1) an absent thumb distal to the carpometacarpal joint with 4 relatively normal fingers (**Fig. 2**); (2) an absent thumb with only 1 or 2 fingers remaining on the ulnar border of the hand; and (3) complete absence of the thumb and all 4 fingers. Their indications for toe transfers for the reconstruction of congenital absent fingers are (1) absence of all 4 fingers but with a normal thumb remaining and (2) complete absence of all 5 digits. In a study by Kaplan and Jones,[36] the investigators showed good patient outcomes in children with congenital or traumatic

missing or hypoplastic digits who underwent reconstruction by microsurgical toe-to-hand transfer. Children regained function, sensation, and ability to perform daily activities. More recent results from Nikkhah and colleagues[41] noted poor active range of motion (ROM) in the transferred digits, but all children were able to perform large object grip and recovery of 2-point discrimination was excellent (5-mm 2-point discrimination). Kay and Wiberg[42] also noted poor active ROM of the toes following transfer; however, even with poor active ROM following surgery, children were still able to grip, which provided an improvement in baseline function. Digit stability appears to be the key factor for function following toe transfer, as digit stability allows force transmission through the transferred toes to the objects that are grasped.

Second toe transfer may also be used in the stabilization of the wrist in cases of radial hypoplasia. Vilkki[43] has described the use of the second metatarsal and proximal phalanx as a means of re-establishing the radial column in cases of Bayne type III and IV radial hypoplasia. The procedure is performed in 2 stages. In the first stage, the wrist and tight radial soft tissues are gradually distracted with and external fixator to establish proper hand alignment before placement of the toe transfer. Once the wrist has straightened, the second toe metatarsal and proximal phalanx are transferred to the radial aspect of the wrist. The metatarsal is stabilized against the ulnar shaft, and the distal end of the proximal phalanx is placed against the remaining base of the scaphoid, trapezium, or second metacarpal. In comparison to centralization and radialization (the standard techniques for wrist stabilization in radial hypoplasia), the Vilkki procedure allows for preservation of wrist flexion and extension, while allowing for ongoing growth of the ulna. Hand alignment as the child develops is dependent on the balanced growth rate of the metatarsal physis and the distal ulnar physis (**Fig. 3**).[43–45] This procedure has also recently been shown to be valuable in cases of failed centralization.[46] Using a similar concept, Yang and colleagues[47] in a recent report showed successful long-term outcomes in 4 children with Bayne and Klug type III radial longitudinal deficiency using a vascularized proximal fibular epiphyseal transfer.

Congenital pseudoarthrosis represents the final area where free tissue transfer has been shown to provide substantial improvement over standard treatment methods. Pseudoarthrosis is a rare bone condition that can result in impaired bone development and fracture healing. It is thought to be caused by neurofibromatosis or fibrous

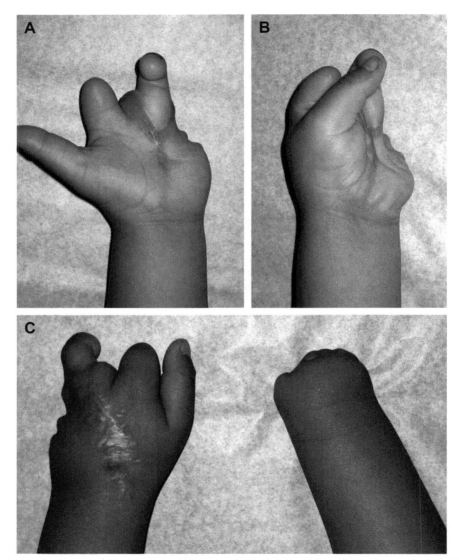

**Fig. 1.** Postoperative images following second toe transfer to left hand in a child with atypical cleft hand. The addition of a third finger to an index finger stump allows the child to pinch and perform chuck grip and key pinch (*A, B*). The child has a congenital amputation of the right hand (*C*).

dysplasia and leads to persistent nonunions in the radius and/or ulna with associated bony atrophy and deformity. Historic treatment with nonvascularized bone grafting has led to poor outcomes. A literature review[48] showed that bone union was obtained in only 36% of cases treated with casting, nonvascularized bone grafting, and adjunct electrical stimulation. In 1981, Allieu and colleagues[49] reported 2 cases successfully treated with vascularized fibular grafts. The use of a vascularized fibula graft allows for larger resections of all diseased bone and allows for the use of plate and screw fixation, which provides enhanced stability over historic pin or fixator stabilization. In addition,

the fibula provides a similar size match for the ulna and radial diaphysis. Recent reports by Bae and colleagues[50] and El Hage and colleagues[51] have noted excellent results with preserved arm growth and bony healing (**Fig. 4**).

## Traumatic Injuries

### Lower extremity trauma

Trauma is one of the most common causes for hospital admissions in children.[52,53] Motor vehicle collisions (MVC) represent a frequent cause of soft tissue trauma in both adults and children. In adults, multiple studies have pointed to the benefits of

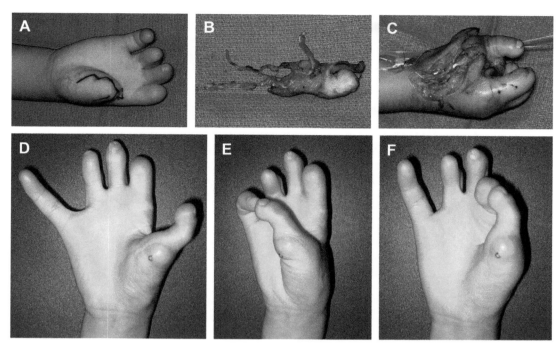

**Fig. 2.** A 2-year-old child with amniotic band syndrome. The thumb is missing (A). A second toe transfer was performed to restore thumb function. (B) The toe before transfer. (C) The toe inset at the base of the remaining thumb metacarpal. K-wires are used for initial fixation, and an implantable Doppler probe is used to assist with postoperative monitoring. It is important to ensure adequate length and oppositional pinch to all digits. Long-term function 4 years following transfer (D–F).

free tissue coverage for lower-third and middle-third Gustio type IIIb and IIIc injuries following MVC; however, these types of defects occur at a much lower incidence in children secondary to their age-dependent bone plasticity, car-seat restraints, and their placement in the rear passenger compartment. Only 10% of pediatric tibial fractures are open, and only 7% are IIIb injuries.[54] In a decade-long retrospective study, Laine and colleagues[54] only identified 8 cases of Gustilo type IIIb and IIIc injuries in children that required free tissue transfer and bony reconstruction. The low numbers of patients reported in this study emphasizes the infrequency of pediatric trauma requiring free tissue transfer for middle- and upper-third coverage in the lower extremity; however, multiple papers have pointed to the need for free tissue transfer in cases of foot and ankle trauma in children following lawnmower or vehicular injury.[5,7,55–58] Serletti and colleagues[7] reported that 63% of their pediatric free flaps were performed for traumatic injury to the foot or ankle region.

Historically, free muscle, myocutaneous flaps, and radial forearm flaps have been transferred most frequently to cover large defects of the lower extremities in children[5,7]; however, the authors

think that the ALT is now the best option for lower-extremity coverage in the pediatric patient due to its size and favorable donor site.[59] The flap may be neurotized for sensation and harvested with the tensor fascia lata or iliotibial band for reconstruction of the Achilles tendon or toe extensors.[56,60] The smooth fasciocutaneous deep surface provided by the ALT is ideal for tendon gliding.[8] In addition, failure rates for this flap in pediatric patients have been reported to be low.[8]

Use of super-microsurgery and perforator-based flaps in pediatric free tissue transfers are becoming more common.[3] Iida and colleagues[61] report on the use of SCIP with a vessel diameter less than 0.7 mm in a 1-year-old child after correction of valgus foot deformity. The SCIP flap represents another perforator flap with an ideal donor site for children producing minimal functional and cosmetic morbidity.

*Facial trauma*
In a review of 433 pediatric soft issue transfers by Upton and Guo,[53] the greatest number of flaps were performed in the head and neck region; however, only 15 cases were performed for trauma. Most large traumatic defects are the result of burns, which are amenable to free soft tissue

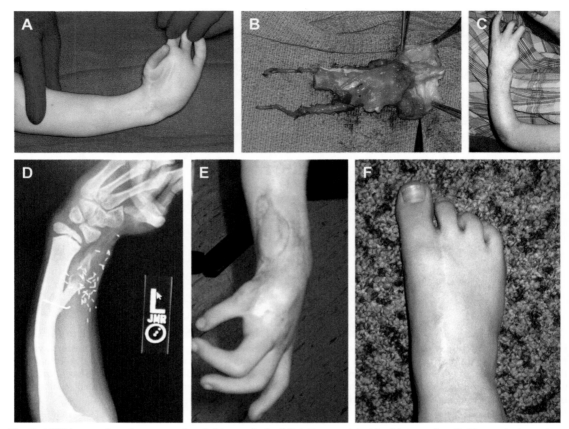

**Fig. 3.** Vilkki procedure in a case of radial hypoplasia. (*A*) A 5-year-old girl with type 4 radial hypoplasia and severe radial deviation of the wrist. (*B*) The second metacarpal head and proximal phalanx are transferred to the radial aspect of the ulna, creating a new radial column for the wrist. Four-year result with good position of the wrist clinically and radiographically (*C, D*). (*E*) Clinical image of skin island. (*F*) Foot 4 years following procedure.

transfer.[62,63] Although the use of free tissue transfer has been clearly established for neck contracture and large scalp burns, the development of newer skin substitutes has allowed many centers to avoid the use of free tissue transfers in situations that were not previously correctable without the use of microsurgical techniques.[64]

### Upper extremity trauma

There are 2 major categories of upper limb trauma that consistently benefit from microsurgical intervention in children, and these include digital replantation and free functioning muscle transfers. Although there is no consensus for when pediatric replantation should be performed, an attempt at replant should be made in most cases of pediatric amputation. Early correction of digital amputation may enhance future functional and psychosocial adaptation of these patients. The success rate of large pediatric replantation series ranges from 63% to 97%.[65–68] Despite these results, pediatric replantation may not be attempted as frequently

as it should. In a recent analysis by Berlin and colleagues,[69] examining 455 pediatric patients undergoing replantation, pediatric patients had a lower likelihood of developing a complication requiring an amputation and had a shorter hospital stay than adult patients. Unfortunately, Berlin also noted that the rate of pediatric replantation was relatively low, being only 27% at most in a given year. Berlin's overall conclusions were that short-term outcomes are better in children than for adults, justifying replantation attempts in this age group.

Success has also been seen in the use of free functioning muscle transfer for restoration of loss of elbow flexion, finger flexor, and finger extensor. Loss of function may be the result of brachial plexus injury or compartment syndrome. The use of gracilis, semitendinosus, pectoralis major, or latissimus dorsi muscles has been described for restoration of function. The first case of pediatric free gracilis transfer was reported by Manktelow[32] in 1984 in a 4-year-old boy suffering from loss of finger flexion following a Volkmann contracture.

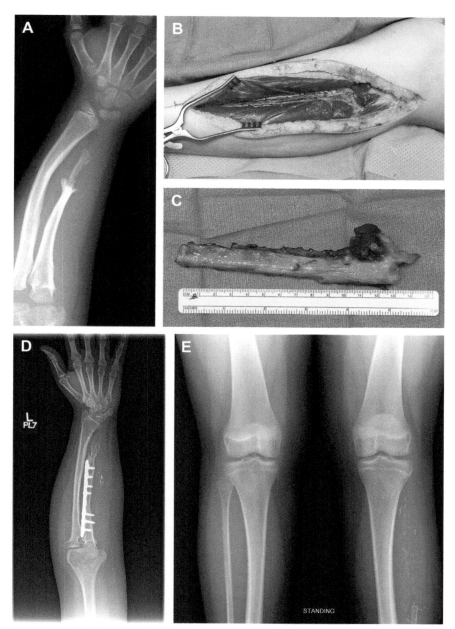

**Fig. 4.** Use of a vascularized proximal fibular graft with intact growth plate for reconstruction of the distal ulna in a girl with pseudoarthrosis of the ulna. (*A*) Anteroposterior (AP) radiograph of the ulnar pseudoarthrosis. (*B*) The proximal fibula harvested based on the blood supply of the anterior tibial vessel. Long-term results 5 years following transfer (*C–E*). The patient has normal gait and full pronation and supination of the forearm.

Since then, numerous reports of gracilis functional transfers have been published for various conditions including polio.[70–72] Most recently, in a review by Upton and Guo,[53] the authors reported successful outcome after 10 free functional muscle transfers for the treatment of Volkmann contracture using gracilis in 7 patients and latissimus in 3 patients.

## Cancer Reconstruction

The quality of life after limb preservation has been shown to be superior to amputation.[70] In children, limb preservation is considered the goal following tumor resection. To provide the patient with an adequate oncologic margin during the tumor resection, large osseous defects can be created that hamper functional limb salvage. Traditionally, structural allografts have been used to fill these defects, providing structural support using cortical bone; however, they are associated with a high complication rate, including fracture and infection.[71,72] Free vascularized fibular grafts have been shown to provide an osteogenic environment and remain viable even in cases of infection, chemotherapy, and radiotherapy.[73] Although fibular grafts have the ability to undergo hypertrophy and remodel, they lack the structural strength of large cortical allografts. Long bone reconstruction with fibular grafts alone may be prone to fracture, and prolonged times to fibular hypertrophy can limit physical activities. To circumvent the complications associated with allograft or fibular grafts alone, Capanna and colleagues[72] supplemented cortical allografts with intramedullary free fibular grafts. The combination of the osteogenic potential of the vascularized free fibula and the structural support of the cortical allograft makes the use of these grafts particularly attractive in the reconstruction of bony defects in children. Moran and colleagues[74] have noted better than 93% long-term limb salvage rates with this technique in pediatric patients (**Fig. 5**). This technique has become the gold standard for lower-limb preservation in cases of intercalary bone defects following tumor extirpation.[75]

### Vascularized Composite Allograft

In 1964, the first hand transplant was performed by Dr Gilbert in Ecuador.[76] Unfortunately, the patient experienced acute rejection and underwent amputation 3 weeks after transplant. Since then, scientific focus shifted toward the development of effective immunosuppressive regimens and improvement of solid organ transplant. In 1998, the first modern hand transplant was performed by Dr Jean-Michel Dubernard and colleagues in Lyon.[77] This hand transplant was followed by the first hand transplant in the United States in 1999 by Dr Breidenbach and his colleagues.[76] Until recently, any extremes of age (<18 or >69 years old) were considered exclusion criteria for hand transplantation in most US transplant centers; however, in June 2014, Dr Gurnaney and his team[78] performed the first successful bilateral pediatric hand transplant in an 8-year-old boy with a previous history of renal transplant and 4-limb amputation at an early age.

Vascularized composite allograft (VCA) is an innovative surgical technique that attempts to improve quality of life while balancing the risks associated with life-long immunosuppression. Unlike solid organ transplantation, hand transplantation is not considered lifesaving and can be challenging to justify in a healthy pediatric population. In this first case, the child already had undergone a kidney transplant and was thus taking immunosuppression. There are several questions to be answered following this first pediatric case, including the ability of the physis to grow, the ability of the muscles to grow, and the long-term risks of subsequent hand rejection episodes on the function of the transplanted kidney.[79]

## SPECIAL CONSIDERATIONS
### Growth

A unique aspect of free tissue transfers in children is the requirement for ongoing growth in the area of reconstruction. Myocutaneous and fasciocutaneous flaps have the potential for expansion with associated skeletal growth. Fasciocutaneous flaps, unlike skin grafts, do not contract after transfer. Muscle, when transferred alone or in a myocutaneous flap, usually undergoes atrophy and fibrosis unless it is innervated at the time of transfer. Innervated muscles can grow and can increase in bulk, whereas denervated muscle tends to fibrosis and may limit growth or produce contractures if placed over areas of rapid growth (such as joints).[34]

Bone flaps, unless they are transferred with an intact physis, will not elongate spontaneously. If transferred into an intercalary defect with an intact physis above and below the defect, there may be little long-term problems associated with growth.[75] Innocenti and colleagues[80] in 2008 published a report on the use of proximal fibular epiphysis, including the physis. This flap could maintain the growth potential in its new heterotopic locations. The original research examining the possibility of preserving an active physis following revascularization dates back to the 1980s.[81] In recent years, Innocenti and colleagues[80,82–84] have noted continued growth in the proximal fibula when used for reconstruction of the radius, humerus, and femur for the treatment pediatric bony defects. The upper fibular physis is supplied by 3 main arterial branches: the inferior genicular artery, a recurrent branch of anterior tibial artery, and an unnamed artery arising from the popliteal vessel. The anterior tibial vascular bundle compared with the peroneal vessel seems to be the best choice to provide blood supply to both the epiphysis and the diaphysis, with a single pedicle allowing continued growth after transfer.[80,82,84] This technique has substantially simplified the surgical procedure and provides a longer pedicle length for more complicated reconstructions (see **Fig. 3**).

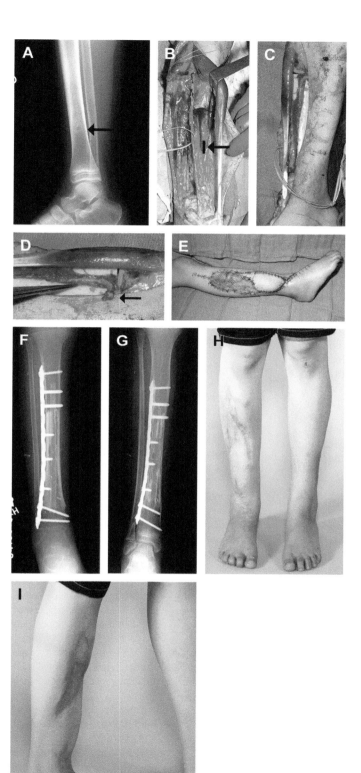

**Fig. 5.** Capanna technique for limb salvage and reconstruction of the tibia in an 8-year-old girl with Ewing sarcoma. (A) Lateral radiograph with arrow pointing to lytic area in the bone, representing the tumor. (B) Bony resection extending from proximal tibial metaphysis through the diaphysis (*arrow*). (C) Medial image of the leg with allograft and fibula construct inset. (D) Close-up with arrow pointing to peroneal vessels exiting tibial allograft in preparation for anastomosis to the native posterior tibial vessels. (E) Lateral image of the leg showing Capanna construct inset with fibular skin paddle exiting construct to assist with skin closure. (F) Initial AP radiograph showing allograft and fibula construct. (G) AP radiograph 4 years after initial procedure showing incorporation of fibula into allograft and ongoing growth at distal physis of tibia. (H, I) The leg following reconstruction showing successful limb salvage 4 years after tumor resection.

## Pediatric Centers

Performing pediatric free tissue transfers in a tertiary pediatric care facility has not been shown to effect the outcomes of pediatric free tissue transfer in cases of trauma[52]; however, tertiary pediatric centers can offer needed expertise in cases of limb salvage for cancer, cases of severe infection, and with the administration and monitoring of pediatric anesthesia. The authors have found the administration of axillary and spinal blocks beneficial in cases of pediatric supra-microsurgery where sympathectomy is beneficial.[85] Indwelling catheters can also substantially aid in postoperative pain management. Recent studies have pointed to improved outcomes in pediatric patients when surgery is performed in centers with high operative volumes.[86]

## SUMMARY

Reconstructive microsurgery and free tissue transfers are commonly used techniques in the modern era for treatment of a broad range of defects in children. The concept of the reconstruction elevator should be considered in situations where a free tissue transfer would give better functional and cosmetic outcomes despite being a more complicated procedure. The advances in microsurgical instrumentation allow for these flaps to be performed with the same flap failure rates as seen in adults.

## REFERENCES

1. Gilbert A. Reconstruction of congenital hand defects with microvascular toe transfers. Hand Clin 1985;1: 351–60.
2. Yildirim S, Calikapan GT, Akoz T. Reconstructive microsurgery in pediatric population—a series of 25 patients. Microsurgery 2008;28:99–107.
3. Van Landuyt K, Hamdi M, Blondeel P, et al. Free perforator flaps in children. Plast Reconstr Surg 2005;116:159–69.
4. Trost O, Kadlub N, Malka G, et al. Microvascular free flap reconstruction in pediatric lower extremity trauma. Plast Reconstr Surg 2006;118:570–1.
5. Rinker B, Valerio IL, Stewart DH, et al. Microvascular free flap reconstruction in pediatric lower extremity trauma: a 10-year review. Plast Reconstr Surg 2005;115:1618–24.
6. Aboelatta YA, Aly HM. Free tissue transfer and replantation in pediatric patients: technical feasibility and outcome in a series of 28 patients. J Hand Microsurg 2013;5:74–80.
7. Serletti JM, Schingo VA Jr, Deuber MA, et al. Free tissue transfer in pediatric patients. Ann Plast Surg 1996;36:561–8.
8. Gharb BB, Salgado CJ, Moran SL, et al. Free anterolateral thigh flap in pediatric patients. Ann Plast Surg 2011;66:143–7.
9. Siebert JW, Anson G, Longaker MT. Microsurgical correction of facial asymmetry in 60 consecutive cases. Plast Reconstr Surg 1996;97:354–63.
10. Longaker MT, Siebert JW. Microsurgical correction of facial contour in congenital craniofacial malformations: the marriage of hard and soft tissue. Plast Reconstr Surg 1996;98:942–50.
11. Fisher J, Jackson IT. Microvascular surgery as an adjunct to craniomaxillofacial reconstruction. Br J Plast Surg 1989;42:146–54.
12. Hemmer KM, Marsh JL, Clement RW. Pediatric facial free flaps. J Reconstr Microsurg 1987;3: 221–9, 231.
13. La Rossa D, Whitaker L, Dabb R, et al. The use of microvascular free flaps for soft tissue augmentation of the face in children with hemifacial microsomia. Cleft Palate J 1980;17:138–43.
14. Inigo F, Jimenez-Murat Y, Arroyo O, et al. Restoration of facial contour in Romberg's disease and hemifacial microsomia: experience with 118 cases. Microsurgery 2000;20:167–72.
15. Brent B, Byrd HS. Secondary ear reconstruction with cartilage grafts covered by axial, random, and free flaps of temporoparietal fascia. Plast Reconstr Surg 1983;72:141–52.
16. Shintomi Y, Ohura T, Honda K, et al. The reconstruction of progressive facial hemi-atrophy by free vascularised dermis-fat flaps. Br J Plast Surg 1981;34:398–409.
17. Upton J, Mulliken JB, Hicks PD, et al. Restoration of facial contour using free vascularized omental transfer. Plast Reconstr Surg 1980;66:560–9.
18. Yamamoto Y, Minakawa H, Sugihara T, et al. Facial reconstruction with free-tissue transfer. Plast Reconstr Surg 1994;94:483–9.
19. Balaji SM. Subdermal fat grafting for Parry-Romberg syndrome. Ann Maxillofac Surg 2014;4:55–9.
20. Zanelato TP, Marquesini G, Colpas PT, et al. Implantation of autologous fat globules in localized scleroderma and idiopathic lipoatrophy–report of five patients. An Bras Dermatol 2013;88:120–3.
21. Moghari A, Macleod ZR, Mohebbi H, et al. The use of split metatarsal osteocutaneous free flaps in palatal and alveolar defects. J Reconstr Microsurg 1989;5:307–10.
22. Futran ND, Haller JR. Considerations for free-flap reconstruction of the hard palate. Arch Otolaryngol Head Neck Surg 1999;125:665–9.
23. MacLeod AM, Morrison WA, McCann JJ, et al. The free radial forearm flap with and without bone for closure of large palatal fistulae. Br J Plast Surg 1987;40:391–5.
24. Bianchi B, Copelli C, Ferrari S, et al. Facial animation in children with Moebius and Moebius-like syndromes. J Pediatr Surg 2009;44:2236–42.

25. Zuker RM, Goldberg CS, Manktelow RT. Facial animation in children with Mobius syndrome after segmental gracilis muscle transplant. Plast Reconstr Surg 2000;106:1–8.

26. Champion R. Re-animation of facial paresis in children. Plast Reconstr Surg Transplant Bull 1958;22:188–93.

27. Bae YC, Zuker RM, Manktelow RT, et al. A comparison of commissure excursion following gracilis muscle transplantation for facial paralysis using a cross-face nerve graft versus the motor nerve to the masseter nerve. Plast Reconstr Surg 2006;117:2407–13.

28. Goldberg C, DeLorie R, Zuker RM, et al. The effects of gracilis muscle transplantation on speech in children with Moebius syndrome. J Craniofac Surg 2003;14:687–90.

29. Zuker RM, Egerszegi EP, Manktelow RT, et al. Volkmann's ischemic contracture in children: the results of free vascularized muscle transplantation. Microsurgery 1991;12:341–5.

30. Manktelow RT, Zuker RM. The principles of functioning muscle transplantation: applications to the upper arm. Ann Plast Surg 1989;22:275–82.

31. Manktelow RT, Zuker RM. Muscle transplantation by fascicular territory. Plast Reconstr Surg 1984;73:751–7.

32. Manktelow RT, Zuker RM, McKee NH. Functioning free muscle transplantation. J Hand Surg Am 1984;9A:32–9.

33. Hadlock TA, Malo JS, Cheney ML, et al. Free gracilis transfer for smile in children. Arch Facial Plast Surg 2011;13:190–4.

34. Terzis JK, Olivares FS. Long-term outcomes of free muscle transfer for smile restoration in children. Plast Reconstr Surg 2009;123:543–55.

35. Giele H, Giele C, Bower C, et al. The incidence and epidemiology of congenital upper limb anomalies: a total population study. J Hand Surg Am 2001;26:628–34.

36. Kaplan JD, Jones NF. Outcome measures of microsurgical toe transfers for reconstruction of congenital and traumatic hand anomalies. J Pediatr Orthop 2014;34:362–8.

37. Moran SL, Jensen M, Bravo C. Amniotic band syndrome of the upper extremity: diagnosis and management. J Am Acad Orthop Surg 2007;15:397–407.

38. Jones NF, Hansen SL, Bates SJ. Toe-to-hand transfers for congenital anomalies of the hand. Hand Clin 2007;23:129–36.

39. Moran SL, Berger RA. Biomechanics and hand trauma: what you need. Hand Clin 2003;19:17–31.

40. Jones NF, Kaplan J. Indications for microsurgical reconstruction of congenital hand anomalies by toe-to-hand transfers. Hand (N Y) 2013;8:367–74.

41. Nikkhah D, Martin N, Pickford M. Paediatric toe-to-hand transfer: an assessment of outcomes from a single unit. J Hand Surg Eur Vol 2016;41:281–94.

42. Kay SP, Wiberg M. Toe to hand transfer in children. Part 1. Technical aspects. J Hand Surg Br 1996;21:723–34.

43. Vilkki SK. Distraction and microvascular epiphysis transfer for radial club hand. J Hand Surg Br 1998;23:445–52.

44. Vilkki SK. Vascularized joint transfer for radial club hand. Tech Hand Up Extrem Surg 1998;2:126–37.

45. de Jong JP, Moran SL, Vilkki SK. Changing paradigms in the treatment of radial club hand: microvascular joint transfer for correction of radial deviation and preservation of long-term growth. Clin Orthop Surg 2012;4:36–44.

46. Morsey M, Perry J, Moran SL. Vascularized second metatarsophalangeal joint transfer for salvage of failed centralization in radial longitudinal deficiency: case report. Ann Plast Surg 2017;78:195–7.

47. Yang J, Qin B, Li P, et al. Vascularized proximal fibular epiphyseal transfer for Bayne and Klug type III radial longitudinal deficiency in children. Plast Reconstr Surg 2015;135:157e–66e.

48. Witoonchart K, Uerpairojkit C, Leechavengvongs S, et al. Congenital pseudarthrosis of the forearm treated by free vascularized fibular graft: a report of three cases and a review of the literature. J Hand Surg Am 1999;24:1045–55.

49. Allieu Y, Gomis R, Yoshimura M, et al. Congenital pseudarthrosis of the forearm—two cases treated by free vascularized fibular graft. J Hand Surg Am 1981;6:475–81.

50. Bae DS, Waters PM, Sampson CE. Use of free vascularized fibular graft for congenital ulnar pseudarthrosis: surgical decision making in the growing child. J Pediatr Orthop 2005;25:755–62.

51. El Hage S, Ghanem I, Dagher F, et al. Free vascularized fibular flap for congenital ulnar pseudarthrosis: a report of two cases and review of the literature. Ann Plast Surg 2009;62:329–34.

52. Hallock GG. Efficacy of free flaps for pediatric trauma patients in an adult trauma center. J Reconstr Microsurg 1995;11:169–74.

53. Upton J, Guo L. Pediatric free tissue transfer: a 29-year experience with 433 transfers. Plast Reconstr Surg 2008;121:1725–37.

54. Laine JC, Cherkashin A, Samchukov M, et al. The management of soft tissue and bone loss in type IIIB and IIIC pediatric open tibia fractures. J Pediatr Orthop 2016;36:453–8.

55. El-Gammal TA, El-Sayed A, Kotb MM, et al. Dorsal foot resurfacing using free anterolateral thigh (ALT) flap in children. Microsurgery 2013;33:259–64.

56. Demirtas Y, Neimetzade T, Kelahmetoglu O, et al. Free anterolateral thigh flap for reconstruction of

car tire injuries of children's feet. Foot Ankle Int 2010; 31:47–52.

57. Acar MA, Güleç A, Aydin BK, et al. Reconstruction of foot and ankle defects with a free anterolateral thigh flap in pediatric patients. J Reconstr Microsurg 2015;31:225–32.

58. Erdmann D, Lee B, Roberts CD, et al. Management of lawnmower injuries to the lower extremity in children and adolescents. Ann Plast Surg 2000;45: 595–600.

59. Demirtas Y, Kelahmetoglu O, Cifci M, et al. Comparison of free anterolateral thigh flaps and free muscle-musculocutaneous flaps in soft tissue reconstruction of lower extremity. Microsurgery 2010;30:24–31.

60. Hu R, Ren YJ, Yan L, et al. A free anterolateral thigh flap and iliotibial band for reconstruction of soft tissue defects at children's feet and ankles. Injury 2015;46:2019–23.

61. Iida T, Yamamoto T, Yoshimatsu H, et al. Supermicrosurgical free sensate superficial circumflex iliac artery perforator flap for reconstruction of a soft tissue defect of the ankle in a 1-year-old child. Microsurgery 2016;36:254–8.

62. Bilkay U, Tiftikcioglu YO, Temiz G, et al. Free-tissue transfers for reconstruction of oromandibular area in children. Microsurgery 2008;28:91–8.

63. Pallua N, Demir E. Postburn head and neck reconstruction in children with the fasciocutaneous supraclavicular artery island flap. Ann Plast Surg 2008;60: 276–82.

64. Hunt JA, Moisidis E, Haertsch P. Initial experience of Integra in the treatment of post-burn anterior cervical neck contracture. Br J Plast Surg 2000;53:652–8.

65. Ikeda K, Yamauchi S, Hashimoto F, et al. Digital replantation in children: a long-term follow-up study. Microsurgery 1990;11:261–4.

66. Taras JS, Nunley JA, Urbaniak JR, et al. Replantation in children. Microsurgery 1991;12:216–20.

67. Jaeger SH, Tsai TM, Kleinert HE. Upper extremity replantation in children. Orthop Clin North Am 1981;12:897–907.

68. Cheng GL, Pan DD, Zhang NP, et al. Digital replantation in children: a long-term follow-up study. J Hand Surg Am 1998;23:635–46.

69. Berlin NL, Tuggle CT, Thomson JG, et al. Digit replantation in children: a nationwide analysis of outcomes and trends of 455 pediatric patients. Hand (N Y) 2014;9:244–52.

70. Mason GE, Aung L, Gall S, et al. Quality of life following amputation or limb preservation in patients with lower extremity bone sarcoma. Front Oncol 2013;7:210.

71. Berrey BH Jr, Lord CF, Gebhardt MC, et al. Fractures of allografts. Frequency, treatment, and end-results. J Bone Joint Surg Am 1990;72:825–33.

72. Capanna R, Campanacci DA, Belot N, et al. A new reconstructive technique for intercalary defects of long bones: the association of massive allograft with vascularized fibular autograft. Long-term results and comparison with alternative techniques. Orthop Clin North Am 2007;38:51–60.

73. Canosa R, Gonzalez del Pino J. Effect of methotrexate in the biology of free vascularized bone grafts. A comparative experimental study in the dog. Clin Orthop Relat Res 1994;301:291–301.

74. Moran SL, Shin AY, Bishop AT. The use of massive bone allograft with intramedullary free fibular flap for limb salvage in a pediatric and adolescent population. Plast Reconstr Surg 2006;118:413–9.

75. Houdek MT, Wagner ER, Stans AA, et al. What is the outcome of allograft and intramedullary free fibula (Capanna technique) in pediatric and adolescent patients with bone tumors? Clin Orthop Relat Res 2016;474:660–8.

76. MacKay BJ, Nacke E, Posner M. Hand transplantation–a review. Bull Hosp Jt Dis (2013) 2014;72: 76–88.

77. Dubernard JM, Owen E, Herzberg G, et al. The first transplantation of a hand in humans. Early results. Chirurgie 1999;124:358–65.

78. Gurnaney HG, Fiadjoe JE, Levin LS, et al. Anesthetic management of the first pediatric bilateral hand transplant. Can J Anaesth 2016;63:731–6.

79. Bartlett SP, Chang B, Levin LS. Discussion: ethical issues in pediatric face transplantation: should we perform face transplantation in children? Plast Reconstr Surg 2016;138:455–7.

80. Innocenti M, Delcroix L, Balatri A. Vascularized growth plate transfer for distal radius reconstruction. Semin Plast Surg 2008;22:186–94.

81. Bowen V. Experimental free vascularized epiphyseal transplants. Orthopedics 1986;9:893–8.

82. Innocenti M, Delcroix L, Manfrini M, et al. Vascularized proximal fibular epiphyseal transfer for distal radial reconstruction. J Bone Joint Surg Am 2004; 86-A:1504–11.

83. Innocenti M, Delcroix L, Manfrini M, et al. Vascularized proximal fibular epiphyseal transfer for distal radial reconstruction. J Bone Joint Surg Am 2005; 87:237–46.

84. Innocenti M, Delcroix L, Romano GF, et al. Vascularized epiphyseal transplant. Orthop Clin North Am 2007;38:95–101.

85. Inberg P, Kassila M, Vilkki S, et al. Anaesthesia for microvascular surgery in children. A combination of general anaesthesia and axillary plexus block. Acta Anaesthesiol Scand 1995;39:518–22.

86. Evans C, van Woerden HC. The effect of surgical training and hospital characteristics on patient outcomes after pediatric surgery: a systematic review. J Pediatr Surg 2011;46:2119–27.

# Innovations and Future Directions in Head and Neck Microsurgical Reconstruction

Marissa Suchyta, BA, Samir Mardini, MD*

## KEYWORDS

- Craniofacial reconstruction • Innovation • Face transplant • Regenerative medicine
- Virtual surgical planning • 3D printing • Perfusion monitoring

## KEY POINTS

- Integration of virtual surgical planning and three-dimensional printing has enabled improved surgical accuracy, efficiency, and dealing with more complex reconstructions.
- Novel intraoperative navigation, imaging, and perfusion assessment have led to ease of flap design, avoidance of vital structures, and innovative flap monitoring.
- The development of minimally invasive reconstructive microsurgery has advanced oncological head and neck reconstruction.
- The integration of regenerative medicine, tissue engineering, and stem cell biology presents novel methods of osteogenic flap prefabrication as well as research in ex vivo generation of patient-specific craniofacial bone and tissue.
- Facial composite tissue allotransplant is an innovation in craniofacial surgery for patients who have exhausted the traditional reconstructive plastic surgery armamentarium.

## INTRODUCTION

"Pourquoi pas?" Paul Tessier, known as the father of modern craniofacial surgery, would often answer questions about his innovative procedures with this response of "Why not?"[1] This expression, which eventually became the motto of the International Society of Craniofacial Surgery, should continue to drive this field of innovation and multidisciplinary advances, encouraging craniofacial and head and neck reconstructive surgeons to think creatively and outside the confines of the discipline. In few other surgical fields do advances in science, technology, and surgical ingenuity combine to better patient outcomes in such dramatic and visible ways.

Large-scale innovations often occur when there is a convergence of knowledge across disciplines, leading to new ideas or the coalescence of ideas to make advances. The development of microsurgery is an example of this. The combination of a series of advances in different fields in the early twentieth century led to the innovation of clinical microsurgery. This innovation includes advancement in surgical technique, with the reporting of the triangulation method of end-to-end anastomosis in 1902.[2] However, advances in basic science were also needed to aid in

The authors have nothing to disclose.
Division of Plastic and Reconstructive Surgery, Mayo Clinic, MA1244W, 200 First Street Southwest, Rochester, MN 55905, USA
* Corresponding author.
E-mail address: Mardini.samir@mayo.edu

Clin Plastic Surg 44 (2017) 325–344
http://dx.doi.org/10.1016/j.cps.2016.11.009
0094-1298/17/

anticoagulation, and the 1916 discovery of heparin thus enabled the patency of microvascular anastomoses.[3] Perhaps most vitally, in the early 1920s, the introduction of the operating microscope as well as fine microsurgical suture and instruments provided necessary bioengineering advances.[4] These multidisciplinary innovations led to the first successful microvascular anastomosis in 1960, thus dramatically changing reconstructive surgery.

In the current era of head and neck microsurgical reconstruction, clinicians again have embraced the coalescence of multidisciplinary fields leading to innovation and future advances, including the integration of virtual surgical planning and three-dimensional (3D) printing technologies in craniofacial surgery, enabling planning of complex procedures before entering the operating room as well as the creation of patient-specific surgical guides and implants. Novel imaging methods enable assessment of flap design and immediate perfusion outcomes intraoperatively. Innovations in postoperative perfusion monitoring incorporate technological advances, including infrared thermography and oxygenation. In addition, smartphone capabilities have also led to dramatic advances in early detection of flap problems, thereby decreasing flap failure rates. Innovation in surgical technique has led to minimally invasive reconstructive procedures, including transoral reconstructive capabilities for oropharyngeal cancer and endoscopic skull base reconstruction. Advances in regenerative medicine and tissue engineering show the potential of merging stem cell biology with reconstructive craniofacial microsurgery, which has already shown advances in prefabrication techniques. In addition, face transplant provides an ideal example of disruptive innovation in craniofacial surgery for patients who have exhausted the armamentarium of plastic surgery options.

## THE INTEGRATION OF VIRTUAL SURGICAL PLANNING AND THREE-DIMENSIONAL PRINTING WITH CRANIOFACIAL RECONSTRUCTION

The ability to plan and virtually execute complex craniofacial surgical procedures has revolutionized head and neck reconstruction. Virtual surgical planning starts with a high-resolution computed tomography (CT) scan with thin cuts; the potential for virtual surgical planning depends on the ability to obtain such scans (**Fig. 1**).[5] The 3D reconstruction is then performed in one of the US Food and Drug Administration (FDA)–approved computer-aided design or computer-aided modeling software environments. A Web conference is conducted between the surgeon and biomedical engineers to virtually plan the surgery, including osteotomy placement, resection margins (in the case of oncological surgery), bone graft placement, and positional alignment. This virtual conference allows the surgeon to plan the procedure in a less time-sensitive environment before surgery rather than relying on intraoperative judgement as the main method of deciding on osteotomies. Virtual surgical planning also requires the declaration of surgical intention, allowing a lower-stress environment in which to decide on recipient vessel choice as well as osteotomy placement. Furthermore, in the case of oncological head and neck reconstruction, virtual surgical planning can avoid any potential conflicts between the resection and reconstruction teams caused by uncertainty or change of plans in the operating room. Most importantly, virtual surgical planning enables surgeons to attempt multiple approaches and reconstructive options in a virtual environment, thereby determining the optimal surgical outcome before entering the operating room.

The integration of virtual surgical planning with 3D printing furthers the frontier of craniofacial

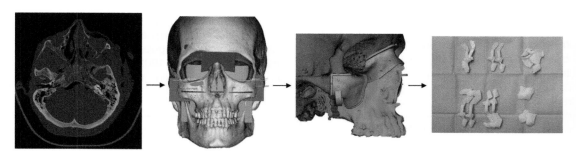

**Fig. 1.** The process of planning a Le Fort III–based face transplant. The process of virtual surgical planning begins with a high-resolution CT scan. This scan is then 3D reconstructed and, in a virtual planning session between engineers and the surgeon, osteotomy locations are planned. Then 3D printed guides are designed to guide these osteotomies, which are then printed, sterilized, and used in the surgery.

reconstruction. Using 3D printed models of patient-specific craniofacial anatomy enables hands-on evaluation of the surgical approach. Models of a defect site and transferred bone can be created so that surgeons can evaluate positioning, aesthetic outcomes, and fixation methods in a 3D manner. In the past, this has proved important in congenital cardiothoracic surgery and is now also another innovative tool for craniofacial surgeons.[6] In particular, using 3D printed models for prebending fixation plates has been shown to reduce operative time and improve reconstruction outcomes. In addition, these models are invaluable to medical education so residents, as well as the rest of the surgical team, can fully understand the operative plan.

Virtual surgical planning can also be used to generate patient-specific cutting guides, templates, and implants that enable surgeons to accurately transform plans into operative reality. Stereolithographic snap-fit guides are 3D printed for osteotomies, thereby enabling accurate recapitulation of the planned cut site. Fibula-to-mandible reconstruction has greatly benefited from this technology because the surgical success largely depends on restoration of facial symmetry. A systematic review of fibula-to-mandible oncological reconstruction showed that, in 93% of cases, virtual surgical planning increased the accuracy of the reconstruction and, in 80% of cases, operative time decreased.[7]

Virtual surgical planning and 3D guide creation has also greatly innovated craniosynostosis surgery, in which reconstruction is often solely based on the surgeon's vision of a normal head shape and subjective intraoperative decisions (**Fig. 2**).[8] Using virtual surgical planning, the child's skull can be overlaid to a normative skull of the same age group. Osteotomies and positional reorganization can then be virtually planned to yield the best aesthetic results (**Fig. 3**), and 3D printed osteotomy and positional alignment plating guides are then created to enable this plan to be executed in a straightforward manner intraoperatively (**Fig. 4**).

The combination of virtual surgical planning and 3D printing also enables patient-specific implants for head and neck reconstruction. Patient-specific polyetheretherketone (PEEK) implants have been designed virtually and 3D printed to reconstruct cranial, frontal, malar, and mandibular defects.[9] Recently, the FDA approved the first 3D printed titanium craniofacial implant, which additionally adds to the armamentarium of implant options.[10] In the case of orbital floor reconstruction, free-hand manipulation of implants is challenging because of the constrained location, potential damage to the eye, and complexity of bone

anatomy. Using 3D printed porous polyethylene custom-created implants now offers alternatives to intraoperative manipulation of titanium mesh implants.[11] Furthermore, custom orbital implants may offer a more aesthetically pleasing, symmetric result, because the contour of the implant generally matches that of the patient's uninjured orbit. In addition, 3D printed models can be used to shape arch forms or titanium spacers to provide optimal shape while bone integration takes place in mandible reconstruction.[12] These implants thus reduce operative time as well as contributing to a more successful functional and aesthetic reconstructive outcome.

## NOVEL INTRAOPERATIVE NAVIGATION AND IMAGING

Intraoperative navigation has greatly improved the accuracy of craniofacial reconstruction as well as preventing damage of vital structures in complex reconstructions. Neurosurgery was the first discipline to adopt intraoperative navigation because of the technology's ability to minimize trauma and surgical perturbation of the brain.[13] Navigation was originally stereotactic, and although this greatly improved outcomes in brain biopsy, electrode placement, and small tumor resection, it did not allow real-time monitoring of operative location, required more invasive fixation of the stereotactic frame, and reduced the operative working space.[14] The advent of frameless navigation led to the adoption of intraoperative navigation in other surgical fields, including craniofacial reconstruction.[15]

In modern frameless intraoperative navigation, reference structures (commonly reflective marker spheres) are placed on the patient.[16] Preoperative imaging is obtained with the markers present. In the operating room, a stereoscopic camera emits infrared light that tracks the 3D position of the marker spheres (**Fig. 5**). These marker spheres are correlated with the markers shown on the CT scan as well as in relation to the stereotactic probe, which also contains a marker sphere. Using the marker sites, the computer can determine the location of the probe and correlate this in real time with the CT scan, thereby enabling visualization of location. This technology is similar to how a car may navigate using GPS; metaphorically, the car is the probe and the satellites in space are the marker probes on the patient. The created map in this analogy is the CT scan with the probe shown in real time.

Intraoperative navigation has broad innovative applications in head and neck reconstruction. Navigation has improved surgical outcomes in

# Preoperative    # Postoperative

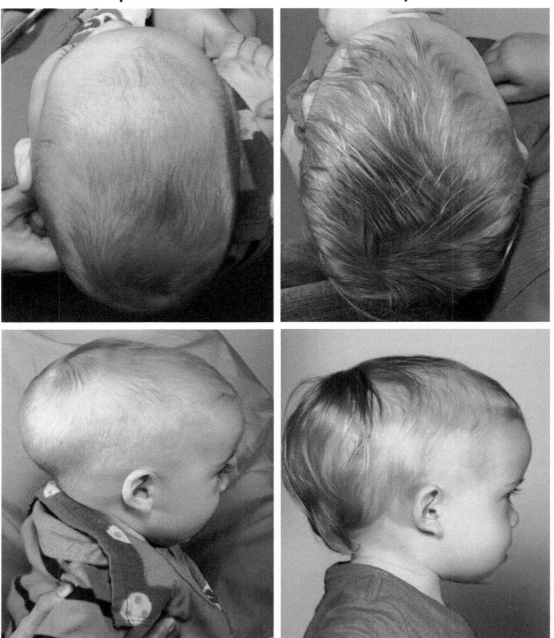

**Fig. 2.** Preoperative and postoperative views of a child with sagittal suture craniosynostosis whose operation was planned and performed using virtual surgical planning and 3D-printed surgical and positional guides.

orthognathic surgery, including ensuring the optimal osteotomy placement for aesthetic outcomes.[17] Navigation has also proved effective in midface distraction for facial deformities, including midface hypoplasia caused by cleft lip/palate or Crouzon syndrome, allowing the avoidance of vital structures as well as ensuring that vectors and tracking of internal distraction devices follow the surgical plan.[18] Furthermore, navigation has improved outcomes in setback of the anterior table of the frontal sinus for pneumosinus dilatans as well as midface reconstruction for Treacher

# Preoperative

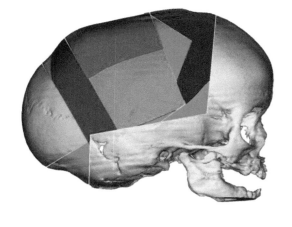

# Postoperative

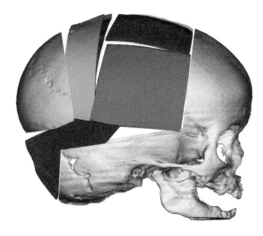

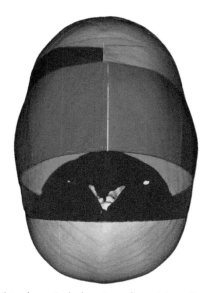

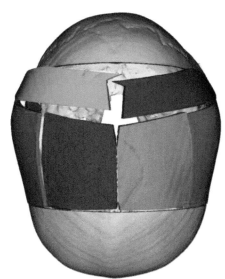

**Fig. 3.** Virtual surgical planning of cranial vault remodeling surgery of sagittal suture craniosynostosis. The preoperative views show osteotomy placement, and postoperative views show the planned rearrangement of cranial segments.

Collins syndrome.[19] In addition, intraoperative navigation has enabled the reconstruction of a delayed orbitozygomaticomaxillary fracture, which allowed anatomic reduction without an otherwise necessary coronal incision and zygomatic arch exposure (**Fig. 6**).[20] Intraoperative navigation has been used as an alternative to stereolithographic osteotomy guides in fibula free-flap reconstruction, thus following the operative plan by determining osteotomy placement and subsequent mandible inset using the stereotactic probe.[21] This method provides another means to ensure operative planning success if 3D printing is not available, too time intensive, or cost prohibitive.

Furthermore, intraoperative navigation has been used to ensure correct placement of 3D printed osteotomy guides and custom implants intraoperatively when snap-fit guides are not possible or reliable because of complex bony anatomy. Navigation has been shown to improve orbital reconstruction following posttraumatic and postablative defects; using this technology to identify correct implant placement led to excellent restoration of the orbit and globe.[22]

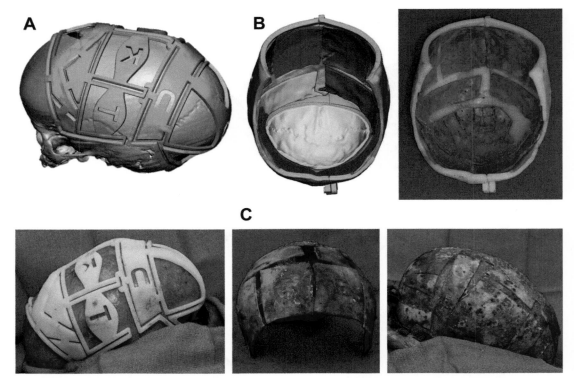

**Fig. 4.** A 3D osteotomy guide for cranial vault remodeling (*A*). The osteotomized cranial segments are then repositioned in a positioning guide (*B*), in which they are internally plated to ensure correct positional alignment according to virtual surgical plan (*C*). The rearranged, plated segments are then plated externally.

The future and potential increase in popularity of intraoperative navigation in craniofacial and head and neck surgery depends on the advancement of this system's capabilities. In a commentary on

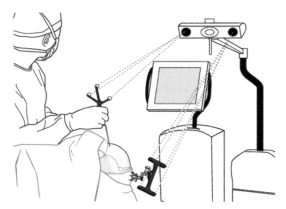

**Fig. 5.** Intraoperative navigation. Before surgery, preoperative imaging is obtained with markers in place. A stereoscopic camera in the operating room (OR) then emits infrared light that tracks the position of the markers on both the patient and the navigation probe, which correlate with position on the CT scans, enabling real-time feedback about probe position. (Copyright © by AO Foundation, Switzerland. Source: AO Surgery Reference, www.aosurgery.org.)

navigation in craniofacial surgery, Gordon and colleagues[23] note that, if modern GPS (global positioning system) was limited to simply showing where a car is on the map, it most likely would not be as popular. However, GPS now offers directions, route planning, and even avoidance of traffic. Modern intraoperative navigation is similar to the limited capability of early GPS. In the future, the authors foresee navigational tools integrating the operative plan, craniofacial cephalometrics, and the surgeon's end goal into an interactive interface that enables real-time feedback on intraoperative decisions. This potential has begun in the innovation of the Computer-Assisted Planning and Execution (CAPE) system in face transplant, an intraoperative navigation system that incorporates the surgical plan with intraoperative guide placement and desired outcome analysis (**Fig. 7**).[24] This system is in early large-animal testing, and provides a hopeful insight into the future of intraoperative navigation in complex craniofacial procedures.

An alternative to intraoperative navigation is intraoperative imaging, made possible by the advent of advanced imaging technology in head and neck reconstruction. CT scans have long been the standard for presurgical planning.

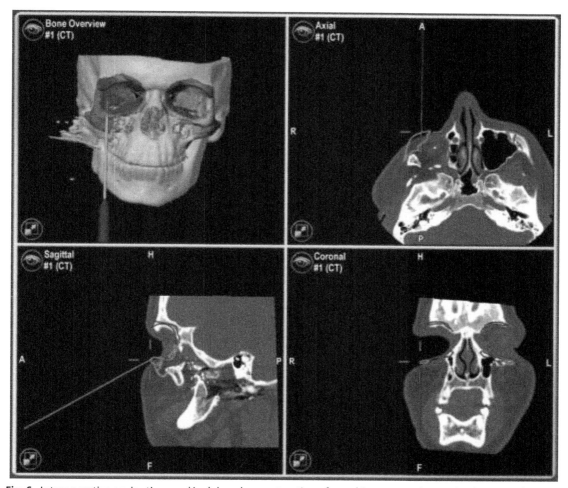

**Fig. 6.** Intraoperative navigation used in delayed reconstruction of an orbitozygomatic complex fracture. This technology enables accurate, real-time feedback about positional information, preventing the need for zygomatic arch exposure. (*From* Morrison CS, Taylor HO, Sullivan SR. Utilization of intraoperative 3D navigation for delayed reconstruction of orbitozygomatic complex fractures. J Craniofac Surg 2013;24(3):e284–6; with permission.)

However, the innovation of cone-beam CT (CBCT) systems (such as the C-arm), which were originally developed for dental practices, has enabled high-quality intraoperative imaging (**Fig. 8**).[25] CT scans can present high radiation exposure to both patient and health care providers in the operating room (OR) and are not cost-effective for intraoperative imaging. Mobile CBCT systems enable immediate 3D imaging analysis of operative results so that any necessary corrections can be made before the patient leaves the OR. This ability is particularly important in the reduction of craniofacial fractures, which have high postsurgical complication rates if reduction is not complete.[26] It was shown that such intraoperative imaging improved outcomes in zygomaticomaxillary complex fractures, mandibular angle fractures, and bimaxillary repositioning osteotomies.[27]

Therefore, the innovation of CBCT systems for intraoperative imaging may improve craniofacial reconstructive outcomes and prevent subsequent returns to the OR.

## INNOVATIONS IN PERFUSION ASSESSMENT AND MONITORING

Innovations in both intraoperative and postoperative monitoring of free flaps have broad implications in head and neck reconstruction. Reconstructive success in these cases depends on both quality perfusion of the flap and rapid identification and salvage of failing flaps.[28,29] Microvascular reconstruction has always depended on a thorough understanding of subvisible human anatomy. Innovations such as Doppler ultrasonography and angiography dramatically

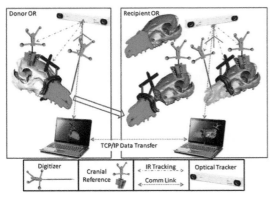

**Fig. 7.** The newly developed CAPE workstation was created to assist with planning and execution of facial transplants. The system enables real-time assessment of reality versus surgical plan because of intraoperative navigation. In addition, Transmission Control Protocol/Internet Protocol (TCP/IP), the basic communication language of the internet, enables seamless communication between donor and recipient surgical teams. (*From* Gordon CR, Murphy RJ, Coon D, et al. Preliminary development of a workstation for craniomaxillofacial surgical procedures: introducing a computer-assisted planning and execution system. J Craniofac Surg 2014;25(1):273–83.)

improved surgeons' abilities to make decisions regarding each patient's unique anatomy and options for microvascular reconstruction. In particular, head and neck reconstruction presents large challenges to reconstructive surgeons because patients often have oncological or traumatic abnormalities affecting standard clinical anatomy. Angiosome size, cutaneous perforator perfusion, and periosteal perfusion (in osteocutaneous flaps) all affect the potential for partial and complete flap loss.

Laser-assisted fluorescent angiography (SPY Elite) offers an innovative means for perfusion monitoring intraoperatively.[30] In this system, indocyanine green (ICG) is injected intravenously, which then binds to plasma proteins circulating in the bloodstream. ICG fluoresces on exposure to laser light emitted by the SPY machine, and is detected by a high-speed imaging system that is sensitive to the ICG wavelength (**Fig. 9**). A perfusion map is then constructed, which allows assessment of perforator vasculature as well as an evaluation of venous and arterial flow. Thus, SPY can be used to aid in free-style flap design and harvest, in which SPY can be used to center the design over the angiosome perfusion center.[31] In addition, in the anterolateral thigh flap, a disadvantage is that the pedicle's septocutaneous or myocutaneous perforating vessels often have irregular derivations from the descending branch

of the lateral circumflex artery.[32] SPY enables reliable raising of this workhorse flap as well as other free flaps for head and neck reconstruction.

In addition, SPY also enables an immediate assessment of vascular anastomoses, thus identifying thrombi and assessing the quality of perfusion intraoperatively. This ability gives the surgeon an early assessment of potential flap necrosis. SPY monitoring intraoperatively has been shown to improve free-flap complications in head and neck reconstruction, including determining early flap necrosis.[30] In addition, the technique has also proven effective in monitoring free jejunum flaps following circumferential pharyngolaryngectomy reconstruction.[33] This technique provides an innovative tool for both operative planning and early intraoperative monitoring.

Postoperative perfusion monitoring advances have proved invaluable in head and neck reconstruction. A systematic review showed that the overall free-flap success in head and neck reconstruction is at least 95% using any type of monitoring.[34] The innovation of the hand-held and then implantable Doppler led to instrumental tools for bedside assessment of anastomotic patency. In addition, new methods of perfusion monitoring now add to the toolbox of postoperative flap assessment. This toolbox includes assessment of tissue oxygenation by near-infrared spectroscopy, which has been shown to be a sensitive, specific, and noninvasive method for postoperative free tissue transfer monitoring.[35] Despite these advantages, this method continues to be cost prohibitive at most institutions because of the high cost of the device, although it may reduce long-term monitoring costs by decreasing specialized nursing Doppler assessment.[36] Visible white light spectroscopy, which measures the hemoglobin saturation at the capillary level, is also a novel mechanism of monitoring.[37] Advancements and increased portability of infrared thermography cameras (including smartphone-compatible cameras) have furthered their potential for noninvasive flap monitoring based on temperature, although this technique is less reliable with buried flaps (**Fig. 10**).[38,39]

The increased use of smartphones and cellular technology has ushered a new era of potential flap monitoring techniques. This era includes the use of telemedicine; a study of 113 consecutive free flaps showed that the accuracy rate of free-flap failure assessment based on in-person examination versus smartphone photograph was 98.7% and 94.2% respectively, which shows the potential future power of the telemedicine consult, which was impossible only a decade ago.[40] The most dramatic example of the impact of smartphone

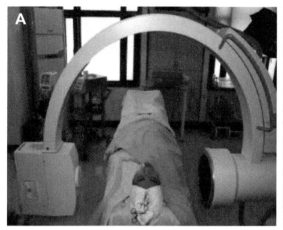

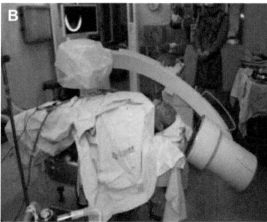

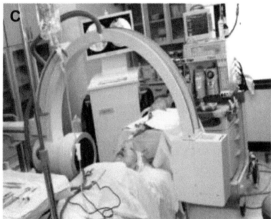

**Fig. 8.** How the C-Arm system can be used to aid in facial fracture reduction. The system can be used to obtain nasal bone on lateral view (*A*), zygoma view at 70° to 90° to the skull's coronal plane and 0° to the skull's sagittal plane (*B*), and mandibular subcondyle on lateral view (*C*). (*From* Hwang SM, Kim JH, Kim HD, et al. C-arm fluoroscopy for accurate reduction of facial bone fracture. Arch Craniofac Surg 2013;14:96–101.)

communication on free-flap outcomes was shown when a hospital altered its monitoring communication strategy (but not monitoring schedule) from a telephone-based report from resident to attending to a mobile app method (**Fig. 11**).[41] This alteration enabled the resident to share all flap information as well as photographs with the team. This simple change led to a reduction in time from flap failure recognition to OR from 4 to 1.4 hours and an increase in flap salvage rate from 50% to 100%, demonstrating the power of smartphone technology in improving postoperative flap monitoring. In addition, there is a new drive to integrate conventional flap monitoring, such as Doppler or oxygenation measurements, with mobile alert systems to enable real-time feedback to the surgical team, thus decreasing time to flap failure recognition.[42] It is clear that technology will continue advancing, and it is our prediction that the future of free-flap monitoring will be seamless detection and communication of perfusion changes that enable quick take-back to the OR.

## RECENT MINIMAL INVASIVE TECHNIQUES IN CRANIOFACIAL RECONSTRUCTIVE MICROSURGERY

The coalescence of new technology with microsurgical techniques has led to the innovation of minimally invasive head and neck surgery. In particular, advances in transoral endoscopic techniques have revolutionized the treatment pathway of patients with oropharyngeal cancer. Advancements in binocular microscopy as well as surgical lasers have enabled a transoral laser microsurgery (TLM) approach, initially to laryngeal papillomas and, more recently, early-stage laryngeal squamous cell carcinoma.[43] In 2003, the role of TLM expanded to also be used in the pharynx and oral cavity.[44] TLM uses a carbon dioxide ($CO_2$) laser that is passed through an endoscope; the laser beam is absorbed by water at the tissue-laser interface, which then transforms it into thermal energy and allows precision tissue cutting (**Fig. 12**). The laser is coupled to an operating microscope, which enables close visualization of the tumor. In the past,

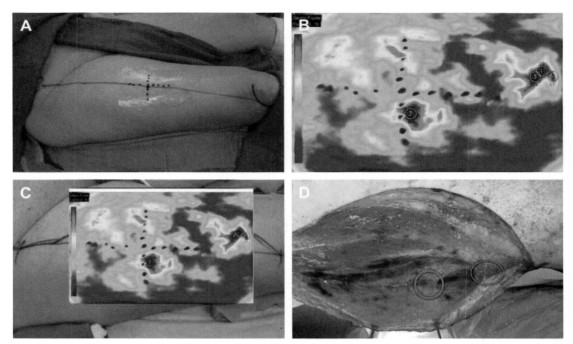

**Fig. 9.** The effectiveness of using SPY to optimize placement of the anterolateral thigh flap. The center of the planned flap is marked in standard fashion (*A*). SPY is used to identify perforator perfusion, with the marked lines shown (*B, C*). These perfusion zones correlate with the perforators circled in *D* on flap harvest. (*From* Gurtner GC, Jones GE, Neligan PC, et al. Intraoperative laser angiography using the SPY system: review of the literature and recommendations for use. Ann Surg Innov Res 2013;7(1):1.)

there were difficulties with requiring direct line of sight because of the rigidity of the laser. However, recent advances have led to fiberoptic laser systems and flexible delivery instruments, which enable better approach angles to tumor resection and the larger adoption of this technique.

Recent innovation has also led to robotic surgery for head and neck applications. In 2003, robotically assisted neck dissection and salivary gland surgery was shown to be feasible in a porcine model.[45] In 2006, 3 patients successfully underwent robot transoral tongue base resection, which enabled straightforward identification of the glossopharyngeal, hypoglossal and lingual nerves, and lingual artery.[46] Since this initial case, the use of transoral robotic-assisted surgery (TORS) has only grown in head and neck oncological surgery. As this application increases, the reconstructive needs and techniques following such resection also need to be addressed in the confined oropharyngeal space. The concept of transoral robotic-assisted reconstruction has thus been presented to enable the reconstruction of this confined space, because the robotic arm flexibility enables suturing of structures in areas of low visibility, which would not be possible with standard technique.

An early case report of TORS microvascular reconstruction involved radial forearm free flaps following TORS resection.[47] In these cases, the flaps were inset robotically, but microanastomosis to the transverse cervical vessels was performed using standard nonrobotic technique. A later report of 5 patients showed the potential of robotic-assisted surgery in the oral cavity, including in cases ranging from local flaps, free flaps, and prior extensive radiation.[48] In these cases, the robot performed flap inset in all cases, showing reconstruction of regions that are impossible to reach manually intraorally and preventing the need for lip-splitting incisions and mandibulectomies. The robot also performed the first microvascular anastomosis, successfully suturing 2-mm vessels (**Fig. 13**). Robot-assisted microsurgery shows clear advantages in intraoral reconstruction by enabling flap inset and microvascular anastomosis in a confined space without the need for larger incisional exposure.[49]

Endoscopic skull base surgery has also led to immense innovation in neuro-oncology, offering patients a minimally invasive technique through the sinuses to avoid an alternative craniotomy, facial incisions, tracheotomy, and extended recovery time. However, this has then required innovation to reconstruct these defects, ideally

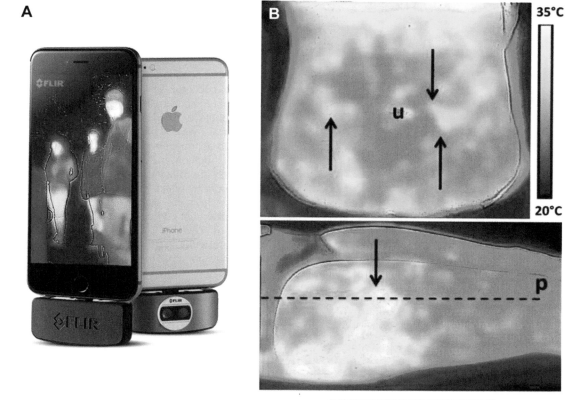

**Fig. 10.** Novel portable smartphone-enabled thermal imaging cameras have expanded the potential of this modality in perforator mapping and, the authors foresee, free flap monitoring. This new device (*A*) can be used to create a thermogram mapping perforator locations (*arrows*) in the anterior abdominal wall and lateral thigh (*B*) (u, the umbilicus; p, the lateral patella). (*Courtesy of* FLIR Systems, Inc., Wilsonville, OR. *From* Hardwicke JT, Osmani O, Skillman JM. Detection of perforators using smartphone thermal imaging. Plast Reconstr Surg 2016;137(1):39–41; with permission.)

using minimally invasive techniques to separate the cranial and sinonasal cavities to prevent cerebrospinal fluid (CSF) leakage and intracranial infection.[50] Previously, endoscopic skull base reconstruction dealt only with small defects arising from trauma, sinus surgery, or spontaneous CSF leaks. Endoscopic skull base resection leads to larger defects and thus has required innovation to meet these more challenging reconstructive goals. These defects have been successfully repaired endoscopically using a layering technique of fascial grafts, fat grafts, and supportive packing. These innovations thus show the future of minimally invasive techniques in head and neck reconstruction.

## THE INTERFACE OF REGENERATIVE MEDICINE, BIOENGINEERING, AND CRANIOFACIAL RECONSTRUCTION

Current standard techniques in craniofacial reconstruction largely depend on autologous tissue transfer. In facial reconstruction, free flaps may succeed in covering defects, but still often lack the optimal aesthetic or functional outcomes. Rather than transferring patient tissue, regenerative medicine seeks to regenerate native tissue or recreate transplantable tissue. This field has large implications in craniofacial and head and neck reconstruction and provides some of the most exciting innovations in the specialty.

A novel recent innovation is the use of stem cells to prefabricate bone for craniofacial reconstruction, thus avoiding the resorption of nonvascularized bone grafts or donor site morbidity of vascularized bone flaps. Adipose-derived stem cells (ASCs) are regenerative tools to aid craniofacial surgeons in bone replacement.[51] These cells can easily be harvested through liposuction and are multipotent, meaning they can differentiate into different cell lineages, including adipogenic, osteogenic, chondrogenic, neurogenic, and myogenic cell types. In

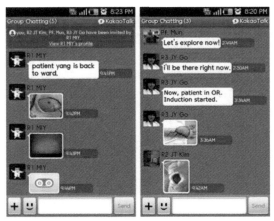

**Fig. 11.** The use of a mobile app–based messaging system versus a telephone-based assessment altered 1 hospital's flap salvage rate from 50% to 100% and flap failure recognition to OR time from 4 to 1.4 hours. This method enabled more streamlined communication between all team members and the sharing of images between the team. (*From* Hwang JH, Mun GH. An evolution of communication in postoperative free flap monitoring: using a smartphone and mobile messenger application. Plast Reconstr Surg 2012;130(1):125–9; with permission.)

addition, bone marrow–derived stem cells are also a potential source of stem cells in clinical practice.[52] Bioactive proteins and materials, including bone morphogenetic protein (BMP-2), also add to the potential of these cells.

In 2009, Mesimäki and colleagues[53] published a case report of implanting a preformed titanium mesh cage filled with autologous ASCs, β-tricalcium phosphate, and BMP-2 into the rectus muscle of a patient who had undergone hemimaxillectomy (**Fig. 14**). Eight months later, these cells formed a vascularized bone piece of the size and morphology needed to reconstruct the craniofacial

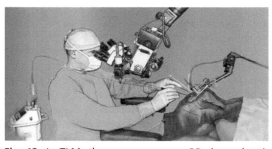

**Fig. 12.** In TLM, the surgeon uses a $CO_2$ laser that is passed through an endoscope. Using a surgical microscope, the surgeon is able to direct precision tissue cutting. (Copyright © Mayo Foundation for Medical Education and Research. All rights reserved.)

defect, which was harvested along with the rectus muscle as a free flap and then successfully inset into the defect (**Fig. 15**). The created bone had the strength to host dental implants and the patient showed excellent outcomes. This method of cell-driven prefabrication was also conducted by Warnke and colleagues,[54] who implanted a similar titanium mesh seeded with bone marrow stem cells, hydroxyapatite, and BMP-2 into the latissimus dorsi muscle. After 7 weeks, this newly created bone flap was able to be transferred to fill a 4-cm mandibular defect. In addition, ASCs have been shown to dramatically improve the retention of nonvascularized bone grafts; when ASCs were combined with bone chips from the iliac crest, a large calvarial defect was almost completely continuously regenerated in a 7-year-old patient.[55] These reports show the potential of multipotent stem cells in ushering in a new generation of bone prefabrication and combined stem cell therapy for craniofacial defects.

Another option to reconstruct large craniofacial defects is through tissue engineering and bioscaffolds. In tissue engineering, cells and biologically active molecules are grown on tissue scaffolds to create functional transplantable tissue to fill defects. The goal of the tissue scaffold is to mimic the extracellular matrix, which affects the ways that cells seeded onto the scaffold migrate, proliferate, and differentiate. However, the main issue with tissue engineering strategies is achieving vascularization of the engineered tissue. Original attempts to create vascularized tissue ex vivo involved using biocompatible material, including collagen and hyaluronic acid as well as synthetic polymers.[56] However, more recent innovative methods of tissue engineering have taken advantage of naturally formed extracellular matrix topology by creating scaffolds through decellularization.[57] In this method, a detergent is used to remove all cells from cadaver tissue, leaving behind a scaffold with anatomic geometry and decellularized vasculature. This scaffold is then reseeded with cells to repopulate the tissue and transferred to a bioreactor, where media is pumped through the tissue through the native vasculature to enable nutrient exchange as the cells grow.

This method of decellularization led to the first tissue-engineered transplanted trachea in 2008.[58] Decellularized scaffolds have become an innovative aspect of craniofacial research, and have included the successful decellularization of a whole ear[59] and temporomandibular joint (**Figs. 16** and **17**).[60] Furthermore, there is also research investigating the decellularization and reseeding of entire soft tissue free flaps for creation of ex vivo engineered tissue to transplant into patients. However, the chief issue with this research

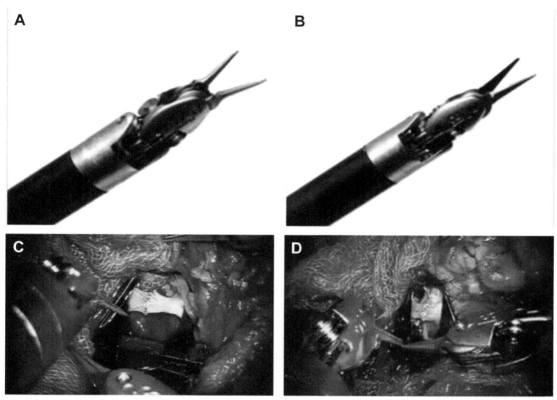

**Fig. 13.** Specialty instruments were used for robot microsurgery (*A, B*). The first example of a robot performing a microvascular anastomosis, successfully suturing 2-mm vessels (*C, D*). Using a robot in this case prevented the need for lip-splitting incisions and mandibulectomies. (*From* Song HG, Yun IS, Lee WJ, et al. Robot-assisted free flap in head and neck reconstruction. Arch Plast Surg 2013;40(4):353–8.)

is the challenge of perfusion and vitality of the reseeded cells. By analyzing real-time perfusion flow in the bioreactor, the creators of the decellularized temporomandibular joint were able to determine optimal nutrient flow and achieved high vitality of reseeded cells, giving insight into innovations in computer technology that can aid in solving this problem. In addition, research

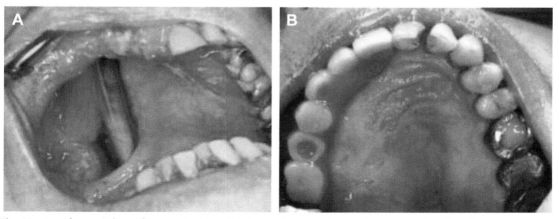

**Fig. 14.** Use of ectopic bone formation through adipose stem cells for maxillary reconstruction. Preoperative clinical status 28 months after removal of keratocyst by hemimaxillectomy (*A*). Final result 1 year after implantation of ectopically formed bone from adipose stem cells along with dental implants (*B*). (*From* Mesimäki K, Lindroos B, Törnwall J, et al. Novel maxillary reconstruction with ectopic bone formation by GMP adipose stem cells. Int J Oral Maxillofac Surg 2009;38(3):201–9; with permission.)

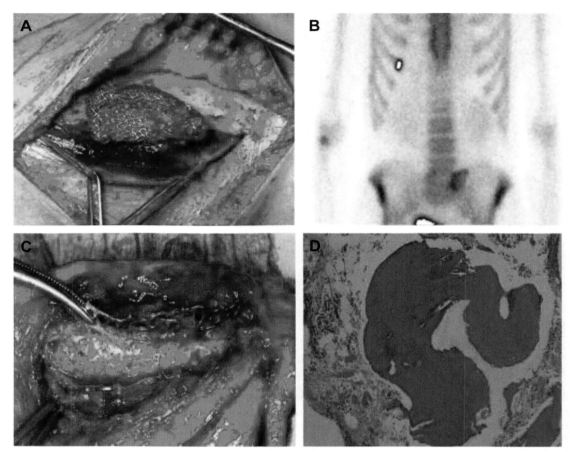

**Fig. 15.** The process of stem cell ectopic bone formation for maxillary defect reconstruction. A preformed titanium mesh cage was filled with adipose stem cells, B-tricalcium phosphate, and BMP-2 and implanted in the rectus muscle (*A*). Eight months later, bone appeared on radiograph (*B*). The vascularized piece of bone was harvested (*C*) and then implanted into the defect. Histologic analysis of the ectopic bone with 0.3% Oil Red O-solution showed normal morphology (*D*). (*From* Mesimäki K, Lindroos B, Törnwall J, et al. Novel maxillary reconstruction with ectopic bone formation by GMP adipose stem cells. Int J Oral Maxillofac Surg 2009;38(3):201–9; with permission.)

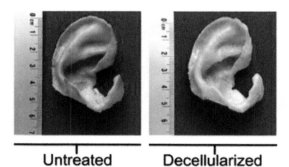

Untreated            Decellularized

**Fig. 16.** Untreated and decellularized ear cartilage. This decellularized scaffold can then be used as a scaffold for stem cell expansion. (*From* Utomo L, Pleumeekers MM, Nimeskern L, et al. Preparation and characterization of a decellularized cartilage scaffold for ear cartilage reconstruction. Biomed Mater 2015;10(1):015010; with permission.)

regarding growth factor and developmental signaling within the scaffolds is also furthering the field, leading to innovative solutions to craniofacial reconstruction.

The interface of bioengineering and craniofacial surgery also has implications for facial reanimation surgery, which depends on the success of facial nerve regeneration to muscle targets or through cross-face nerve grafts. One proposed method of restoring facial animation is through neural interface technologies.[61] These technologies use implantable electrodes to read from nerves on the healthy side of the face, then respond to these readings to stimulate the muscles on the opposing side that lack proper innervation. One such device has recently been developed for patients with hemiparalysis to restore eye blink (**Fig. 18**).[62] The device reads electromyographic signals from an electrode

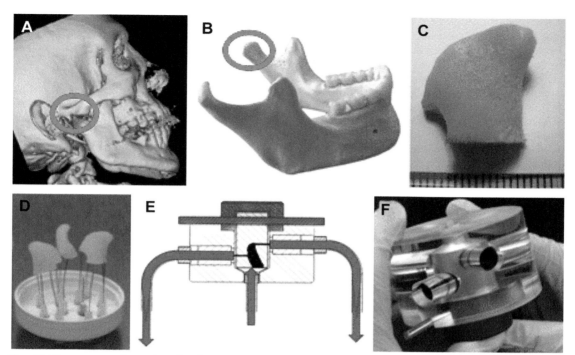

**Fig. 17.** The process of creating the decellularized temporomandibular joint. Clinical CT images were used to reconstruct the joint (*circled* in *A* and *B*) and to form a 3D printed scaffold (*C*). The complexity of the scaffold is shown in *D*. This scaffold was then seeded with human mesenchymal stem cells within a bioreactor that enabled controlled perfusion (*E, F*). (*From* Grayson WL, Fröhlich M, Yeager K, et al. Engineering anatomically shaped human bone grafts. Proc Natl Acad Sci U S A 2010;107:3299–304.)

implanted into the orbicularis oculi muscle on the healthy side of the face. On reading a signal, the device delivers electric stimulation to surface electrodes on the paralyzed side of the face, leading

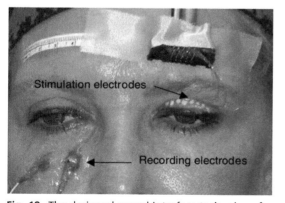

**Fig. 18.** The designed neural interface technology for blink restoration involves recording electrodes on the contralateral unimpaired hemiface, which interface with stimulation electrodes on the paretic upper eyelid. (*From* McDonnall D, Guillory KS, Gossman MD. Restoration of blink in facial paralysis patients using FES. Neural Engineering, 2009., NER '09. 4th International IEEE/EMBS Conference on Neural Engineering, 2009. p. 76–9; with permission.)

to eye closure. The device still faces challenges; the restored blink often appears as a spasm. However, the device does maintain protection and lubrication of the eye. On further electrode development, including creation of implantable electrodes, the method shows promise and may be integrated with free-muscle transfer for other facial paralysis indications, including smile restoration.

## FACE TRANSPLANT: FROM AUTOGRAFT TO ALLOGRAFT

Facial vascularized composite tissue allotransplantation (VCA) is an evolving new frontier in reconstructive regenerative surgery for complex and serious facial injuries not amenable to conventional techniques.[63] This surgical innovation has filled an unmet clinical need as a single procedure capable of restoring facial functions and aesthetic appearance by replacing missing tissue with like tissue. Since the first face transplant in 2005, the field has dramatically moved forward, with a total of 37 transplants performed (20 partial and 17 full faces) from 2005 to December 2015.[64] The procedure, although originally questioned by ethicists for its risk-benefit balance, has now become a more ethically accepted clinical practice. Facial composite tissue allotransplantation is also one of the most innovative areas of craniofacial reconstruction because it combines multidisciplinary fields and pushes the boundaries of reconstructive surgery.

One area of intense research in face transplantation is bettering immunosuppressive protocols. The current standard of care for these patients is tacrolimus, which is based on experience in solid organ transplantation. Tacrolimus has also shown benefits in improving nerve regeneration in animal models, adding a benefit to facial nerve reinnervation following transplant.[65] However, tacrolimus,

as a broad repressor of T-cell activity, also targets T-regulatory ($T_{reg}$) cells, which are thought to have a role in preserving VCA transplants.[66] One potential option being investigated is using low-dose interleukin (IL)-2, which redirects the pathway of activated T cells to $T_{reg}$ cells. This option has been attempted in a pilot program through low-dose skin injections of IL-2 in facial VCA patients.[67] Another, more risky, option is to pair VCA with a bone marrow transplant using the VCA donor's bone marrow (**Fig. 19**). This option has been used in VCA transplant in pigs and is

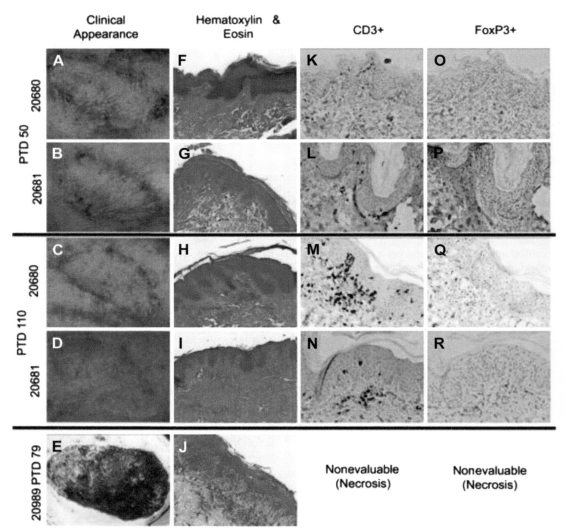

**Fig. 19.** Swine that received a hematopoietic stem cell transplant (HCT) along with a VCA displayed no clinical signs of rejection at post-transplant day (PTD) 50 or 100 (A–D). Banff stage 1 or 2 rejection was diagnosed at day 50 (F, G), but resolved by day 100 (H, I). In contrast, in an animal that did not receive HCT but still was under immunosuppression, complete rejection and necrosis occurred by day 79 (E, J). The authors noted the presence of CD3+ infiltrates (K, L), which persisted beyond day 100 (M, N) but which were not associated with histological evidence of tissue damage. (O–R) FoxP3+ cells could be identified co-localized with the CD3+ cells at all time points tested. (*From* Leonard DA, Kurtz JM, Mallard C, et al. Vascularized composite allograft tolerance across MHC barriers in a large animal model. Am J Transplant 2014;14(2):343–55; with permission.)

currently in preclinical trial in nonhuman primates.[68] This protocol has already proved successful in kidney transplant recipients, who have been weaned off immunosuppressants.[69] Another avenue of research is to combine donor and recipient bone marrow stem cells before transferring them into recipients; the thought behind this research is that the cells will train the immune system to accept the graft. In a rat model, this protocol improved immune tolerance following face transplant.[70] The main concern about facial VCA is the risk/benefit ratio of immunosuppression

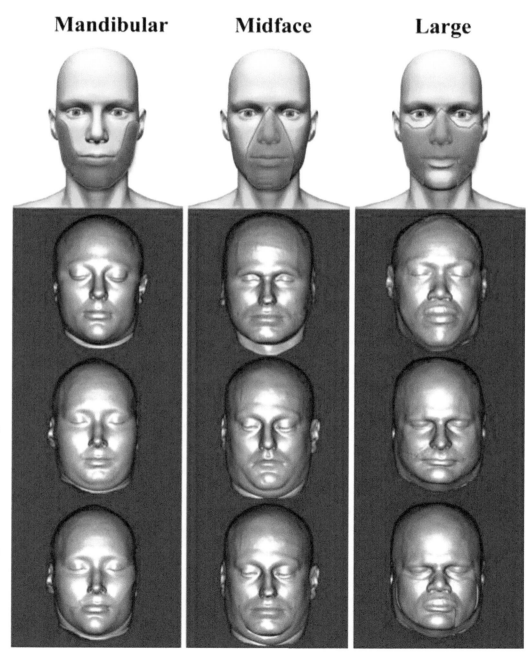

**Fig. 20.** Novel computer modeling enables virtual face transplants, enabling studies on donor suitability, aesthetic and functional outcomes, and preoperative planning before entering the operating room. (*From* Chandawarkar AA, Diaz-siso JR, Bueno EM, et al. Facial appearance transfer and persistence after three-dimensional virtual face transplantation. Plast Reconstr Surg 2013;132(4):957–66; with permission.)

versus the quality of life increases caused by the transplant, so research in this realm is vital to improving transplant outcomes and the acceptability of the procedure.

Advances in computer-assisted technology as well as 3D printing capabilities have particularly affected facial VCA. The ability to plan the complete surgery before entering the OR, including the inset of donor allograft and mitigation of potential size mismatches, enables a more seamless surgery and the ability to perform greater surgical complexity. Furthermore, the ability to perform virtual face transplants also enables studies on donor-recipient suitability, including the suitability of gender, age, and dramatic size mismatches in the context of cephalometric outcomes (**Fig. 20**).[71] This research thus informs clinical face transplant programs as they move forward.

Face transplant is a frontier of innovation in craniofacial microsurgical reconstruction. Its future advancement depends on improving outcomes and decreasing immunosuppressive side effects. This advancement includes furthering facial nerve regeneration to better postoperative graft function; current small animal models do not recapitulate the time or distance needed for facial nerve regeneration in a human model and large-animal models have not shown sufficient long-term survival to evaluate nerve function. So many aspects of return of neural function in face transplant patients are still not understood, including return of vasovagal response in the graft as well as patterns of sensory reinnervation. Furthermore, there needs to be a more complete understanding of patient quality-of-life outcomes in response to face transplant to fully show the risk/benefit ratio of this procedure. Facial VCA is an exciting area of craniofacial reconstruction, and much remains unknown in this growing field.

## SUMMARY

Head and neck reconstructive microsurgery is pushing the boundaries of innovation because of a coalescence of advances in bioengineering, technology, regenerative medicine, and surgical ingenuity. Advances in computing technology now enable complex surgical planning, and 3D printing allows these plans to be performed intraoperatively. This progress has enabled large advances in surgical technique, most notably the ability to conduct complex facial composite tissue transplants. Technology now enables intraoperative navigation and imaging, as well as novel mechanisms for perfusion monitoring. These advances lead to better patient outcomes and the ability to salvage failing flaps quickly and effectively. Technological advances have also led to minimally invasive techniques for head and neck oncological reconstruction. The integration of craniofacial surgery with regenerative medicine, stem cell biology, and tissue engineering has not only already created prefabricated, stem cell–derived bone but continues to pave the way for future innovation. It is vital that craniofacial microsurgeons think creatively and seek multidisciplinary viewpoints when assessing potential future advances. This willingness to seek challenges and embrace new ideas has led clinicians to the forefront of this growing field. After all, as Paul Tessier would proclaim, "Pourquoi pas?"

## REFERENCES

1. Jones BM. Paul Louis Tessier. J Plast Reconstr Aesthet Surg 2008;61:1005–7.
2. Dutkowski P, De Rougemont O, Clavien PA. Alexis Carrel: genius, innovator and ideologist. Am J Transplant 2008;8:1998–2003.
3. Wardrop D, Keeling D. The story of the discovery of heparin and warfarin. Br J Haematol 2008;141:757–63.
4. Tamai S. History of microsurgery. Plast Reconstr Surg 2009;124:e282–94.
5. Zhao L, Patel PK, Cohen M. Application of virtual surgical planning with computer assisted design and manufacturing technology to craniomaxillofacial surgery. Arch Plast Surg 2012;39:309–16.
6. Costello JP, Olivieri LJ, Su L, et al. Incorporating three-dimensional printing into a simulation-based congenital heart disease and critical care training curriculum for resident physicians. Congenit Heart Dis 2015;10:185–90.
7. Rodby KA, Turin S, Jacobs RJ, et al. Advances in oncologic head and neck reconstruction: systematic review and future considerations of virtual surgical planning and computer aided design/computer aided modeling. J Plast Reconstr Aesthet Surg 2014;67:1171–85.
8. Mardini S, Alsubaie S, Cayci C, et al. Three-dimensional preoperative virtual planning and template use for surgical correction of craniosynostosis. J Plast Reconstr Aesthet Surg 2014;67:336–43.
9. Parthasarathy J. 3D modeling, custom implants and its future perspectives in craniofacial surgery. Ann Maxillofac Surg 2014;4:9–18.
10. Available at: http://www.meddeviceonline.com/doc/world-s-first-d-printed-titanium-cranial-implant-cleared-by-fda-0001. Accessed October 12, 2016.
11. Podolsky DJ, Mainprize JG, Edwards GP, et al. Patient-specific orbital implants: development and implementation of technology for more accurate

orbital reconstruction. J Craniofac Surg 2016;27: 131–3.

12. Hou JS, Chen M, Pan CB, et al. Application of CAD/CAM-assisted technique with surgical treatment in reconstruction of the mandible. J Craniomaxillofac Surg 2012;40:e432–7.

13. Mezger U, Jendrewski C, Bartels M. Navigation in surgery. Langenbecks Arch Surg 2013;398:501–14.

14. Zrinzo L. Pitfalls in precision stereotactic surgery. Surg Neurol Int 2012;3:S53–61.

15. Hassfeld S, Mühling J. Computer assisted oral and maxillofacial surgery–a review and an assessment of technology. Int J Oral Maxillofac Surg 2001;30: 2–13.

16. Chauhan H, Rao SG, Chandramurli BA, et al. Neuronavigation: an adjunct in craniofacial surgeries: our experience. J Maxillofac Oral Surg 2011;10: 296–300.

17. Lin HH, Lo LJ. Three-dimensional computer-assisted surgical simulation and intraoperative navigation in orthognathic surgery: a literature review. J Formos Med Assoc 2015;114:300–7.

18. Bell RB. Computer planning and intraoperative navigation in cranio-maxillofacial surgery. Oral Maxillofac Surg Clin North Am 2010;22:135–56.

19. Taub PJ, Narayan P. Surgical navigation technology for treatment of pneumosinus dilatans. Cleft Palate Craniofac J 2007;44:562–6.

20. Morrison CS, Taylor HO, Sullivan SR. Utilization of intraoperative 3D navigation for delayed reconstruction of orbitozygomatic complex fractures. J Craniofac Surg 2013;24:e284–6.

21. Bell RB, Weimer KA, Dierks EJ, et al. Computer planning and intraoperative navigation for palatomaxillary and mandibular reconstruction with fibular free flaps. J Oral Maxillofac Surg 2011;69:724–32.

22. Baumann A, Sinko K, Dorner G. Late reconstruction of the orbit with patient-specific implants using computer-aided planning and navigation. J Oral Maxillofac Surg 2015;73:S101–6.

23. Gordon CR, Murphy RJ, Grant G, et al. Commentary on "a multicenter experience with image-guided surgical navigation: broadening clinical indications in complex craniomaxillofacial surgery". J Craniofac Surg 2015;26:1140–2.

24. Gordon CR, Murphy RJ, Coon D, et al. Preliminary development of a workstation for craniomaxillofacial surgical procedures: introducing a computer-assisted planning and execution system. J Craniofac Surg 2014;25:273–83.

25. Sukovic P. Cone beam computed tomography in craniofacial imaging. Orthod Craniofac Res 2003;6: 31–6.

26. Klatt JC, Heiland M, Marx S, et al. Clinical indication for intraoperative 3D imaging during open reduction of fractures of the mandibular angle. J Craniomaxillofac Surg 2013;41:e87–90.

27. Heiland M, Schmelzle R, Hebecker A, et al. Intraoperative 3D imaging of the facial skeleton using the SIREMOBIL Iso-C3D. Dentomaxillofac Radiol 2004;33:130–2.

28. Salgado CJ, Chim H, Schoenoff S, et al. Postoperative care and monitoring of the reconstructed head and neck patient. Semin Plast Surg 2010;24:281–7.

29. Chen KT, Mardini S, Chuang DC, et al. Timing of presentation of the first signs of vascular compromise dictates the salvage outcome of free flap transfers. Plast Reconstr Surg 2007;120:187–95.

30. Green JM, Thomas S, Sabino J, et al. Use of intraoperative fluorescent angiography to assess and optimize free tissue transfer in head and neck reconstruction. J Oral Maxillofac Surg 2013;71:1439–49.

31. Wei FC, Mardini S. Free-style free flaps. Plast Reconstr Surg 2004;114:910–6.

32. Gurtner GC, Jones GE, Neligan PC, et al. Intraoperative laser angiography using the SPY system: review of the literature and recommendations for use. Ann Surg Innov Res 2013;7:1.

33. Murono S, Ishikawa N, Ohtake H, et al. Intraoperative free jejunum flap monitoring with indocyanine green near-infrared angiography. Eur Arch Otorhinolaryngol 2014;271:1335–8.

34. Novakovic D, Patel RS, Goldstein DP, et al. Salvage of failed free flaps used in head and neck reconstruction. Head Neck Oncol 2009;1:33.

35. Steele MH. Three-year experience using near infrared spectroscopy tissue oximetry monitoring of free tissue transfers. Ann Plast Surg 2011;66:540–5.

36. Pelletier A, Tseng C, Agarwal S, et al. Cost analysis of near-infrared spectroscopy tissue oximetry for monitoring autologous free tissue breast reconstruction. J Reconstr Microsurg 2011;27:487–94.

37. Fox PM, Zeidler K, Carey J, et al. White light spectroscopy for free flap monitoring. Microsurgery 2013;33:198–202.

38. Yamamoto T, Todokoro T, Koshima I. Handheld thermography for flap monitoring. J Plast Reconstr Aesthet Surg 2012;65:1747–8.

39. Hardwicke JT, Osmani O, Skillman JM. Detection of perforators using smartphone thermal imaging. Plast Reconstr Surg 2016;137:39–41.

40. Engel H, Huang JJ, Tsao CK, et al. Remote real-time monitoring of free flaps via smartphone photography and 3G wireless Internet: a prospective study evidencing diagnostic accuracy. Microsurgery 2011;31:589–95.

41. Hwang JH, Mun GH. An evolution of communication in postoperative free flap monitoring: using a smartphone and mobile messenger application. Plast Reconstr Surg 2012;130:125–9.

42. Ricci JA, Vargas CR, Lin SJ, et al. A novel free flap monitoring system using tissue oximetry with text message alerts. J Reconstr Microsurg 2016;32: 415–20.

43. Rubinstein M, Armstrong WB. Transoral laser microsurgery for laryngeal cancer: a primer and review of laser dosimetry. Lasers Med Sci 2011;26:113–24.

44. Li RJ, Richmon JD. Transoral endoscopic surgery: new surgical techniques for oropharyngeal cancer. Otolaryngol Clin North Am 2012;45:823–44.

45. Haus BM, Kambham N, Le D, et al. Surgical robotic applications in otolaryngology. Laryngoscope 2003; 113:1139–44.

46. O'Malley BV, Weinstein GS, Sneyder W, et al. Transoral robotic surgery (TORS) for base of the tongue neoplasms. Laryngoscope 2006;116:1465–72.

47. Mukhija VK, Sung CK, Desai SC, et al. Transoral robotic assisted free flap reconstruction. Otolaryngol Head Neck Surg 2009;140:124–5.

48. Song HG, Yun IS, Lee WJ, et al. Robot-assisted free flap in head and neck reconstruction. Arch Plast Surg 2013;40:353–8.

49. Selber JC, Sarhane KA, Ibrahim AE, et al. Transoral robotic reconstructive surgery. Semin Plast Surg 2014;28:35–8.

50. Snyderman CH, Kassam AB, Carrau R, et al. Endoscopic reconstruction of cranial base defects following endonasal skull base surgery. Skull Base 2007;17:73–8.

51. Mizuno H, Tobita M, Uysal AC. Concise review: adipose-derived stem cells as a novel tool for future regenerative medicine. Stem Cells 2012;30: 804–10.

52. Koźlik M, Wójcicki P. The use of stem cells in plastic and reconstructive surgery. Adv Clin Exp Med 2014; 23:1011–7.

53. Mesimäki K, Lindroos B, Törnwall J, et al. Novel maxillary reconstruction with ectopic bone formation by GMP adipose stem cells. Int J Oral Maxillofac Surg 2009;38:201–9.

54. Warnke PH, Wiltfang J, Springer I, et al. Man as living bioreactor: fate of an exogenously prepared customized tissue-engineered mandible. Biomaterials 2006;27:3163–7.

55. Lendeckel S, Jodicke A, Christophis P, et al. Autologous stem cells (adipose) and fibrin glue used to treat widespread traumatic calvarial defects: case report. J Craniomaxillofac Surg 2004;32:370–3.

56. Ward BB, Brown SE, Krebsbach PH. Bioengineering strategies for regeneration of craniofacial bone: a review of emerging technologies. Oral Dis 2010;16: 709–16.

57. Gilbert TW, Sellaro TL, Badylak SF. Decellularization of tissues and organs. Biomaterials 2006;27: 3675–83.

58. Macchiarini P, Jungebluth P, Go T, et al. Clinical transplantation of a tissue-engineered airway. Lancet 2008;372:2023–30.

59. Utomo L, Pleumeekers MM, Nimeskern L, et al. Preparation and characterization of a decellularized cartilage scaffold for ear cartilage reconstruction. Biomed Mater 2015;10:015010.

60. Grayson WL, Fröhlich M, Yeager K, et al. Engineering anatomically shaped human bone grafts. Proc Natl Acad Sci U S A 2010;107:3299–304.

61. Langhals NB, Urbanchek MG, Ray A, et al. Update in facial nerve paralysis: tissue engineering and new technologies. Curr Opin Otolaryngol Head Neck Surg 2014;22:291–9.

62. McDonnall D, Guillory KS, Gossman MD. Restoration of blink in facial paralysis patients using FES. 4th International Conference on Neural Engineering, 2009. p. 76–9.

63. Chim H, Amer H, Mardini S, et al. Vascularized composite allotransplant in the realm of regenerative plastic surgery. Mayo Clin Proc 2014;89:1009–20.

64. Sosin M, Rodriguez ED. The face transplantation update: 2016. Plast Reconstr Surg 2016;137: 1841–50.

65. Gold BG. FK506 and the role of immunophilins in nerve regeneration. Mol Neurobiol 1997;15:285–306.

66. Swearingen B, Ravindra K, Xu H, et al. Science of composite tissue allotransplantation. Transplantation 2008;86:627–35.

67. Keener AB. Saving face: the search for alternatives to life-long immunosuppression for face transplants. Nat Med 2016;22:448–9.

68. Leonard DA, Kurtz JM, Mallard C, et al. Vascularized composite allograft tolerance across MHC barriers in a large animal model. Am J Transplant 2014;14: 343–55.

69. Sayegh MH, Fine NA, Smith JL, et al. Immunologic tolerance to renal allografts after bone marrow transplants from the same donors. Ann Intern Med 1991; 114:954–5.

70. Hivelin M, Klimczak A, Cwykiel J, et al. Immunomodulatory effects of different cellular therapies of bone marrow origin on chimerism induction and maintenance across MHC barriers in a face allotransplantation model. Arch Immunol Ther Exp (Warsz) 2016;64:299–310.

71. Chandawarkar AA, Diaz-siso JR, Bueno EM, et al. Facial appearance transfer and persistence after three-dimensional virtual face transplantation. Plast Reconstr Surg 2013;132:957–66.

# Microsurgical Tissue Transfer in Breast Reconstruction

Nakul Gamanlal Patel, MBBS (Lond), FRCS (Plastic Surgery)[a],*,
Venkat Ramakrishnan, MS, FRCS, FRACS (Plastic Surgery)[b]

## KEYWORDS

- Breast reconstruction • Deep inferior epigastric flap (DIEP) flap
- Transverse upper gracilis (TUG) flap • Profunda artery perforator (PAP) flap
- Inferior gluteal artery perforator (IGAP) flap • Superior gluteal artery perforator (SGAP) flap

## KEY POINTS

- Autologous breast reconstruction provides durable and symmetric breast reconstruction without the need for longer-term revisions.
- The deep inferior epigastric flap remains the flap of choice, if available, given the potential for aesthetic improvement at the donor site.
- Secondary autologous options include transverse upper gracilis, profunda artery perforator, lumbar artery perforator, gluteal artery perforator, and latissimus dorsi flaps.
- A single autologous flap can be augmented with secondary flaps, fat transfer, and implants.
- Flap planning can be made easier with imaging modalities, including computed tomography angiography, magnetic resonance angiography, and duplex.

## INTRODUCTION

The first publication of free tissue transfer for breast reconstruction was in 1978 by Serafin and Georgiade.[1] A groin flap with an implant was used to reconstruct the breast following a radical mastectomy with an acceptable result (**Fig. 1**).[1] A year later, Hans Holmstrom[2] produced an article well ahead of its time and directed our attention to the availability of the abdominal pannus for breast reconstruction using microsurgical techniques (**Fig. 2**). They have made some profound comments about the superficial inferior epigastric veins and the venous problems associated with such a transfer. The microsurgical reconstruction as it is practiced today owes its beginning to the pioneers of flap surgery. Professor Taylor's[3] work on the angiosomes concept followed by Koshima and Soeda's[4] first deep inferior epigastric perforator (DIEP) flap were key to what we are practicing today.[3–5] Allen and Treece[6] published the first report of using DIEPs to transfer the abdominal planus to reconstruct the breast. Although pedicle transverse rectus abdominis myocutaneous (TRAM), free TRAM, and muscle-sparing TRAM (MS-TRAM) were being practiced at the time, this article on the DIEP flap caught the imagination of the microsurgeon and an explosion of microsurgical breast reconstruction started. The concept of trunk to leaves versus foliage to roots discussed by Taylor[3] summarized a

The authors have nothing to disclose.
<sup>a</sup> Department of Plastic Surgery & Burns, The Royal Infirmary Hospital, University Hospitals of Leicester, Infirmary Square, Leicester LE1 5WW, UK; <sup>b</sup> St. Andrew's Centre for Plastic Surgery & Burns, Broomfield Hospital, Court Road, Chelmsford, Essex CM1 7ET, UK
* Corresponding author.
*E-mail address:* nakul9@gmail.com

plasticsurgery.theclinics.com

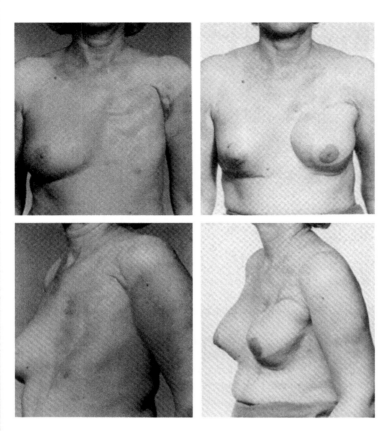

**Fig. 1.** First publication of a delayed breast reconstruction with a groin flap and implant. (*From* Serafin D, Georgiade NG. Transfer of free flaps to provide well-vascularized, thick cover for breast reconstructions after radical mastectomy. Plast Reconstr Surg 1978;62(4):528; with permission.)

microsurgeon's view on perforator flaps used in breast microsurgery.

There 3 broad options for microsurgical breast reconstruction can be grouped as follows (**Fig. 3**):

1. Abdominal flaps
2. Thigh flaps
3. Buttock and lower back flaps

## ABDOMINAL FLAPS
### Evolution of Abdominal Flaps

Abdominal based flaps have seen the most significant evolution from the TRAM flap, MS-TRAM, the DIEP flap, and the superficial inferior epigastric artery (SIEA) flap. The DIEP flap remains the gold standard and most widely used method of transferring the abdominal pannus to reconstruct the breast. In a suitable patient, with adequate hospital infrastructure, this is a routine operation that can achieve excellent results. It can be used in both immediate and delayed breast reconstruction to provide adequate volume of soft malleable tissue with minimal donor morbidity and can often lead to an improved abdomen.

The abdominal donor site has evolved from muscle flap to perforator flap, or TRAM to DIEP,

to limit potential donor site morbidity, including hernia and weakness. Perforator flaps subtly compromise the blood supply when compared to muscle flaps and the latter part of this chapter addresses how to combat this.

### Vascular Anatomy of the Abdomen

A thorough understanding of the macrovascular and microvascular anatomy of the abdomen has become essential in flap design.

The original description of the lower abdomen zones of perfusion were described for the pedicled TRAM flap by Hartrampf and colleagues[7] in which the abdomen is divided into 4 zones of perfusion: zone I comprises the area directly over the ipsilateral pedicled rectus abdominis muscle; zone II is the adjacent area across the midline over the contralateral muscle; zone III is lateral to the ipsilateral muscle; and zone IV is the remaining area lateral to the contralateral rectus abdominis muscle. Perfusion was though to be greatest in zones I and II, with lesser perfusion in III and least perfusion in IV (**Fig. 4**).

Holm and colleagues[8] reexamined the zones of perfusion for the DIEP flap and revised Hartrampf and colleagues'[7] concept of a centrally perfused skin ellipse with declining perfusion at the

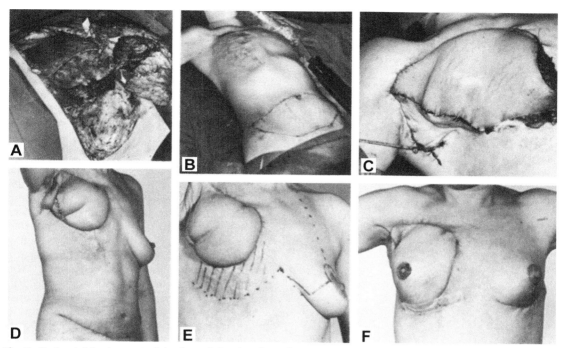

**Fig. 2.** First published report of the free abdominoplasty flap. (*A*) The free abdominoplasty flap raised and based on the right inferior epigastric vessels and the left superficial epigastric vein. The flap was resutured and delayed. (*B*) The viability of the flap 5 days later was not disturbed. (*C*) The flap sutured to the defect on the mastectomy area. (*D*) 2 weeks later the flap and the lower abdomen are well healed. (*E*) The planning of the final reconstruction 2 months later with reduction of the left breast and spreading of the flap on the right side with removal of the residual scarring. (*F*) Final result. The areola was formed by using the circumference of the areola on the left side. (*From* Holmstrom H. The free abdominoplasty flap and its use in breast reconstruction. An experimental study and clinical case report. Scand J Plast Reconstr Surg 1979;13(3):426; with permission.)

peripheral ends. They found that the lower abdominal flap should be described as 2 halves separated by the midline. The ipsilateral half has an axial pattern of perfusion; the contralateral half shows a random-pattern, individually variable blood supply. Therefore, the classic Hartrampf zones should be rearranged, switching zones II and III.[8]

Finally, Wong and colleagues[9] demonstrated that both the Hartrampf and Holm's zones of perfusion were correct depending on the location of the perforator. Hartrampf's zones of perfusion are correct for medial row perforators and Holm's for lateral row perforators, which effect flap design and harvest. They introduce a concept of perforasomes to the DIEP flap.

The most important points about the abdominal vasculature are

1. *Superficial and deep vascular systems*: There are 2 main vascular systems, which perfuse the abdominal pannus. Because of the hydrostatic pressure in the arteries the dominance of either system may not play a significant part in the arterial perfusion. However, there could be variations in the venous drainage of the abdominal pannus in patients depending on dominance of one or other system.

2. *Limited midline vascular connections*: The main obstacle for the transfer of blood is across the midline along the median raphe of the abdomen. It is well understood that the connections across the midline are limited, especially in the venous system.

3. *Superficial and deep system interconnections*: The main crossover of the venous drainage across the midline happens within the superficial system in the subumbilical region. The importance of the communication within the veins of the deep system and the superficial system plays a crucial part in promoting venous drainage across the midline and may have a role limiting fat necrosis within these flaps.

## Imaging Modalities

An understanding of the vascular tree facilitates faster operating times, improved operative

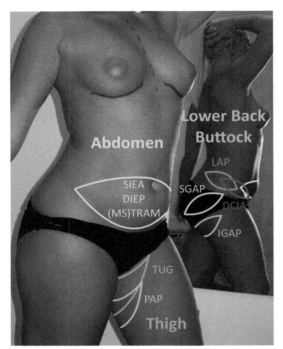

**Fig. 3.** Options for microsurgical breast reconstruction. DCIA, deep circumflex iliac artery; IGAP, inferior gluteal artery perforator; LAP, lumbar artery perforator; PAP, profunda artery perforator; SGAP, superior gluteal artery perforator; SIEA, superficial inferior epigastric artery; TUG, transverse upper gracilis.

the best parts of the flap with a chosen vascular tree (**Fig. 5**).[10]

### Strategies to Optimize Reconstruction

In addition, these imaging modalities provide the opportunity for presurgical planning that can further enhance flap vascularity. Broadly, they can be divided into

1. Use of multiple pedicles
2. Venous augmentation techniques

The use of multiple pedicles to perfuse the DIEP flap could be classified into stacked and bipedicled DIEP flaps. The technique is useful when reconstructing a relatively large breasted patient who has a small abdomen.[11–13] The flap can be anastomosed in series or parallel, the former requiring intraflap anastomosis. The abdominal pannus can be molded by dividing and layering, folding, or coning in order to best achieve symmetry to match a breast of varying shape, ptosis, and projection (**Fig. 6**).[14] Occasionally, the DIEP flap can be augmented with another autologous flap with a view to providing well-vascularized tissue to reconstruct the breast (**Fig. 7**).[15]

Significant effort has been made to better understand venous drainage from the DIEP flap, because this can be variable and lead to poor circulation. In cases with superficial venous system dominance, noted on preoperative imaging or intraoperatively, primary venous augmentation can be performed. The superficial inferior epigastric vein or the superficial circumflex iliac vein from the ipsilateral or the contralateral side of the DIEP vessels can be anastomosed to another

outcomes, and reduced morbidity. Various vascular imaging modalities, including duplex Doppler, computed tomography angiography (CTA), and magnetic resonance angiography (MRA), have provided a definite route map to recruit

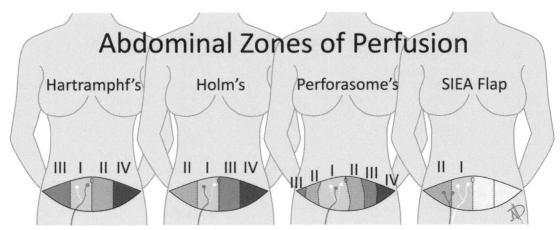

**Fig. 4.** Abdominal zones of perfusion: (I) Hartrampf's pedicled TRAM, (II) Holm's DIEP, (III) Wong's perforasome concept, (IV) SIEA.

**A**

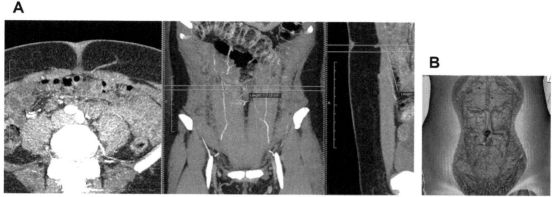

**B**

**Fig. 5.** (A) CTA showing the deep inferior epigastric artery perforators from left to right 3 images showing the perforator in cross-section, vertical section, and anterior-posterior section of the abdominal wall. (B) An image after 3-dimensional reconstruction.

recipient or to the cranial extension of the DIEP pedicle (**Fig. 8**).

There are other nonvascular strategies that would also support the use of abdominal tissue while limiting vascular problems, such as the following:

1. Reduction of the tissue required with a wise pattern reduction of the skin-sparing mastectomy envelope and primary or secondary contralateral breast reduction[16]
2. Transfer of vascular matrix that is a smaller, well-perfused flap followed with staged lipofilling
3. Primary lipofilling of the donor site that is the pectoralis muscle[17]
4. Use of implants along with free tissue transfers[18]

The advent of the perforator concept and the understanding that the subdermal plexus forms the main spine of any of these flaps allows us to shape these flaps with deep sutures that could be placed under the inferior surface of the flap to contour the flap without compromising the vascularity of these flaps (**Fig. 9**). The work on understanding the shaping of the flap to mold a breast from Blondeel and colleagues[19] has refined the aesthetic outcomes in microsurgical breast reconstructions (**Fig. 10**).

### Short Pedicle Transfers

A further advancement in DIEP flap breast reconstruction is the short pedicle transfers. The capability of the reconstructive surgeon to anastomose smaller vessels predictably increases options to use perforators from the intercostal system as

recipient vessels, when these are available. Short pedicle transfers limit donor site morbidity by limiting both the fascial incision and intramuscular dissection while accelerating flap harvest time (**Fig. 11**).

## SUPERFICIAL INFERIOR EPIGASTRIC ARTERY FLAP

The abdominal donor site has evolved from TRAM to DIEP to significantly reduce donor site morbidity; nevertheless, it does require incision through the anterior rectus sheath and dissection through the muscle with possible injury to the nerves. The SIEA flap is advantageous given that it does not involve dissection through these structures and is complete suprafascial. Anita and Buch[20] introduced this in 1971 for facial reconstruction given its favorable pedicle orientation, given it arises from the border of the flap. It was 2 decades later that Grotting[21] first used this flap for breast reconstruction and coined the term *free abdominoplasty flap*. Arnez and colleagues[22] then reported their experience in a series of 20 patients. Despite its obvious advantages, the flap has failed to advance popularity over the DIEP flap given the smaller caliber of pedicle vessels, shorter pedicle length, and questionable vascular territory across the midline. It is generally accepted that the SIEA supplies the ipsilateral hemiabdomen (see **Fig. 4**).

## THIGH FLAPS

The upper medial thigh is a reliable option for autologous breast reconstruction in those patients whereby the abdomen is not available. The transverse upper gracilis (TUG) flap is well

FOLDED

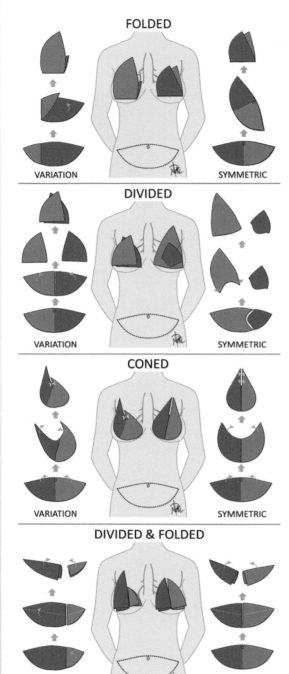

VARIATION                    SYMMETRIC

DIVIDED

VARIATION                    SYMMETRIC

CONED

VARIATION                    SYMMETRIC

DIVIDED & FOLDED

VARIATION                    SYMMETRIC

**Fig. 6.** Shaping of the abdominal pannus for stacked and bipedicle DIEP flaps.

established, with the profunda artery perforator (PAP) flap being a more recent introduction (**Fig. 12**). The scars are relativity concealable, and the flap raise is consistent with vessel caliber sufficient for reliable breast reconstruction.[23–25]

## The Transverse Upper Gracilis Flap

### History and nomenclature

The myocutaneous gracilis flap can be designed with various skin paddles, including a transverse, vertical, and diagonal pattern. There are various acronyms, including TUG, transverse myocutaneous gracilis (TMG), diagonal upper gracilis (DUG), vertical upper gracilis (VUG), and bilateral stacked VUG (BUG).[25–28]

Yousif and colleagues[29] first described the TUG flap for breast reconstruction in 1992. They noticed significantly more reliability of the transverse skin paddle compared with the vertical skin paddle, which suffered distal tip necrosis. They mapped out musculocutaneous perforators, which favored the transverse skin paddle within the upper third of the muscle.[30] Schoeller and Wechselberger[23,31] have popularized this flap for breast reconstruction.

### Flap harvest

The TUG flap is harvested from the upper medial thigh. This is not a perforator flap, but a true musculocutaneous flap and is useful in smaller sized breast reconstructions. Flap raise is consistent and vessel caliber is sufficient for reliable breast reconstruction.[23–25] Several refinements, including the preservation of the great saphenous vein, fascial resuspension to avoid distortion of the labia, and effective fat recruitment, have improved outcomes.[32] The flap is a melon slice shape of fat with a small muscle component that lends itself for coning into a breast mound. The peak of the cone also allows a standing cone deformity to be used to reconstruct the nipple in a single stage (**Fig. 13**). Up to 250 to 400 g of tissue could be harvested from the upper thigh with a relatively well-concealed donor site scar. In slimmer patients, especially those who require bilateral reconstructions, this is the favored option in many centers (**Fig. 14**). In larger-breasted patients, primary or secondary lipofilling and implants can be added.

### Double transverse upper gracilis

Double TUG breast reconstruction can be useful for reconstruction of larger-breasted patients.[26,32,33] These flaps can be inset in a yin-yang orientation and anastomosed in parallel to 2 separate recipients, such as the thoracodorsal and internal mammary systems, or in series when a sufficient adductor branch of the gracilis pedicle is available.[33]

### Complications

Seroma, delayed wound healing, infection, and sensory changes are recognized complications.

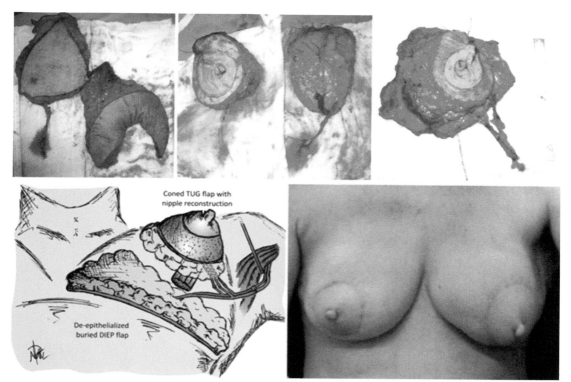

**Fig. 7.** Bilateral DIEP flaps with transverse upper gracilis (TUG) flaps.

The most difficult issue is a low scar that is not concealable in swimwear. A serious complication of temporary or permanent lymphedema is possible if the lymphatics of the groin are injured.[34] Appropriate patient selection and minimizing harvest volumes have led to decreased donor site morbidity.[35]

### The Profunda Artery Perforator Flap

The profunda artery perforator (PAP) flap uses tissue similar to the TUG flap to reconstruct the breast. However, the source of vascular supply is from the first perforating artery of the profunda

femoris artery. The island of skin, which is harvested from the upper medial thigh, tends to be skewed more posteriorly compared with the TUG flap. In addition, the PAP flap provides a longer pedicle with larger-caliber vessels to match the internal mammary vessels (**Fig. 15**). As the skin paddle is more posterior, it does not violate the femoral triangle and has less interference with the lymphatic system and its potential complications. The position of the scar, however, may be more caudal, as it depends on the location of the perforator and so may be more visible. The PAP flap may prove to be an alternative to the TUG flap, which avoids harvesting muscle.[36–41]

### Comparison with Buttock and Abdominal Donor Sites

The medial thigh donor site provides a natural crescent-shaped skin, which lends itself to coning and resembles a natural breast shape compared with a relatively flat abdominal flap.[23] In comparison with buttock tissues, the thigh provides a softer, more natural consistency to a breast reconstruction.

The thigh flap can be harvested supine and allow parallel operating in comparison with the buttock flaps, which require an operative turn and, hence, increase the length and complexity of the surgery.

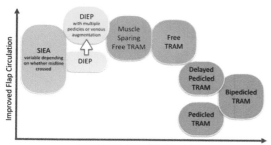

**Fig. 8.** Comparing the vascularity and abdominal donor site morbidity for abdominal free flaps.

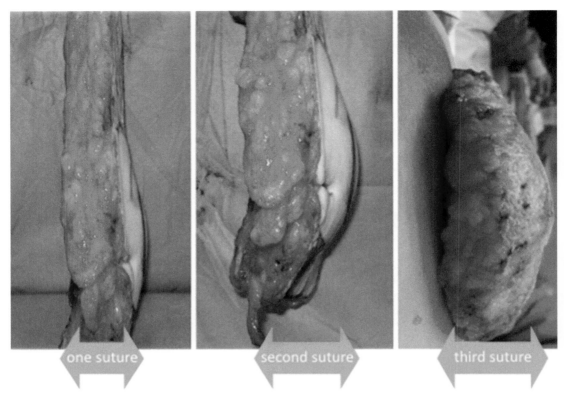

**Fig. 9.** Coning sutures to increase projection of the DIEP flap.

### Buttock and Lower Back Flaps

We have 4 different options in this area (see **Fig. 3**):

1. Inferior gluteal artery perforator (IGAP) flap
2. Superior gluteal artery perforator (SGAP) flap
3. Lumbar artery perforator (LAP) flap
4. Ruben flap based on the deep circumflex iliac artery and its branches

These options are reserved as secondary options if the abdominal and thigh donor site are unavailable.

### Gluteal Artery Perforator Flaps

The IGAP and SGAP flaps use the tissue from the inferior and superior buttock, respectively.[42,43] The flaps can be raised without muscle sacrifice or significant contour change of the buttock. The gluteal region is an excellent donor site particularly when there is redundant adiposity in these areas as it can enhance the buttock contour.[44] The main issues with raising the flap include a short vascular pedicle, exposure of the sciatic nerve, and recipient vessel size discrepancy requiring

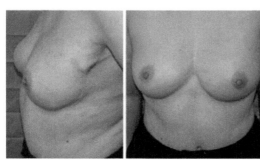
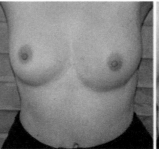
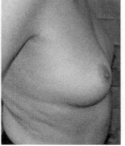

**Fig. 10.** Left breast reconstruction with a DIEP flap via a nipple-preserving, lateral envelope mastectomy approach.

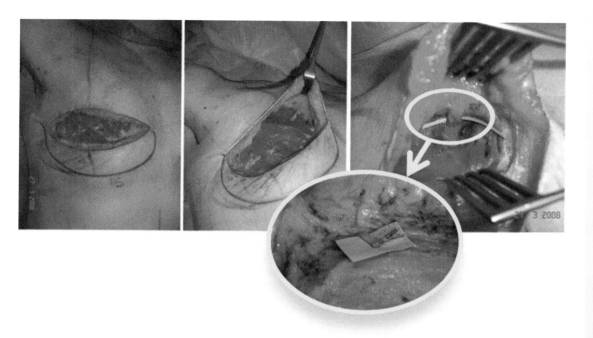

**Fig. 11.** Internal mammary artery and vein perforator allow for short pedicle transfer.

vein grafts.[43] These flaps are technically challenging to raise and provide tissue that is much firmer in consistency than a normal breast and result in microsurgeons exploring other areas.

### Lumbar Artery Perforator Flaps

The LAP flap is a new addition to the reconstructive surgeon's armamentarium having first been described in 2003.[45] The advantage of this flap is

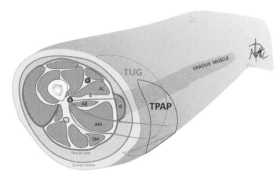

**Fig. 12.** The TUG and PAP flap anatomy. AB, adductor brevis muscle; AL, adductor longus muscle; AM, adductor magnus muscle; G, gracilis muscle; SM, semimembranosus muscle; TPAP, transverse profunda artery perforator flap; TUG, transverse upper gracilis flap.

the consistency of the vascular pedicle and the ease of flap elevation. It provides softer fat, which is more akin to the breast tissue, compared with the IGAP flaps. It also provides a donor site, which settles with very minimal contour defect despite a large harvest from this area. The significant issue with the LAP flap is its very short pedicle, which usually requires a vascular extension. Furthermore, the donor site is prone to seroma accumulation and may require prolonged drainage. It is common practice to plan these flaps with a CTA and plan for an extension of the vascular pedicle using either vein grafts or the deep inferior epigastric artery and vein pedicle, which is harvested through a separate lower transverse abdominal incision (**Figs. 16–18**).[46]

### Comparison with Abdominal and Thigh Donor Sites

Buttock and lower back flaps require patients to be either in the lateral decubitus or prone position. Hence, these operations tend to take longer, given that they involve patient repositioning and are not amenable to parallel operating. In addition, the GAP flaps are technically more challenging to raise, and the LAP flap adds complexity with the need of artery and vein extension grafts for the pedicle.[46]

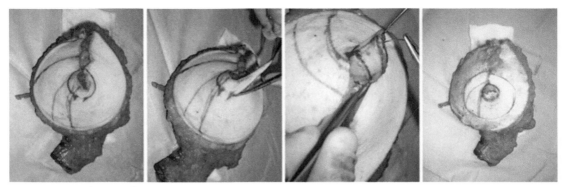

**Fig. 13.** Coning the TUG flap with immediate nipple reconstruction.

## COMBINATION FREE FLAPS

In select cases whereby patients would prefer a totally autologous reconstruction but have a paucity of tissue at each donor site, then 2 different free flaps can be combined to reconstruct the breast. A DIEP flap with a TUG flap, for example, can significantly increase the volume of a breast reconstruction.[16]

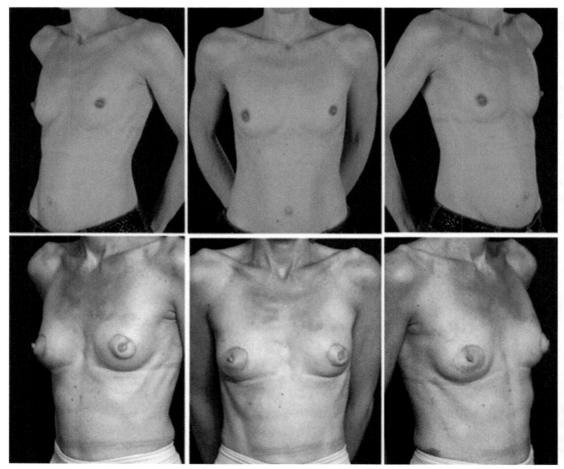

**Fig. 14.** Bilateral skin-sparing mastectomy with TUG flap reconstructions.

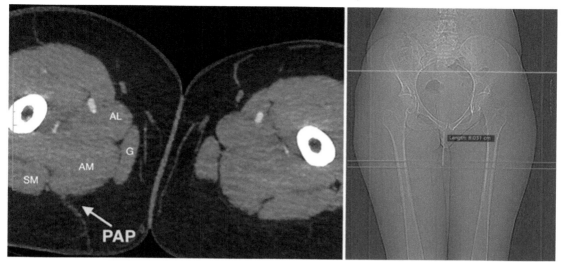

**Fig. 15.** CTA showing the PAP. AL, adductor longus muscle; AM, adductor magnus muscle; G, gracilis muscle; SM, semimembranosus muscle.

## FREE FLAP IN LOCALLY ADVANCED BREAST CANCERS

The consistency of the perforator flaps and the predictability of their transfer have spurred reconstructive microsurgeons toward using these for palliative reconstruction to significantly improve patients' quality of life. Locally advanced breast cancers with fungating lesions are rare but require management in these occasions. With chest wall resections and skeletal reconstruction of the chest, a free tissue transfer using a DIEP flap or an anterolateral thigh flap (ALT) flap can provide excellent palliation for these unfortunate patients (**Fig. 19**). This area is being explored with great benefit to our patients today.[47]

## LYMPHATIC SURGERY

The advent of lymph node transfers and lymphovenous anastomosis has opened new avenues for patients with lymphedema. There is an increasing demand for microsurgical reconstruction because of the obvious advantages, including excellent aesthetic outcomes, consistency of reconstruction, durability of reconstruction, and above all, availability of these reconstructions today. There is also an increasing interest in reconstructive breast surgery amid the younger plastic surgeons in view of its microsurgical and aesthetic challenges. The addition of lymphatic surgery to the armamentarium of the reconstructive breast surgeon has opened new vistas. With further technological advances, such as indocyanine green

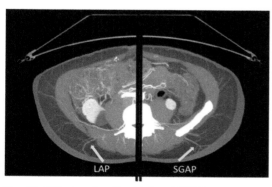

**Fig. 16.** CTA showing the LAP and SGAP.

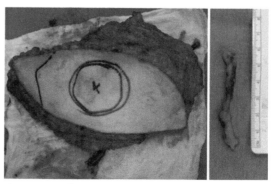

**Fig. 17.** LAP flap with a short pedicle and deep inferior epigastric vessels bridging graft.

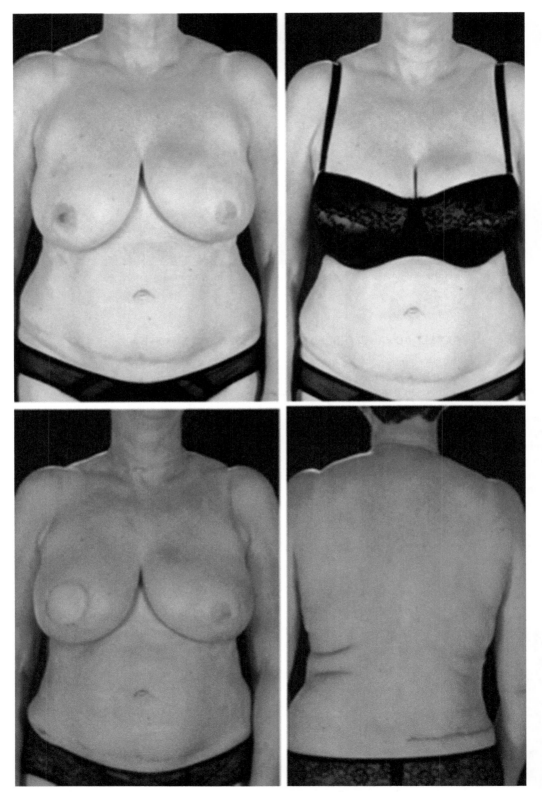

**Fig. 18.** Right skin-sparing mastectomy and reconstruction with LAP flap.

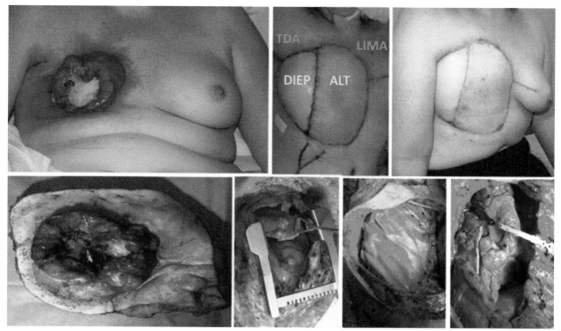

**Fig. 19.** Chest wall tumor resection including pleural and rib reconstruction and resurfacing with ALT and DIEP flaps. LIMA, left internal mammary artery; TDA, thoracodorsal artery.

(ICG), assessment of vascularity of flaps, refined tests for assessing the vascular tree using CTA, MRA, and Osiris reformatting of images, we are set to see further development in these areas.

## SUMMARY

Microsurgical breast reconstruction offers reliable, durable, and aesthetically superior reconstructions. The abdominal donor remains the mainstay of the reconstructive microsurgeons work. The TUG and LAP flaps are a useful second choice when the abdomen is not available. The GAP flaps remain a lifeboat when other options are exhausted. With increasing numbers of patients requesting autologous reconstruction, and those with failed implant-based reconstruction, the breast microsurgeon has a definite role in future years. Their focus should not only be on achieving high-quality results but also to ensure efficiency in operating to allow these microsurgical reconstructions to become routine practice in all breast surgery centers.

## REFERENCES

1. Serafin D, Georgiade NG. Transfer of free flaps to provide well-vascularized, thick cover for breast reconstructions after radical mastectomy. Plast Reconstr Surg 1978;62:527–36.
2. Holmstrom H. The free abdominoplasty flap and its use in breast reconstruction. An experimental study and clinical case report. Scand J Plast Reconstr Surg 1979;13:423–7.
3. Taylor GI. The angiosomes of the body and their supply to perforator flaps. Clin Plast Surg 2003;30: 331–42.
4. Koshima I, Soeda S. Inferior epigastric artery skin flaps without rectus abdominis muscle. Br J Plast Surg 1989;42:645–8.
5. Taylor GI, Palmer JH. The vascular territories (angiosomes) of the body: experimental study and clinical applications. Br J Plast Surg 1987;40:113–41.
6. Allen RJ, Treece P. Deep inferior epigastric perforator flap for breast reconstruction. Ann Plast Surg 1994;32:32–8.
7. Hartrampf CR, Scheflan M, Black PW. Breast reconstruction with a transverse abdominal island flap. Plast Reconstr Surg 1982;69:216–25.
8. Holm C, Mayr M, Hofter E, et al. Perfusion zones of the DIEP flap revisited: a clinical study. Plast Reconstr Surg 2006;117:37–43.
9. Wong C, Saint-Cyr M, Mojallal A, et al. Perforasomes of the DIEP flap: vascular anatomy of the lateral versus medial row perforators and clinical implications. Plast Reconstr Surg 2010;125:772–82.
10. Rozen WM, Ashton MW, Stella DL, et al. Stereotactic image-guided navigation in the preoperative imaging of perforators for DIEP flap breast reconstruction. Microsurgery 2008;28:417–23.

11. Rabey NG, Erel E, Malata CM. Double-pedicled abdominal free flap using an entirely new microvascular combination of DIEP and SIEA vascular pedicles for unilateral breast reconstruction: a novel addition to the Hamdi classification. Plast Reconstr Surg 2012;130:767e–9e.

12. Hamdi M, Khuthaila DK, Van Landuyt K, et al. Double-pedicle abdominal perforator free flaps for unilateral breast reconstruction: new horizons in microsurgical tissue transfer to the breast. J Plast Reconstr Aesthet Surg 2007;60:904–12.

13. Murray A, Wasiak J, Rozen WM, et al. Stacked abdominal flap for unilateral breast reconstruction. J Reconstr Microsurg 2015;31:179–86.

14. Patel NG, Rozen WM, Chow WT, et al. Stacked and bipedicled abdominal free flaps for breast reconstruction: considerations for shaping. Gland Surg 2016;5:115–21.

15. Rozen WM, Patel NG, Ramakrishnan VV. Increasing options in autologous microsurgical breast reconstruction: four free flaps for 'stacked' bilateral breast reconstruction. Gland Surg 2016;5:255–60.

16. Cheng A, Losken A. Essential elements of the preoperative breast reconstruction evaluation. Gland Surg 2015;4:93–6.

17. Locke MB, Zhong T, Mureau MA, et al. Tug 'O' war: challenges of transverse upper gracilis (TUG) myocutaneous free flap breast reconstruction. J Plast Reconstr Aesthet Surg 2012;65:1041–50.

18. Figus A, Canu V, Iwuagwu FC, et al. DIEP flap with implant: a further option in optimising breast reconstruction. J Plast Reconstr Aesthet Surg 2009;62:1118–26.

19. Blondeel PN, Hijjawi J, Depypere H, et al. Shaping the breast in aesthetic and reconstructive breast surgery: an easy three-step principle. Plast Reconstr Surg 2009;123:455–62.

20. Antia NH, Buch VI. Transfer of an abdominal dermofat graft by direct anastomosis of blood vessels. Br J Plast Surg 1971;24:15–9.

21. Grotting JC. The free abdominoplasty flap for immediate breast reconstruction. Ann Plast Surg 1991;27:351–4.

22. Arnez ZM, Khan U, Pogorelec D, et al. Breast reconstruction using the free superficial inferior epigastric artery (SIEA) flap. Br J Plast Surg 1999;52:276–9.

23. Schoeller T, Wechselberger G. Breast reconstruction by the free transverse gracilis (TUG) flap. Br J Plast Surg 2004;57:481–2.

24. McCulley SJ, Macmillan RD, Rasheed T. Transverse upper gracilis (TUG) flap for volume replacement in breast conserving surgery for medial breast tumours in small to medium sized breasts. J Plast Reconstr Aesthet Surg 2011;64:1056–60.

25. Bodin F, Schohn T, Dissaux C, et al. Bilateral simultaneous breast reconstruction with transverse musculocutaneous gracilis flaps. J Plast Reconstr Aesthet Surg 2015;68:e1–6.

26. Park JE, Alkureishi LW, Song DH. TUGs into VUGs and friendly BUGs: transforming the gracilis territory into the best secondary breast reconstructive option. Plast Reconstr Surg 2015;136:447–54.

27. Dayan ESM, Sultan M, Samson W, et al. The diagonal upper gracilis (DUG) flap: a safe and improved alternative to the TUG flap. Plast Reconstr Surg 2013;132:33–4.

28. Natoli NB, Wu LC. Vascular variations of the transverse upper gracilis flap in consideration for breast reconstruction. Ann Plast Surg 2015;74:528–31.

29. Yousif NJ, Matloub HS, Kolachalam R, et al. The transverse gracilis musculocutaneous flap. Ann Plast Surg 1992;29:482–90.

30. Yousif NJ. The transverse gracilis musculocutaneous flap. Ann Plast Surg 1993;31:382.

31. Schoeller T, Huemer GM, Wechselberger G. The transverse musculocutaneous gracilis flap for breast reconstruction: guidelines for flap and patient selection. Plast Reconstr Surg 2008;122:29–38.

32. Fattah A, Figus A, Mathur B, et al. The transverse myocutaneous gracilis flap: technical refinements. J Plast Reconstr Aesthet Surg 2010;63:305–13.

33. Hunter JE, Mackey SP, Boca R, et al. Microvascular modifications to optimize the transverse upper gracilis flap for breast reconstruction. Plast Reconstr Surg 2014;133:1315–25.

34. Hallock GG. The conjoint medial circumflex femoral perforator and gracilis muscle free flap. Plast Reconstr Surg 2004;113:339–46.

35. Buchel EW, Dalke KR, Hayakawa TE. The transverse upper gracilis flap: efficiencies and design tips. Can J Plast Surg 2013;21:162–6.

36. Hunter JE, Lardi AM, Dower DR, et al. Evolution from the TUG to PAP flap for breast reconstruction: comparison and refinements of technique. J Plast Reconstr Aesthet Surg 2015;68:960–5.

37. Saad A, Sadeghi A, Allen RJ. The anatomic basis of the profunda femoris artery perforator flap: a new option for autologous breast reconstruction–a cadaveric and computer tomography angiogram study. J Reconstr Microsurg 2012;28:381–6.

38. Haddock NT, Greaney P, Otterburn D, et al. Predicting perforator location on preoperative imaging for the profunda artery perforator flap. Microsurgery 2012;32:507–11.

39. Allen RJ, Haddock NT, Ahn CY, et al. Breast reconstruction with the profunda artery perforator flap. Plast Reconstr Surg 2012;129:16e–23e.

40. Blechman KM, Broer PN, Tanna N, et al. Stacked profunda artery perforator flaps for unilateral breast

reconstruction: a case report. J Reconstr Microsurg 2013;29:631–4.

41. Mayo JL, Allen RJ, Sadeghi A. Four-flap breast reconstruction: bilateral stacked DIEP and PAP flaps. Plast Reconstr Surg Glob Open 2015;3:e383.

42. Allen RJ, Tucker C Jr. Superior gluteal artery perforator free flap for breast reconstruction. Plast Reconstr Surg 1995;95:1207–12.

43. Allen RJ. The superior gluteal artery perforator flap. Clin Plast Surg 1998;25:293–302.

44. Allen RJ, Levine JL, Granzow JW. The in-the-crease inferior gluteal artery perforator flap for breast reconstruction. Plast Reconstr Surg 2006;118:333–9.

45. de Weerd L, Elvenes OP, Strandenes E, et al. Autologous breast reconstruction with a free lumbar artery perforator flap. Br J Plast Surg 2003;56:180–3.

46. Peters KT, Blondeel PN, Lobo F, et al. Early experience with the free lumbar artery perforator flap for breast reconstruction. J Plast Reconstr Aesthet Surg 2015;68:1112–9.

47. Arya R, Chow WT, Rozen WM, et al. Microsurgical reconstruction of large oncologic chest wall defects for locally advanced breast cancer or osteoradionecrosis: a retrospective review of 26 cases over a 5-year period. J Reconstr Microsurg 2016;32:121–7.

# Anastomosis of the Superficial Inferior Epigastric Vein to the Internal Mammary Vein to Augment Deep Inferior Artery Perforator Flaps

CrossMark

Aparna Vijayasekaran, MBBS, MS[a],*, Anita Mohan, MBBS[a],
Lin Zhu, MD[b], Basel Sharaf, MD, DDS[a], Michel Saint-Cyr, MD, FRCS(C)[c]

## KEYWORDS

- Deep inferior artery perforator flap • Venous congestion • Venous augmentation

## KEY POINTS

- Use of the retrograde limb of the internal mammary vein has been described previously as a lifeboat for venous congestion but not prophylactically.
- Maximizing the length of the deep inferior artery perforator (DIEP) flap pedicle, identifying and dissecting the superficial inferior epigastric vein proximally in every patient, and taking advantage of the retrograde internal mammary vein are all technical details that facilitate the additional venous anastomosis as well as flap inset.
- Performing a second venous anastomosis routinely using the superficial inferior epigastric vein to the retrograde internal mammary vein helps with flap inset by narrowing the width of the breast mound.
- Routine venous augmentation is simple without additional morbidity to the procedure and in the authors' experience has offset the incidence of venous congestion and fat necrosis.

## INTRODUCTION

Venous congestion is a major pitfall in the deep inferior artery perforator (DIEP) flap for breast reconstruction. No clear evidence has supported routine venous augmentation, although several studies have shown a potential clinical benefit leading to decreased venous congestion and fat necrosis. Secondary venous recipients described have included a second internal mammary vein if present, the thoracodorsal vein, cephalic vein, thoracoacromial vein, or external jugular vein turndown. Use of each of these veins as a recipient has been associated with additional dissection beyond

The authors have nothing to disclose.
[a] Division of Plastic and Reconstructive Surgery, Mayo Clinic, 200 First Street Southwest, Rochester, MN 55905, USA; [b] Department of Plastic Surgery, Peking Union Medical College Hospital, Beijing, China; [c] Division of Plastic Surgery, Baylor Scott & White Health, Scott & White Memorial Hospital, MS-01-E443, 2401 South 31st Street, Temple, TX 76508, USA
* Corresponding author.
E-mail address: Vijayasekaran.Aparna@mayo.edu

Clin Plastic Surg 44 (2017) 361–369
http://dx.doi.org/10.1016/j.cps.2016.12.006

what is routinely done for DIEP flap inset, increasing operative time and adding morbidity to the procedure.

Use of the caudal (retrograde) limb of the internal mammary vein (IMV) has been described as a lifeboat for venous congestion but not prophylactically. Also, several studies have evaluated the flow in the retrograde IMV. This anastomosis is feasible due to the fact that the IMV is valveless. Since September 2014, the authors have routinely performed a second venous anastomosis predominantly with the SIEV (superficial inferior epigastric vein) to the caudal IMV. This article reviews the authors' experience using this technique and shares their algorithm for routine venous augmentation of DIEP flap using the SIEV and caudal IMV.

## PATIENTS AND CLINICAL METHODS

The senior author has performed 30 DIEP flaps since September 2014, in which 2 venous anastomoses were performed in each flap irrespective of the presence or absence of intraoperative venous congestion. Thirty flaps prior to September 2014 with 1 anastomosis were included in the control limb. Only single or double perforator DIEP flaps were included in this review. Muscle-sparing transverse rectus abdominis muscle (TRAM) flaps and free TRAM flaps were excluded.

## CLINICAL RESULTS

Patient demographics were comparable between both groups (**Table 1**). The average body mass index (BMI) was around 30 in both groups (30.4 vs 30.1), and the patients were comparable in their co-morbidities, which included diabetics, hyperlipidemia, high blood pressure, and previous abdominal surgeries. Average age was also comparable (47.5 vs 48.5 years old), and there were equal numbers of smokers in both groups.

The average length of the DIEA/DIEV pedicle was comparable in both groups (11.27 vs 11.89 cm). The SIEV length was also similar. Additionally, other flap characteristics were comparable between the 2 groups. Average flap weight was slightly higher in the 2-vein group (830 vs 690 g). There was no flap loss overall in either group. The intraoperative venous congestion rate was 6.7% in the single venous anastomosis group and 13.3% in the venous augmentation group (**Table 2**). There was no postoperative venous congestion or re-exploration in the group in which routine venous augmentation was performed when compared with the single venous anastomosis group (0% vs 6.7%). Clinical rates of fat necrosis were decreased from 10% to 3.3%.

## THE NEEDS AND TECHNICAL POINTS FOR VENOUS AUGMENTATION
### Disadvantages of Current Deep Inferior Artery Perforator Flaps

One of the few disadvantages of the DIEP flap is the greater incidence of venous congestion and fat necrosis. Reported rates of venous congestion in DIEP flaps range from 3% to 25%.[1–3] Venous congestion remains the most common cause of flap loss in DIEP breast reconstruction. The highest incidence of venous congestion is in the intraoperative period.

### Vascular Anatomy and the Reason for Increased Venous Congestion in Deep Inferior Artery Perforator Flaps

The DIEP flap is associated with higher rates of venous congestion when compared with other flaps because of limitations in the intrinsic vascular anatomy of the DIEP flap. In the majority of patients, the DIEA remains the dominant artery. However, the same cannot be said of the venous

**Table 1**
**Patient demographics**

| Patient Demographics | Single Venous Anastomosis | Double Venous Anastomosis |
|---|---|---|
| Average age | 47.5 | 48.53 |
| Average weight | 80.5 kg (54–114) | 83.9 kg (55–120) |
| Average BMI | 30.4 (25.2–40.1) | 30.1 (21.2–43.2) |
| Diabetes | 3 (10%) | 4 (13.3%) |
| Hyperlipidemia | 10 (33.3%) | 8 (26.7%) |
| History of smoking | 4 (13.3%) | 4 (13.3%) |
| Hypertension | 6 (20%) | 8 (26.7%) |
| Previous abdominal surgery or liposuction | 8 (26.7%) | 8 (26.7%) |

**Table 2**
**Comparison of flap characteristics, technical details, and outcomes between single and double venous anastomoses groups**

|  | Single Venous Anastomosis | Double Venous Anastomosis |
|---|---|---|
| Unilateral | 4 (13.3%) | 4 (13.3%) |
| Immediate | 6 (20%) | 8 (26.6%) |
| Single perforator DIEP | 22 (73.3%) | 25 (83.3%) |
| Average pedicle length | 11.27 cm (9–13) | 11.89 cm (10–13) |
| SIEV length | 7.55 cm (6–8) | 7.46 cm (6–12) |
| Average flap weight | 690.9 gm (318–1245) | 830.88 gm (427–2024) |
| Second venous anastomosis | 2 (6.7%) | 100% |
| Intraoperative venous congestion | 2 (6.7%) | 4 (13.3%) |
| Postoperative venous congestion | 2 (6.7%) | 0 (0%) |
| Re-exploration | 2 (6.7%) | 0 (0%) |
| Flap survival | 30 (100%) | 30 (100%) |
| Venous augmentation with second anastomosis | 4 (13.7%) | 30 (100%) |
| Fat necrosis | 3 (10%) | 1 (3.3%) |

anatomy. Carramenha and colleagues[4] reported that the venous drainage of the skin paddle in a DIEP as well as TRAM flap is largely dependent on the SIEV rather than the deep system in the normal state. When the superficial system is divided during the process of flap harvest, this directs the venous drainage caudally via the connecting vascular network between the superficial and the deep system, with the venous return eventually draining via the deep system. This was further studied by Blondeel and colleagues,[2] who examined the interconnecting network between the superficial and deep systems. Variable vascular communicating patterns were noted across subjects, which explain the unpredictable occurrence of venous congestion. The rate of intraoperative venous congestion in Blondeel's series was 2%.[1,2,5] Various studies in the interim have reported varying rates of venous congestion ranging from 2% to 27%.[2,6] This difference could in part be explained by differing flap elevation techniques, adequacy of the primary venous anastomosis, and varying criteria defining venous congestion by different surgeons.[7]

It is difficult to predict the dominance of the superficial system even with preoperative computed tomography (CT) or magnetic resonance (MR) angiography (**Fig. 1**). CT angiography (CTA) allows for a snapshot of the abdominal wall vascular anatomy when the patient is in a supine position and under baseline hemodynamic parameters. However, CTA lacks information on the physiologic flow dynamics after flap elevation, when the patient is under general anesthesia in the flap. Sadik and colleagues[8] found no correlation between the calibers of the SIEV on CTA with superficial system dominance. They recommended judicious harvest of the SIEV in every DIEP flap irrespective of the size of the SIEV. These findings were contradictory to previous data, which supported the correlation between the SIEV caliber and superficial dominance. Hence, although CTA remains a valuable tool to guide perforator selection in flap harvest, it is unreliable in predicting venous system dominance and risk of congestion.

## To Supercharge Versus not Supercharge

Given the lack of a single reliable means or method to predict the occurrence of venous congestion, the questions arise: Should one routinely perform venous augmentation of all DIEP flaps? Given that the stakes are high, with venous congestion being the most common cause of flap loss and with a known 2% incidence of intraoperative venous congestion, should one move toward a practice pattern of routinely augmenting all flaps?

Various options for venous augmentation have been described in the setting of existing venous congestion to improve outcomes.[9–15] The thoracodorsal vein, cephalic vein, basilic vein, and intercostal branches are options for recipient veins for outflow.[1,9,10,13,16–19] The first large series of

A

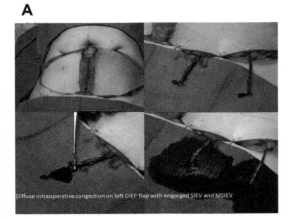

B

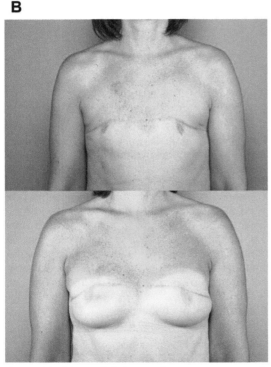

**Fig. 1.** (*A*) This top left image demonstrates immediate diffuse intraoperative venous congestion. 2 large superficial veins were identified in this patient (MSIEV and SIEV) and preserved. Engorged SIEV and MSIEV are noted in the top right and bottom left images, consistent with a superficial dominant system. The bottom right image shows a definite improvement in flap color, confirming resolution of venous congestion by venting the superficial veins. This picture clearly highlights the importance of superdrainage in flap salvage in the setting of venous congestion. (*B*) Pre and postoperative images of patient in whom the flap with intraoperative venous congestion was salvaged with venous augmentation via the SIEV. She has no evidence of fat necrosis at 12 months. MSIEV, medial superficial inferior epigastric vein.

superdrainage for venous congestion was by Wechselberger and colleagues[15] in 2001. More recently, prophylactic venous augmentation was found to decrease partial fat loss and fat necrosis with superdrainage using the SIEV.[20] Enajat and colleagues[21] compared single versus double venous anastomosis and found that venous augmentation significantly decreased the rates of venous congestion with no increase in complication rates. Boutros reported a decrease in operative take backs with routine venous augmentation when compared with single anastomosis.[22]

## Use of the Retrograde Internal Mammary Vein for Venous Outflow

The retrograde limb of the internal mammary vein has been described in the past for venous augmentation of a DIEP flap. Li and colleagues[23] described using the proximal and distal ends of the IMV for pedicled TRAM flap reconstruction. They studied the flow patterns in both the proximal and distal IMV/IMA and concluded that the flow was adequate in both ends to sustain the perfusion patterns of free tissue transfer. There has been a vested interest in evaluating the flow dynamics of the internal mammary venous system over the last decade, but there is not much evidence supporting the routine use of the retrograde IMV. Anatomic studies have reported the IMV system as a valveless low pressure system, which could explain the feasibility of using the retrograde limb for venous outflow. Results from some cadaveric studies have contradicted this theory of valve-less IMV system.[24,25] Studies have demonstrated that there may be diminished perfusion in the retrograde IMV when compared with the antegrade vein, but this flow is enough to sustain flap perfusion and drainage. Mackey and Ramsey[25] reported that a proportion of IMV has valves between the second and third intercostal spaces contrary to popular belief and urged caution in basing the venous outflow entirely on the retrograde system. Various clinical studies have reported small series of patients with the retrograde IMV as venous outflow for flap salvage. Kerr-Valentic and colleagues[26] described the anastomosis of the second DIEV to the retrograde limb and reported good intraoperative patency rates with ultrasound.

Even with all the evidence supporting the safe use of the retrograde IMV, it has not been standard practice thus far.[27–33] No downsides or complications have been reported with the use of the retrograde IMV. The authors have been using the retrograde IMV routinely for venous augmentation with good success, and it is now a standard part of their algorithm to offset venous congestion.

## Technical Details for Harvesting Deep Inferior Artery Perforator Flap with Intention to Augment Venous Outflow with Turbocharging Using the Retrograde Internal Mammary Vein

### Maximizing rib space dissection

The internal mammary vessels are exposed in the standard manner either in the second or third intercostal space. A cuff of pectoralis major muscle can be resected to provide better exposure. Maximizing the length on the internal mammary veins is of prime importance when considering using the caudal limb for venous augmentation.[34] The intercostal muscles on either side of the removed rib can be excised to add some length to the exposed vessels. This maneuver is an underutilized but key technical feature that can add an extra few millimeters to vessel length. Venous side branches and larger perforators if present are identified and preserved.[18] And lastly, a second rib can be removed if all previously described maneuvers do not provide adequate length. Adequate length of the IMV can be described as the minimal length where the exposed vessels can be divided in the middle leaving enough proximal and distal length for performing 2venous anastomoses (**Fig. 2**).

### Harvesting a long pedicle

The pedicle lengths are typically longer in a DIEP flap when compared with a muscle-sparing or free TRAM, especially when the flap is based off a more cephalad perforator. The pedicle dissection is carried up to the origin of the deep inferior epigastric artery and vein from the iliac artery (**Fig. 3**). Usually there are DIEV vena comitantes, which are preserved in all cases. Larger side branches of the vena comitantes are also dissected out to length for possible use as a venous outflow should the need arise. The average

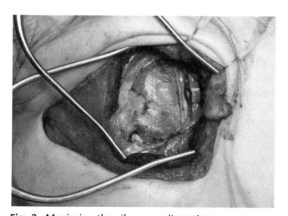

**Fig. 2.** Maximize the rib space dissection.

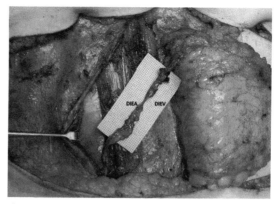

**Fig. 3.** Harvest a long pedicle.

pedicle length in the current series was around 12 cm in both groups (see **Table 2**).

### Dissect and harvest the MSIEV (when present) and the superficial inferior epigastric vein routinely at maximal length

The superficial inferior epigastric vein is located within 8 cm from the midline. Sometime then SIEV branches into a medial and lateral branch, and this bifurcation pattern can be variable. When the medial and lateral branches of the SIEV merge more proximally, medial branch of the SIEV (MSIEV) is the vein that one encounters in dissection, and the MSIEV is usually more medial than the SIEV. Rozen and colleagues[35] described the presence of 2 separate SIEV trunks in almost 40% of their patients, which is almost analogous to the authors' description of the MSIEV. To the authors' knowledge, this is the only paper describing this variation of SIEV. Both MSIEV and the SIEV should be carefully identified and dissected out to gain adequate length (**Fig. 4**). The average pedicle length of the superficial vein in the authors' series is around 7.5 cm in both groups (6–8 cm). Getting adequate length of the SIEV helps with inset, especially in the bulky flaps in an obese patient (see **Fig. 4**B). A vertical inset pattern is preferred in the authors' practice (**Fig. 5**).

An inset pattern should be used when performing venous augmentation of DIEP flap by performing a second venous anastomosis between SIEV and caudal IMV.

### Authors' Algorithm

The authors' algorithm starts with the previously described technique of harvesting a DIEP flap including maximizing pedicle length, dissecting out the SIEV up to 6 to 8 cm in all patients when present, and maximizing intercostal space dissection in anticipation of using the caudal IMV for

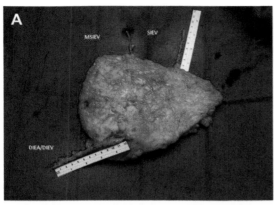

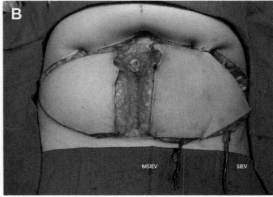

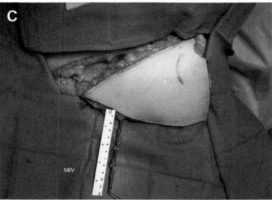

Fig. 4. (*A*) Maximize length of DIEA, SIEV, and MSIEV. (*B*) Dissect and harvest the MSIEV (when present) and the SIEV routinely at maximal length. This image demonstrates the anatomic variation of the SIEV wherein 2 superficial veins are identified. The more medical of the 2 veins is labeled as MSIEV, and the lateral remains the true SIEV. (*C*) A single large SIEV is identified and dissected. The length of SIEV harvested in this patient is almost 11 cm.

routine venous augmentation. Venous augmentation (supercharging) is performed in all flaps routinely when technically feasible irrespective of the incidence of venous congestion. When the SIEV is present and available for a second outflow, the authors prefer to use the SIEV over the second DIEV. This is based on the vascular anatomy of the

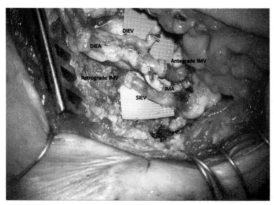

Fig. 5. Intraoperative picture demonstrating the inset pattern with routine anastomosis of the SIEV to the caudal IMV.

DIEP flap that the venous drainage in a DIEP flap is more dependent the superficial system in the normal presurgical state. Although this may not hold true in all patients in whom clear dominance of the DIEP system is noted, it is still the more common phenomenon. The SIEV is coupled to a second IMV if present (presence of second IMV is variable although more frequent on the right side). If only 1 IMV is present, the SIEV is anastomosed to the retrograde IMV (**Fig. 6**).

If the SIEV is not present, the second DIEV is used for outflow. The second DIEV is then anastomosed to the second IMV when present or to the retrograde limb of the IMV. On the rare occasion when the SIEV/MSIEV and SIEV are all absent, the authors perform a single venous anastomosis and assess the flap to for venous congestion. If the flap becomes congested, alternative methods of venous supercharging are explored to help salvage the congested flap. A branch of the DIEV (if identified and preserved during dissection) can be used as an additional outflow. The thoracodorsal vein, cephalic vein turndown, and basilic vein can all be explored as secondary options for venous drainage in the setting of technical issues with the use of the retrograde IMV. Vein grafts may be need.

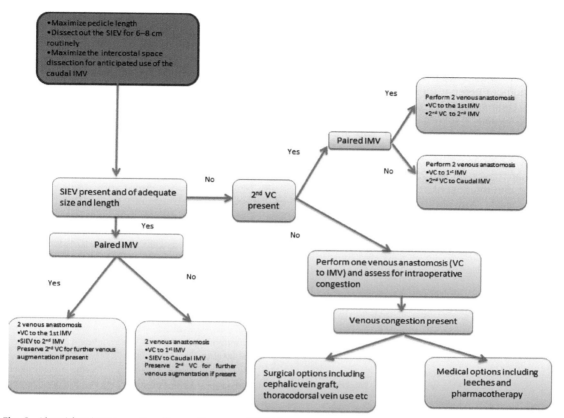

**Fig. 6.** Algorithm incorporating the routine use of SIEV for venous augmentation in a DIEP flap to offset the incidence of intraoperative and postoperative venous congestion.

Rohde and Keller[36] augmented venous drainage by anastomosing the SIEV to the second DIEV, which then drains via a connecting branch to the primary DIEV coupled to the IMV. The authors prefer to use the retrograde IMV over the second vena comitantes, because it is usually readily available and does not need much additional dissection. Pharmacotherapy and leeches are other tools that are valuable in the setting of flap salvage.

## Pitfalls Associated with Performing a Second Anastomosis Routinely

The time for performing a second venous anastomosis may be viewed as a minor disadvantage by some. In the authors' hands, the average time to couple a vein is less than 10 minutes. The retrograde IMV is easily accessible and does not warrant any additional time to dissect. Dissecting out the SIEV adds 10 to 15 minutes to the operative, time but with experience this also has been shown to decrease. Although these few minutes do add to overall operative time, these additional minutes pale in comparison to the time needed for a flap take back or even when compared with the time spent in flap salvage after venous congestion sets in. Performing a second venous anastomosis is much more laborious, technically challenging, and time consuming during a flap take back when compared with routine augmentation at the initial operation. In their experience, the authors have noted less re-exploration since their practice change of routinely augmenting all flaps. No additional morbidity was noted with performing a second anastomosis. Although the authors found no difference in flap loss in 2 methods, overall morbidity was significantly improved with the current method.

## SUMMARY

The use of SIEV for venous augmentation of the DIEP flap has significantly decreased the rates of venous congestion and re-explorations in the authors' patients. Performing a second venous anastomosis routinely using the SIEV to the caudal IMV helps with the inset by narrowing the width of the breast mound and does not add morbidity. The caudal IMV was used as the second outflow channel except in patients who had 2 internal mammary veins. Maximizing the pedicle length during harvest, identifying and dissecting out the SIEV with diligence, and maximizing the intercostal space to enable use of the caudal IMV are keys to the ease of the anastomosis as well as the inset.

The authors present their algorithm for routine venous augmentation in a DIEP flap using the SIEV to the caudal IMV to offset the incidence of venous congestion and overall flap morbidity (see **Fig. 6**). It has been proven that there are really no downsides to routine venous augmentation other than maybe adding 20 minutes to the operative time and the cost of a venous coupler. So the authors ask "…Why not?" In the words of George Bernard Shaw "You see things: and you say; Why? And I dream things that never were; and I say, Why not?"

## REFERENCES

1. Blondeel PN. One hundred free DIEP flap breast reconstructions: a personal experience. Br J Plast Surg 1999;52:104–11.
2. Blondeel PN, Arnstein M, Verstraete K, et al. Venous congestion and blood flow in free transverse rectus abdominis myocutaneous and deep inferior epigastric perforator flaps. Plast Reconstr Surg 2000;106: 1295–9.
3. Selber JC, Serletti JM. The deep inferior epigastric perforator flap: myth and reality. Plast Reconstr Surg 2010;125:50–8.
4. Carramenha e Costa MA, Carriquiry C, Vasconez LO, et al. An anatomic study of the venous drainage of the transverse rectus abdominis musculocutaneous flap. Plast Reconstr Surg 1987;79:208–17.
5. Al-Dhamin A, Bissell MB, Prasad V, et al. The use of retrograde limb of internal mammary vein in autologous breast reconstruction with DIEAP flap: anatomical and clinical study. Ann Plast Surg 2014;72:281–4.
6. Galanis C, Nguyen P, Koh J, et al. Microvascular lifeboats: a stepwise approach to intraoperative venous congestion in DIEP flap breast reconstruction. Plast Reconstr Surg 2014;134:20–7.
7. Kim DY, Lee TJ, Kim EK, et al. Intraoperative venous congestion in free transverse rectus abdominis musculocutaneous and deep inferior epigastric artery perforator flaps during breast reconstruction: a systematic review. Plast Surg (oakv) 2015;23:255–9.
8. Sadik KW, Pasko J, Cohen A, et al. Predictive value of SIEV caliber and superficial venous dominance in free DIEP flaps. J Reconstr Microsurg 2013;29:57–61.
9. Ochoa O, Pisano S, Chrysopoulo M, et al. Salvage of intraoperative deep inferior epigastric perforator flap venous congestion with augmentation of venous outflow: flap morbidity and review of the literature. Plast Reconstr Surg Glob Open 2013;1:e52.
10. Ali R, Bernier C, Lin YT, et al. Surgical strategies to salvage the venous compromised deep inferior epigastric perforator flap. Ann Plast Surg 2010;65: 398–406.
11. Cohn AB, Walton RL. Immediate autologous breast reconstruction using muscle-sparing TRAM flaps with superficial epigastric system turbocharging: a salvage option. J Reconstr Microsurg 2006;22:153–6.
12. Liu TS, Ashjian P, Festekjian J. Salvage of congested deep inferior epigastric perforator flap with a reverse flow venous anastomosis. Ann Plast Surg 2007;59: 214–7.
13. Niranjan NS, Khandwala AR, Mackenzie DM. Venous augmentation of the free TRAM flap. Br J Plast Surg 2001;54:335–7.
14. Tutor EG, Auba C, Benito A, et al. Easy venous superdrainage in DIEP flap breast reconstruction through the intercostal branch. J Reconstr Microsurg 2002;18:595–8.
15. Wechselberger G, Schoeller T, Bauer T, et al. Venous superdrainage in deep inferior epigastric perforator flap breast reconstruction. Plast Reconstr Surg 2001;108:162–6.
16. Blondeel PN. Venous augmentation of the free TRAM flap. Br J Plast Surg 2002;55:87.
17. Guzzetti T, Thione A. The basilic vein: an alternative drainage of DIEP flap in severe venous congestion. Microsurgery 2008;28:555–8.
18. Saint-Cyr M, Chang DW, Robb GL, et al. Internal mammary perforator recipient vessels for breast reconstruction using free TRAM, DIEP, and SIEA flaps. Plast Reconstr Surg 2007;120:1769–73.
19. Saint-Cyr M, Youssef A, Bae HW, et al. Changing trends in recipient vessel selection for microvascular autologous breast reconstruction: an analysis of 1483 consecutive cases. Plast Reconstr Surg 2007;119:1993–2000.
20. Lee KT, Mun GH. Benefits of superdrainage using SIEV in DIEP flap breast reconstruction: a systematic review and meta-analysis. Microsurgery 2017; 37:75–83.
21. Enajat M, Rozen WM, Whitaker IS, et al. A single center comparison of one versus two venous anastomoses in 564 consecutive DIEP flaps: investigating the effect on venous congestion and flap survival. Microsurgery 2010;30:185–91.
22. Boutros SG. Double venous system drainage in deep inferior epigastric perforator flap breast reconstruction: a single-surgeon experience. Plast Reconstr Surg 2013;131:671–6.
23. Li S, Mu L, Li Y, et al. Clinical study of the hemodynamics of both ends (proximal and distal) of internal mammary artery and its following-up. Zhonghua Zheng Xing Wai Ke Za Zhi 2002;18:140–2 [in Chinese].
24. O'Neill AC, Ngan NC, Platt J, et al. A decision-making algorithm for recipient vein selection in bipedicle

deep inferior epigastric artery perforator flap autologous breast reconstruction. J Plast Reconstr Aesthet Surg 2014;67:1089–93.

25. Mackey SP, Ramsey KW. Exploring the myth of the valveless internal mammary vein—a cadaveric study. J Plast Reconstr Aesthet Surg 2011;64:1174–9.

26. Kerr-Valentic MA, Gottlieb LJ, Agarwal JP. The retrograde limb of the internal mammary vein: an additional outflow option in DIEP flap breast reconstruction. Plast Reconstr Surg 2009;124:717–21.

27. Mohebali J, Gottlieb LJ, Agarwal JP. Further validation for use of the retrograde limb of the internal mammary vein in deep inferior epigastric perforator flap breast reconstruction using laser-assisted indocyanine green angiography. J Reconstr Microsurg 2010;26:131–5.

28. Kubota Y, Mitsukawa N, Akita S, et al. Postoperative patency of the retrograde internal mammary vein anastomosis in free flap transfer. J Plast Reconstr Aesthet Surg 2014;67:205–11.

29. Salgarello M, Cervelli D, Barone-Adesi L, et al. Anterograde and retrograde flow anastomoses to the internal mammary vessels in the third intercostal space. J Reconstr Microsurg 2010;26:637–8.

30. Salgarello M, Visconti G, Barone-Adesi L, et al. The retrograde limb of internal mammary vessels as reliable recipient vessels in DIEP flap breast

reconstruction: a clinical and radiological study. Ann Plast Surg 2015;74:447–53.

31. Stalder MW, Lam J, Allen RJ, et al. Using the retrograde internal mammary system for stacked perforator flap breast reconstruction: 71 breast reconstructions in 53 consecutive patients. Plast Reconstr Surg 2016;137:265e–77e.

32. Sugawara J, Satake T, Muto M, et al. Dynamic blood flow to the retrograde limb of the internal mammary vein in breast reconstruction with free flap. Microsurgery 2015;35:622–6.

33. Venturi ML, Poh MM, Chevray PM, et al. Comparison of flow rates in the antegrade and retrograde internal mammary vein for free flap breast reconstruction. Microsurgery 2011;31:596–602.

34. Mohan AT, Zhu L, Wang Z, et al. Techniques and perforator selection in single, dominant DIEP flap breast reconstruction: algorithmic approach to maximize efficiency and safety. Plast Reconstr Surg 2016;138:790e–803e.

35. Rozen WM, Chubb D, Whitaker IS, et al. The importance of the superficial venous anatomy of the abdominal wall in planning a superficial inferior epigastric artery (SIEA) flap: case report and clinical study. Microsurgery 2011;31:454–7.

36. Rohde C, Keller A. Novel technique for venous augmentation in a free deep inferior epigastric perforator flap. Ann Plast Surg 2005;55:528–30.

# Maximizing the Utility of the Pedicled Anterolateral Thigh Flap for Locoregional Reconstruction
## Technical Pearls and Pitfalls

Aparna Vijayasekaran, MBBS, MS[a], Waleed Gibreel, MD[a],
Brian T. Carlsen, MD[a], Steven L. Moran, MD[a],
Michel Saint-Cyr, MD, FRCS(C)[b], Karim Bakri, MBBS[a],
Basel Sharaf, MD, DDS[a],*

## KEYWORDS

- Anterolateral thigh flap (ALT) • Pedicled perforator flap • Perineal reconstruction
- Abdominal reconstruction • Trochanteric reconstruction • ALT flap technique

## KEY POINTS

- The pedicled anterolateral thigh flap (PALT) is reliable, has a good arc of rotation, and can be harvested as a fasciocutaneous flap with or without muscle depending on local anatomy and reconstructive needs. All these features make the flap a versatile option for locoregional reconstruction.
- Understanding the anterolateral thigh (ALT) flap vascular anatomy and its variations helps in flap design and reach.
- When ligating the arterial branch to the rectus femoris muscle, the secondary blood supply to the muscle must be assessed before ligation to avoid muscle necrosis. Also, during ALT flap harvest, care should be taken to preserve the minor pedicles to the rectus femoris muscle and ensure muscle viability.
- Tunneling the flap deep to the rectus femoris and sartorius muscles, ligating the arterial branch to the rectus femoris when deemed necessary and safe, and including the largest distal skin paddle perforator are all key factors in maximizing the reach of the PALT flap for locoregional reconstruction.

## INTRODUCTION

The anterolateral thigh (ALT) flap was initially described as a free flap by Song and colleagues in 1984.[1] It gained popularity after Wei and colleagues[2] published their experience using 672 free ALT flaps over a 14-year period. Since then, the clinical applications of the ALT flap have dramatically increased.[3] The ALT flap was initially heavily used in head and neck reconstruction, and its use has extended to extremity and trunk reconstruction as well. Although primarily described as a free flap, the use of the ALT as a pedicled flap has gained more popularity recently.[4–6] The pedicled anterolateral thigh flap (PALT) has been described for reconstruction of

The authors have nothing to disclose.
[a] Division of Plastic and Reconstructive Surgery, Mayo Clinic, 200 First Street Southwest, Rochester, MN 55905, USA; [b] Division of Plastic Surgery, Baylor Scott & White Health, Scott & White Memorial Hospital, MS-01-E443, 2401 South 31st Street, Temple, TX 76508, USA
* Corresponding author.
*E-mail address:* Sharaf.basel@mayo.edu

Clin Plastic Surg 44 (2017) 371–384
http://dx.doi.org/10.1016/j.cps.2016.12.004

groin and abdominal wounds,[7] perineal,[8,9] peno-scrotal, vaginal, vulvar,[10] trochanteric, ischial,[11] and posterior thigh defects. The PALT reach to reconstruct epigastric and supraumbilical defects has been reported to be reliable in about one-third of the patients.[12] It has also been described as a functional flap for lower abdominal wall recon-struction[13] (**Fig. 1**).

The PALT flap is a versatile flap due to its reliable vascular anatomy, relatively long pedicle, versatile skin paddle, and the feasibility of flap harvest as a chimeric flap based on the profunda artery vascular system. The PALT flap can be harvested as a fasciocutaneous, myocutaneous, or adipofascial flap. In addition, the PALT can be harvested with the rectus femoris (RF), vastus lateralis, or the tensor fascia lata (TFL), depending on the local anatomy and the reconstructive needs. Flap reach can be extended by including a distal perforator when appropriate. Suprafascial harvest has also been described to provide pliable tissue coverage when less flap bulk is needed. Few case series reported the use of PALT flap for locoregional reconstruction, but there is a paucity of technical details pertaining to extending the flap's reach for different anatomic locations. Here the authors review their institutional experience and outcomes using the PALT flap for locoregional reconstruction with an emphasis on technical details pertaining to flap design, elevation, and extending reach.

## PATIENTS AND SURGICAL METHODS
### Patients

Twenty-one consecutive patients underwent PALT for locoregional reconstruction at the Mayo Clinic,

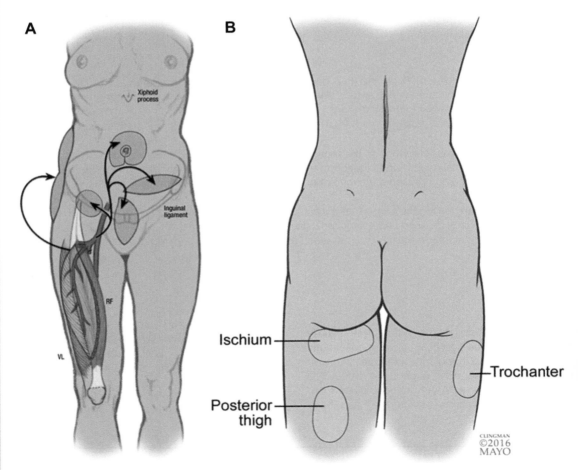

**Fig. 1.** (*A* and *B*) The PALT flap can be used to resurface the lower abdomen, epigastrium, perineum, ipsilateral groin, contralateral groin, trochanter, ischial, posterior thigh, and lower thigh defects. (*A*) Anteriorly, the PALT flap can be extended to reach the ipsilateral groin, suprapubic region/lower abdomen, contralateral groin, and periumbilical region. Laterally, the PALT flap can be extended to reach the lower flank region. (*B*) The PALT flap can reach the posterior thigh via intermuscular tunneling as well the ischial region. The PALT can also be used to resurface the trochanteric region. (Copyright © Mayo Foundation for Medical Education and Research. All rights reserved.)

Rochester, Minnesota from November 2005 to April 2015. Operative details were analyzed including type and number of perforators, flap composition (fasciocutaneous or myofasciocutaneous), flap tunneling methods, intraoperative complications, postoperative complications, and methods of donor site closure. Postoperative complications were divided into early (within 30 days of the operation) and late (after 30 days).

## Data Collection

There were 16 men and 5 women, who underwent PALT flap for locoregional reconstruction at a median age of 41 years. Mean follow-up was 20 months (range 0.4–64). Medical comorbidities were present in 8 (33%) of the patients, with hypertension being the most common medical comorbidity (n = 5), followed by diabetes mellitus (n = 4), hyperlipidemia (n = 4), coronary artery disease (n = 1), and chronic lung disease (n = 1). Only one patient was an active smoker at the time of the operation. Mean body mass index was 26 (range 15–40). In 6 (28%) of the patients, the recipient site received preoperative radiotherapy.

## Indications and Site of the Defect that Needed Coverage

Reconstruction after oncologic resection was the most common indication of PALT flap usage (n = 13), followed by coverage of infected joints/prosthesis (n = 8), and pressure ulcers (n = 3). PALT was used for hip (n = 5), groin (n = 4), proximal thigh (n = 3), trochanteric (n = 3), lower abdomen (n = 2), posterior thigh (n = 2), ischial (n = 1), and vaginal (n = 1) reconstructions.

## Perforator Patterns and Flap Composition

A pattern of septocutaneous and musculocutaneous perforators in the same patient was observed in only 3 patients, and the remaining 18 patients had either septocutaneous (9 patients) or musculocutaneous (9 patients) perforators. Myofasciocutaneous flaps were designed in 16 patients (4 of these were chimeric flaps), fasciocutaneous flaps in 4 patients, and a cutaneous flap in one patient.

## Tunneling Methods

Various tunneling methods were entertained in the authors' series to maximize the effective vascular pedicle length and minimize tension on the pedicle. Passing the flap under the RF muscle was necessary in 5 patients to avoid vascular pedicle compression and maximize length. Division of the sartorius muscle was required in 2 patients for the same reasons.

Tunneling the flap subcutaneously to reach the recipient site was successfully performed in 17 patients. After completion of the subcutaneous tunneling, division of the skin bridge between the donor and recipient sites was performed in 10 of the 17 patients to avoid excessive compression on the PALT vascular pedicle by the skin bridge. This step was not necessary in the remaining 7 patients. In one patient, the flap was passed between the femur and the vastus intermedius muscle to cover a posterior thigh defect. The RF branch of the descending branch of the lateral circumflex femoral artery (LCFA) was divided in 7 patients after confirming rectus muscle viability through secondary perforators after clamping the vessel for 20 minutes. In these cases, the PALT pivot point was proximal to the RF perforator. The remaining patients had the PALT flap pivot point distal to the RF perforator (in these patients, the artery to the RF was preserved). Drain placement at the donor and recipient sites was routine.

## Donor Site Management

The PALT donor site was closed primarily in 11 (52%) patients. Split-thickness skin graft (STSG) was necessary for donor site coverage in the remaining 10 (48%) patients.

## Surgical Outcomes

There were no intraoperative complications. Early postoperative donor site complications occurred in 2 patients (inadequate STSG healing and infected donor site seroma). There were no late (more than 30 days) donor site complications. Two postoperative recipient site complications (one early and one late) occurred during the follow-up period. Both complications were related to recipient site infection of an underlying hip joint. Both complications required reoperation, PALT flap re-elevation, and further bone debridement. During the follow-up duration, no cases of partial or total flap loss were encountered.

## SURGICAL PEARLS AND PITFALLS

The PALT flap is gaining popularity. It is reliable, has a good arc of rotation, has relatively consistent vascular pedicle, and can be elevated as a skin-only flap (suprafascial dissection), fasciocutaneous, or myofasciocutaneous flap. These features make the PALT flap a valuable option for locoregional reconstruction. Various tunneling options to various defect locations and technical pearls to extend flap reach were summarized based on literatures (**Table 1**).

**Table 1**
**Tunneling options for pedicled anterolateral thigh flap to extend its reach to various sites**

| Recipient Site | Options for Tunneling | Technical Pearls and Pitfalls |
|---|---|---|
| Lower abdomen | 1. Divide the skin bridge for inset<br>2. Subcutaneous tunnel over the rectus mainly for lower abdominal defect<br>3. Tunnel under the RF proximal to the rectus branch to increase the medial and superior extent of flap reach<br>4. Alternatively, partially divide the RF laterally to increase reach | • Tunnel proximal to the rectus branch |
| Epigastrium | 1. Tunnel under the RF and sartorius and then change tunneling plane to the suprafascial level to reach the epigastrium | • Usually have to take the rectus branch to reach the epigastrium and lower costal regions |
| Ipsilateral groin | 1. Divide the skin bridge and inset<br>2. Subcutaneous tunnel<br>3. Tunnel under the RF proximal to the rectus arterial branch to increase the medial arc of rotation | |
| Contralateral groin | 1. Medial subcutaneous tunnel extending through the pubic region to the contralateral groin | • Be aware and careful of the medial saphenous vein when tunneling |
| Complex perineal and vaginal reconstruction | 1. Tunnel under the RF and in the medial subcutaneous plane (perineal route)<br>2. Tunnel the flap subcutaneously in the groin and over the inguinal ligament (ligament can be divided lateral to the vessels if needed) to deliver into the pelvis (inguinal route) | • If a large skin paddle is required, the perineal route is preferred for tunneling, although the reach is greater via inguinal region<br>• Inguinal tunneling is usually preferred for an isolated vastus lateralis rather than an ALT |
| Greater trochanteric defects | 1. Lateral subcutaneous tunnel<br>2. Lateral tunnel below the TFL | • Design the flap based on distal perforators to maximize the superior extent of reach of the ALT flap<br>• If a larger skin paddle is needed, divide the skin bridge to help enable inset |
| Ischial defects | 1. Lateral subcutaneous tunnel<br>2. Medial subcutaneous tunnel<br>3. Medial intermuscular pathway<br>4. Directly via the intermuscular septum | • Watch for the saphenous vein when tunneling medially<br>• Consider tunneling via the medial intermuscular pathway when the pedicle length is short |
| Posterior thigh defects | 1. Lateral subcutaneous tunnel<br>2. Medial subcutaneous tunnel<br>3. Intermuscular tunnel via the vastus intermedius muscle | • Decide on tunnel based on where exactly the defect is located in the posterior thigh (posterolateral vs posteromedial). The intermuscular tunnel can be a useful option when the pedicle length is small and a greater reach is needed, especially in an obese patient |

### Vascular Anatomy of the Anterolateral Thigh Flap and Considerations in Flap Design

The descending branch of the LCFA remains the dominant blood supply to PALT flap as well the RF muscle. However, multiple variations have been described in the arterial anatomy of the ALT with the dominant blood supply arising from the ascending (aLCFA), transverse (tLCFA), or oblique branches of the LCFA. The reported incidence of absent skin perforators in the literature ranges from 2% to 10%.[14] In 43% of the cases, the dominant perforator is from the descending branch of the LCFA. Alternatively, the dominant perforator can arise from the ascending, transverse, or oblique branches of the LCFA or on the rare occasion directly from the LCFA, common femoral artery, or the profunda.

The oblique branch of the LCFA is one of the more recently described variants of the profunda system, and it was initially described by Wong and colleagues in 2009[15] with the incidence being 35%. The dominant perforator has classically been described to be in the midthigh within a 3-cm diameter, at a point bisecting a line between the anterior superior iliac spine and the superolateral border of the patella.[16,17] Multiple studies have described the average number of skin perforators to be around 1 to 4.[18,19]

Knowledge of variations in perforator takeoff is critical in safe flap design. Templates and preoperative measurements are useful aids in flap design. Furthermore, flap reach is affected by the patient's body habitus. Leaner patients with longer thighs are better candidates for extended reach PALT flap reconstruction than obese patients with relatively short stature. Including the most reliable distal skin perforator is also necessary to maximize flap reach. The longest ALT pedicle reported was around 37 cm.[20] Although local vascular anatomy of the pedicle and perforators largely dictates flap design and reach, knowledge of these anatomic concepts remains critical in making key flap design changes to optimize reach and outcome.

### Ligating the Arterial Branch to the Rectus Femoris Muscle

Understanding the vascular anatomy of the RF muscle is one of the key factors in extending the PALT flap reach.[14,21] The primary vascular pedicle to the RF can arise from the horizontal branch of the LCFA, from the descending branch of the LCFA, or from the profunda femoris (**Figs. 2 and 3**). When the arterial branch of the RF arises from the LCFA, ligating the RF branch has been shown to extend the reach of the PALT flap as described by Tamai and colleagues.[12]

In the authors' series, 7 out of 21 patients underwent ligation of the arterial branch to the RF muscle to increase flap reach and ease tunneling with no incidence of muscle necrosis. The RF branch is routinely clamped for 20 minutes to evaluate muscle perfusion before ligating the RF branch. SPY angiography can also be used to assess muscle perfusion if necessary. When the RF branch is to

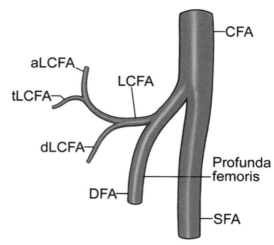

**Fig. 2.** The classic vascular anatomy of the ALT flap. The descending branch of the lateral circumflex femoral artery (dLCFA) remains the dominant blood supply to PALT flap as well the rectus femoris (RF) muscle. However, multiple variations have been described in the arterial anatomy of the ALT with the dominant blood supply arising from the ascending lateral circumflex femoral artery (aLCFA), transverse lateral circumflex femoral artery (tLCFA), or oblique (not demonstrated in picture) branches of the LCFA. CFA, common femoral artery; DFA, deep femoral artery; SFA, superficial femoral artery.

be ligated, distal collateral perforators to the RF from other pedicles should be preserved.

The RF was traditionally described as a type 1 muscle by Mathes and Nahai[22] in 1981 with a single dominant vascular pedicle. However, with the advent of the ALT, many studies have described the existence of an additional codominant oblique branch.[15] Based on recent studies, the vascular anatomy of the RF muscle can be either type A with only one dominant pedicle or type B with a codominant oblique pedicle.[23] The clamping trial of the main RF perforator will help confirm the existence of type B anatomy or other collateral blood supply and allow for safe ligation of the RF branch. Depending on the location of the RF branch along the descending branch of the lateral circumflex femoral axis, ligating the RF branch can extend the reach of the PALT an additional 2 to 5 cm.

### Tunneling Options for Pedicled Anterolateral Thigh Flap to Lower Abdomen and Epigastrium

The PALT has been routinely described for lower abdominal and groin reconstruction.[24] Ting and colleagues[25] reported a case where the PALT was advanced up to the epigastrium. The flap was tunneled under the RF and the sartorius, rotated 180°, and further advanced in the

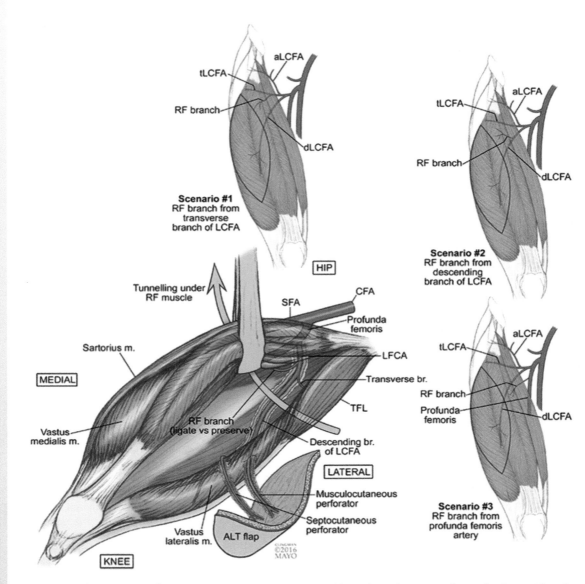

**Fig. 3.** Vascular anatomy of the RF muscle. The primary arterial branch to the RF muscle can be from either the descending branch of the LCFA, transverse branch of the LCFA, or the profundal femoris directly. When the RF branch originates from the LCFA, ligating the arterial branch helps extend the reach of the PALT flap. Br., branch; m., muscle. (Copyright © Mayo Foundation for Medical Education and Research. All rights reserved.)

suprafascial plane. Tamai and colleagues[12] recently published a cadaveric study and concluded that the PALT can reach the umbilicus in less than one-third of the patients.[12] Tunneling the flap below the RF and the sartorius after ligating the arterial branch of the RF was shown to significantly increase flap reach (**Fig. 4**).

### Tunneling Options for Pedicled Anterolateral Thigh Flap to Ipsilateral Groin

The PALT flap is an ideal choice for groin reconstruction and has been increasingly used in

addition to the more traditional RF or vertical rectus abdominis flap.[26–28] The PALT can be tunneled either under or over the RF muscle to reach the ipsilateral groin (**Fig. 5A**). Another option would be to perform lateral myotomy to extend the pedicle reach. Lateral RF myotomy should be reserved only for challenging scenarios because this maneuver weakens the RF muscle, a powerful knee extender. Care should be taken to preserve the RF muscle especially when the vastus lateralis muscle is elevated with the PALT.

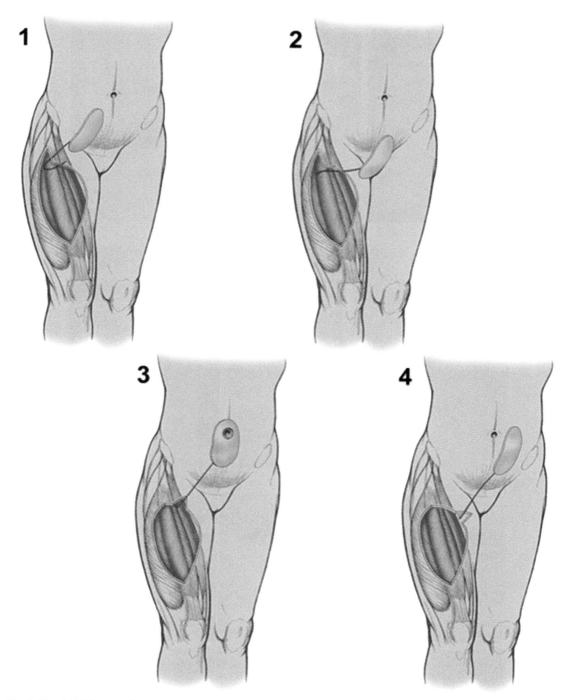

**Fig. 4.** The PALT flap can be tunneled over the RF muscle (1, 2), under the RF and over the sartorius (3), or under both the RF and the sartorius (4). Although tunneling the PALT flap (especially the larger flaps) under both muscles can be technically challenging, this maneuver is necessary to extend flap reach. (Copyright © Mayo Foundation for Medical Education and Research. All rights reserved.)

A

B

C

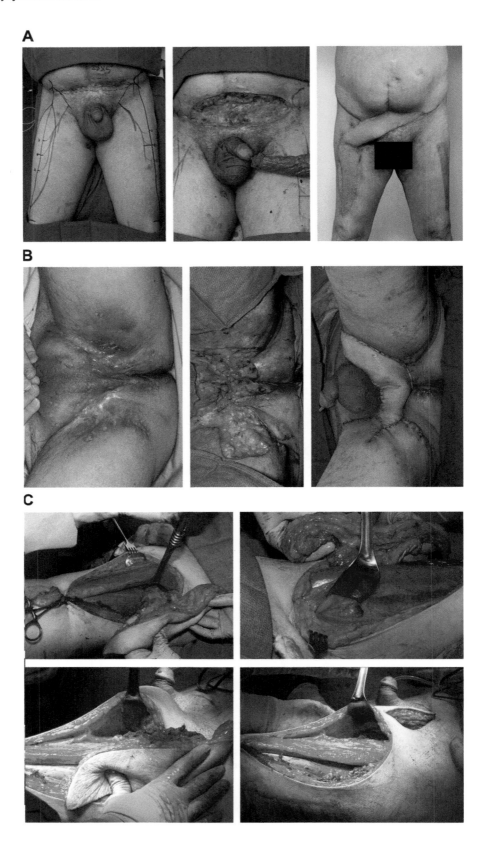

## Tunneling Options for Pedicled Anterolateral Thigh Flap to Contralateral Groin

The PALT flap when designed appropriately can be extended to reach the contralateral groin and anterior superior iliac spine. Designing the flap and incorporating the most distal skin paddle perforator, dissecting the pedicle to its origin from the LCFA, and selective ligation of the arterial branch to the RF are all necessary to increase reach. When tunneling, the flap should be tunneled under the RF whenever possible to increase flap reach. Lateral myotomies of the RF may be necessary also. Care should be taken to identify the vascular anatomy so as to pursue the maximal extent of safe dissection to extend flap reach. In the patient who underwent resection of lower abdominal skin for hidradenitis, the authors designed a large skin paddle extending distally and tunneled the flap under the rectus muscle. They used an endoscopic plastic bag to wrap the flap. Surgical lube was applied to the bag, and the flap was tunneled to facilitate passing under the RF muscle. The authors did not ligate the arterial branch to the RF because the patient had type A anatomy.

## Tunneling Options for Pedicled Anterolateral Thigh Flap to Perineum and Pelvic Floor

The PALT flap is useful for vaginal, perineal, and urologic reconstruction. The options for tunneling a PALT flap to the perineum include (1) subcutaneously in the tissues of the medial thigh, (2) under the RF muscle (with or without ligating the arterial branch), and (3) tunneling under the sartorius muscle. When tunneling subcutaneously in the medial thigh, care must be taken to avoid injury to the saphenous vein. Tunneling under the RF muscle does increase the pedicle reach, but if the vastus lateralis muscle is harvested along with the PALT flap adding to flap bulk, tunneling medially becomes more difficult, and hence, ligating the arterial branch to the rectus muscle must be considered to facilitate tunneling. The other option would be to divide the intervening skin bridge. Tunneling under the sartorius is also needed

sometimes based on the location of the defect. Proximal perforators to the sartorius muscle can be ligated to help tunnel the pedicle under this muscle. This is feasible without sacrificing the muscle given segmental blood supply to this muscle. It is imperative to inset the flap without any tension on the pedicle. In one of the authors' patients, they tunneled the flap under the sartorius to reach the defect, and given the size of the defect, a pedicled gracilis flap for additional resurfacing of the perineal floor was required (**Fig. 6**).

## Tunneling Options for Pedicled Anterolateral Thigh Flap to Posterior Thigh

Tunneling a PALT to the posterior thigh was first described by Batdorf and colleagues[29] in 2013 in 2 patients (**Fig. 7**). The descending branch of the LCFA was dissected all the way to the origin after ligating the arterial branch to the RF. A limited portion of the vastus intermedius was elevated from the femur, and an intermuscular tunnel was created to reach the posterior thigh (**Fig. 8A**). The flap was tunneled transmuscularly, and the patient was repositioned and flap inset completed in the lateral position (**Fig. 8B**). Acland clamps were used to assess the viability of the RF flap with clamping the RF branch before ligating the RF branch as described earlier.

## Tunneling Options of Pedicled Anterolateral Thigh Flap to Greater Trochanteric Defects and Hip Defects

The TFL flap for covering trochanteric defects was initially described by Nahai and colleagues[30,31] and has remained the gold standard for covering trochanteric defects. However, use of the TFL has been limited by flap tip necrosis, dog ear deformities, limited flap size, and lack of bulk. In 2006, Wang and colleagues[32] described their experience in 21 patients using the PALT flap for trochanteric coverage. The lateral subcutaneous tunnel remains the easiest way to tunnel the flap to the defect, and the skin bridge can be divided if necessary to directly transpose the flap into the defect (**Figs. 9 and 10**).

**Fig. 5.** (*A–C*) Staged reconstruction in a 58-year-old male patient with stage 4 hidradenitis suppurativa in proximity to abdominal mesh, necessitating soft tissue coverage of lower abdomen, groin, as well the perineum using bilateral PALT flaps. (*A*) Planned wide local excision of affected skin and flap design. The affected lower abdominal and bilateral groin skin was excised, and the soft tissue defect was resurfaced with a PALT flap (28 × 7 cm) from the right thigh. The flap was tunneled distal to the RF arterial branch to enable reach to the lower abdomen and contralateral groin. (*B*) One year later, the remaining disease in the scrotal/perineal region was excised, and the resulting defect was resurfaced using a PALT flap (33 × 10 cm) from the left side. (*C*) During this procedure, the flap was tunneled under the RF (*top left* and *right*) and then subcutaneously (*bottom left* and *right*) to enable reach to the contralateral perineum and groin. The rectus branch was not ligated during this procedure.

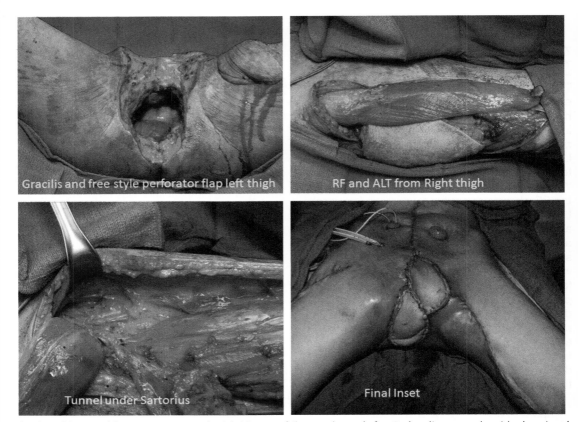

**Fig. 6.** A 39-year-old woman presented with history of ileo-anal pouch for Crohn disease and residual perineal disease and multiple fistulas. She underwent pelvic exenteration. The resulting large perineal defect with significant pelvic empty space required vascular tissue coverage. The vertical rectus abdominis muscle flap was not an option in this patient because the patient had ostomies on both sides of the abdomen. Her extensive defect was reconstructed with a pedicled RF flap and PALT flap from the right thigh, a pedicled gracilis muscle, and freestyle perforator flap from the left thigh. The skin paddle from the PALT was used to resurface the perineum, and the skin paddle from the perforator flap was used to resurface the superior aspect of the defect. The RF and the gracilis flaps were used to obliterate the pelvic cavity.

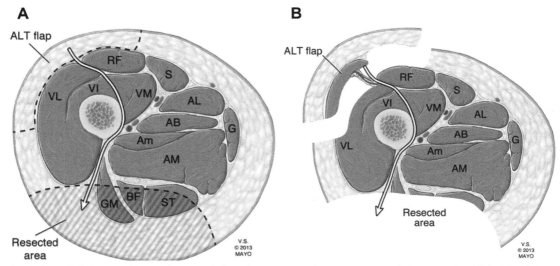

**Fig. 7.** (*A* and *B*) The PALT flap can be tunneled via the intermuscular septum to reach the posterior thigh. AB, adductor brevis; AL, adductor longus; Am, adductor minimus; AM, adductor magnus; BF, biceps femoris; G, gracilis; GM, gluteus maximus; RF, rectus femoris; VI, vastus intermedius; VL, vastus lateralis; VM, vastus medialis; S, sartorius; ST, semitendinosus. (Copyright © Mayo Foundation for Medical Education and Research. All rights reserved.)

**A**

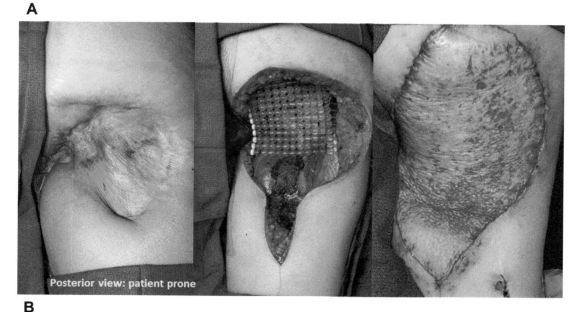

**B**

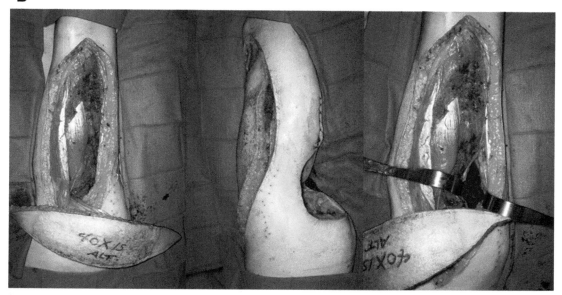

**Fig. 8.** (*A* and *B*) PALT flap for posterior thigh reconstruction. (*A*) A 38-year-old woman presented with a recurrent large epithelioid sarcoma of the upper posterior thigh. She underwent neoadjuvant radiation followed by surgical resection and intraoperative radiation. (*A*) The large defect in the posterior thigh after resection and the final reconstruction using a PALT flap, which was tunneled via the intermuscular septum. (*B*) The anterior view (*left*) where a large ALT (40 × 15 cm) flap was raised. The patient is shown in a lateral decubitus position (*middle*) after flap elevation showing the posterior thigh defect, and (*right*) the intramuscular septum tunnel created.

## Tunneling Options for Pedicled Anterolateral Thigh Flap to Ischial Defects

Traditional options for soft tissue coverage of ischial defects are gluteal flaps, V-Y advancement flaps, and posterior thigh flaps. The PALT flap is valuable for coverage of recurrent defects.[11] Initial

reports described the use of the lateral subcutaneous tunnel for the pathway. Tunneling the flap subcutaneously, however, may make flap reach to the intended defect more difficult even when the descending branch of the LCFA is dissected up to its origin.[11,33] Designing the flap with a distal skin paddle to increase the reach

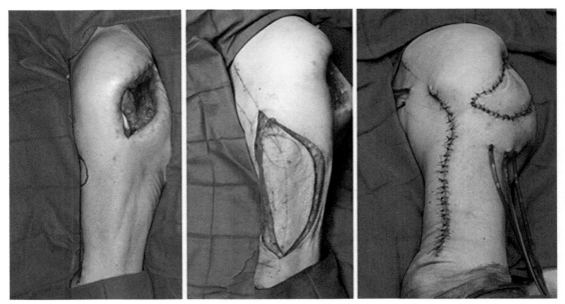

**Fig. 9.** A 64-year-old paraplegic man presented with a stage 4 left greater trochanteric ulcer. After adequate bony debridement, the defect was resurfaced using a PALT flap. The flap was tunneled subcutaneously.

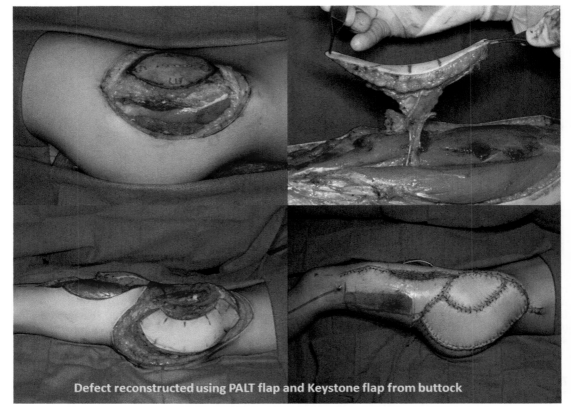

Defect reconstructed using PALT flap and Keystone flap from buttock

**Fig. 10.** An 8-year-old boy presented with large extraskeletal chondrosarcoma of the left gluteal region. The defect was reconstructed using a combination of unilateral PALT flap and keystone flap from the lateral gluteal region. Given the close proximity to the defect, the skin bridge was divided and the flap was then inset without any tension. A posterior gluteal keystone flap was designed and used to resurface the posterior aspect of the defect and minimize tension on PALT flap inset.

of the flap is required. When a distal perforator is not present, however, an increased risk of congestion and flap compromise may be encountered. In 2006, Lee and colleagues[33] reported transmuscular tunneling of the flap via the upper thigh to reach the ischium. They found that the distance between the origin of the LCFA and the ischium is 10 to 15 cm through this pathway, and this is a much shorter route when compared with the lateral subcutaneous tunnel. In the authors' patient series, they were able to use the lateral tunnel to reach the defect in all patients; however, they recognize that the transmuscular pathway will be an important tool to consider especially in more challenging body habitus, such as in morbidly obese patients.

## SUMMARY

Although excellent reconstructive outcomes can be achieved using PALT flaps, the authors' results highlight strategies to maximize the PALT flap reach. Understanding the vascular anatomy of the PALT and RF muscle and incorporating this anatomic knowledge in flap design and tunneling are important to extend flap reach. Tunneling the flap deep to the RF and sartorius muscles, ligating the arterial branch to the RF, and incorporating the most distal perforator to the skin paddle when possible are all key factors in maximizing the utility of the PALT flap for locoregional reconstruction.

## REFERENCES

1. Song YG, Chen GZ, Song YL. The free thigh flap: a new free flap concept based on the septocutaneous artery. Br J Plast Surg 1984;37:149–59.
2. Wei FC, Jain V, Celik N, et al. Have we found an ideal soft-tissue flap? An experience with 672 anterolateral thigh flaps. Plast Reconstr Surg 2002;109: 2219–26.
3. Gedebou TM, Wei FC, Lin CH. Clinical experience of 1284 free anterolateral thigh flaps. Handchir Mikrochir Plast Chir 2002;34:239–44.
4. Lee YC, Chiu HY, Shieh SJ. The clinical application of anterolateral thigh flap. Plast Surg Int 2011; 2011:127353.
5. Neligan PC, Lannon DA. Versatility of the pedicled anterolateral thigh flap. Clin Plast Surg 2010;37: 677–81.
6. Ng RW, Chan JY, Mok V, et al. Clinical use of a pedicled anterolateral thigh flap. J Plast Reconstr Aesthet Surg 2008;61:158–64.
7. Zelken JA, AlDeek NF, Hsu CC, et al. Algorithmic approach to lower abdominal, perineal, and groin reconstruction using anterolateral thigh flaps. Microsurgery 2016;36:104–14.
8. Lannon DA, Ross GL, Addison PD, et al. Versatility of the proximally pedicled anterolateral thigh flap and its use in complex abdominal and pelvic reconstruction. Plast Reconstr Surg 2011;127:677–88.
9. Wong S, Garvey P, Skibber J, et al. Reconstruction of pelvic exenteration defects with anterolateral thigh-vastus lateralis muscle flaps. Plast Reconstr Surg 2009;124:1177–85.
10. Zhang W, Zeng A, Yang J, et al. Outcome of vulvar reconstruction by anterolateral thigh flap in patients with advanced and recurrent vulvar malignancy. J Surg Oncol 2015;111:985–91.
11. Kua EH, Wong CH, Ng SW, et al. The island pedicled anterolateral thigh (pALT) flap via the lateral subcutaneous tunnel for recurrent ischial ulcers. J Plast Reconstr Aesthet Surg 2011;64:e21–3.
12. Tamai M, Nagasao T, Miki T, et al. Rotation arc of pedicled anterolateral thigh flap for abdominal wall reconstruction: how far can it reach? J Plast Reconstr Aesthet Surg 2015;68:1417–24.
13. Vranckx JJ, Stoel AM, Segers K, et al. Dynamic reconstruction of complex abdominal wall defects with the pedicled innervated vastus lateralis and anterolateral thigh PIVA flap. J Plast Reconstr Aesthet Surg 2015;68:837–45.
14. Lakhiani C, Lee MR, Saint-Cyr M. Vascular anatomy of the anterolateral thigh flap: a systematic review. Plast Reconstr Surg 2012;130:1254–68.
15. Wong CH, Wei FC, Fu B, et al. Alternative vascular pedicle of the anterolateral thigh flap: the oblique branch of the lateral circumflex femoral artery. Plast Reconstr Surg 2009;123:571–7.
16. Ribuffo D, Atzeni M, Saba L, et al. Angio computed tomography preoperative evaluation for anterolateral thigh flap harvesting. Ann Plast Surg 2009;62:368–71.
17. Kim EK, Kang BS, Hong JP. The distribution of the perforators in the anterolateral thigh and the utility of multidetector row computed tomography angiography in preoperative planning. Ann Plast Surg 2010;65:155–60.
18. Valdatta L, Tuinder S, Buoro M, et al. Lateral circumflex femoral arterial system and perforators of the anterolateral thigh flap: an anatomic study. Ann Plast Surg 2002;49:145–50.
19. Zhang Q, Qiao Q, Gould LJ, et al. Study of the neural and vascular anatomy of the anterolateral thigh flap. J Plast Reconstr Aesthet Surg 2010;63:365–71.
20. Sananpanich K, Tu YK, Kraisarin J, et al. Flow-through anterolateral thigh flap for simultaneous soft tissue and long vascular gap reconstruction in extremity injuries: anatomical study and case report. Injury 2008;39:47–54.
21. Wong CH, Ong YS, Wei FC. Revisiting vascular supply of the rectus femoris and its relevance in the harvest of the anterolateral thigh flap. Ann Plast Surg 2013;71:586–90.

22. Mathes SJ, Nahai F. Classification of the vascular anatomy of muscles: experimental and clinical correlation. Plast Reconstr Surg 1981;67:177–87.

23. Schaverien M, Saint-Cyr M, Arbique G, et al. Three- and four-dimensional computed tomographic angiography and venography of the anterolateral thigh perforator flap. Plast Reconstr Surg 2008;121:1685–96.

24. Kayano S, Sakuraba M, Miyamoto S, et al. Comparison of pedicled and free anterolateral thigh flaps for reconstruction of complex defects of the abdominal wall: review of 20 consecutive cases. J Plast Reconstr Aesthet Surg 2012;65:1525–9.

25. Ting J, Trotter D, Grinsell D. A pedicled anterolateral thigh (ALT) flap for reconstruction of the epigastrium. Case report. J Plast Reconstr Aesthet Surg 2010;63: e65–7.

26. LoGiudice JA, Haberman K, Sanger JR. The anterolateral thigh flap for groin and lower abdominal defects: a better alternative to the rectus abdominis flap. Plast Reconstr Surg 2014;133:162–8.

27. Chao AH, McCann GA, Fowler JM. Bilateral groin reconstruction with a single anterolateral thigh perforator flap as an alternative to traditional myocutaneous flaps. Gynecol Oncol Case Rep 2014;9:15–7.

28. Aslim EJ, Rasheed MZ, Lin F, et al. Use of the anterolateral thigh and vertical rectus abdominis musculocutaneous flaps as utility flaps in reconstructing large groin defects. Arch Plast Surg 2014;41:556–61.

29. Batdorf NJ, Lettieri SC, Saint-Cyr M. Trans-vastus intermedius transfer of the pedicled anterolateral thigh flap for posterior thigh reconstruction. Plast Reconstr Surg Glob Open 2014;1:e81.

30. Nahai F. The tensor fascia lata flap. Clin Plast Surg 1980;7:51–6.

31. Nahai F, Hill L, Hester TR. Experiences with the tensor fascia lata flap. Plast Reconstr Surg 1979; 63:788–99.

32. Wang CH, Chen SY, Fu JP, et al. Reconstruction of trochanteric pressure sores with pedicled anterolateral thigh myocutaneous flaps. J Plast Reconstr Aesthet Surg 2011;64:671–6.

33. Lee JT, Cheng LF, Lin CM, et al. A new technique of transferring island pedicled anterolateral thigh and vastus lateralis myocutaneous flaps for reconstruction of recurrent ischial pressure sores. J Plast Reconstr Aesthet Surg 2007;60: 1060–6.

# Keystone and Pedicle Perforator Flaps in Reconstructive Surgery
## New Modifications and Applications

Jasson T. Abraham, MD, Michel Saint-Cyr, MD, FRCS(C)*

## KEYWORDS

• Keystone flap • Perforator flap • Reconstruction

## KEY POINTS

• The increase in knowledge of vascular anatomy, including the concept of the perforasome theory and perforator hot-spot versus cold-spot anatomy, has led to significant advances in reconstructive options.
• Pedicle perforator flap (PPF)–based reconstruction benefits patients by using autologous tissue for reconstruction and decreases operative morbidity by limiting transfer of tissue on perforators.
• Freestyle PPF allows greater degrees of freedom in operative planning, because flaps can be based on any dominant perforator.
• Keystone perforator island flap is a multiperforator advancement flap based on musculocutaneous or fasciocutaneous perforators with high rates of flap survival, decreased donor site morbidity and pain, and quick patient recovery.

## INTRODUCTION

Initial descriptions of perforator flaps in 1989 by Koshima and Soeda,[1] by using a musculocutaneous flap with an inferior epigastric artery–based skin island for reconstruction of defects involving the floor of mouth and groin, have led to significant additional advancements in the understanding of perforator flaps and vascular anatomy. Kroll and Rosenfield[2] reported that perforator flaps had vascular reliability comparable with musculocutaneous flaps, but limited donor site morbidity by avoiding muscle harvest. The transfer of tissues therefore is not limited by the requirement to include muscle or underlying deep fascia for adequate tissue perfusion. Milton[3] showed that the inclusion of a pedicle with a large vessel was critical for flap survival, and also dictated the viable length of harvest for islanded flaps.

Further modifications of the perforator flap led to the advent of the propeller flaps, first introduced in 1991 by Hyakusoku and colleagues,[4] with later modifications by Hallock[5] and Teo.[6] Propeller flaps allow significant tissue reconstruction with ideal like-for-like tissue, and maintain similar complication rates to free flap reconstruction.[7–12] Recent advances in the understanding of vascular anatomy have led to significant advancements and freedom in perforator-based reconstruction. Taylor and Palmer[13] introduced the angiosome concept, which was further detailed in many additional studies evaluating the static vascular territories of every source vessel and their perforators.[13–26] Further anatomic studies by Saint-Cyr and colleagues[27–29] and other investigators[30–34] introduced the perforasome concept of distinct vascular territories of individual perforators, which

The authors have nothing to disclose.
Division of Plastic Surgery, Baylor Scott & White Health, Scott & White Memorial Hospital, Temple, TX, USA
* Corresponding author. Division of Plastic Surgery, Baylor Scott & White Health, 2401 South 31st Street, Temple, TX 76508.
E-mail address: Michel.SaintCyr@BSWHealth.org

plasticsurgery.theclinics.com

are dynamic and have significant interactions with adjacent perforating vessels or perforasomes.

The keystone perforator island flap (KPIF) is a versatile flap that was originally described by Behan[35] for reconstruction of defects after excision of skin cancer, and has since been used for the reconstruction of defects located on the head and neck, trunk, and extremities.[35–38] Modifications in planning, design, and execution of the KPIF by relying on a sound understanding of vascular anatomy and the perforasome theory by Saint-Cyr and colleagues have allowed large defect reconstruction after tumor resection, with high rates of flap survival, low risk of significant complications, decreased pain, and quicker postoperative recovery.[39]

## PERFORASOME PRINCIPLES

The ability of a single arterial perforator to adequately vascularize large volumes of soft tissue for reconstruction can only be understood with a comprehensive understanding of the perforasome theory. A perforasome is described as the unique vascular territory of a single arterial perforator from an underlying source vessel. Four major principles elucidate the ability of a single perforator to sustain a large volume of soft tissue, and the consistent preferential direction of vascular flow.[29,40]

1. Perforasomes are linked with adjacent perforasomes by direct and indirect linking vessels (**Fig. 1**). Direct linking vessels are larger vessels that directly connect one perforator to another in the suprafascial plexus, whereas indirect perforators connect one perforator to another through the subdermal plexus.[29] In addition, there are communicating branches that connect direct linking vessels to indirect linking vessels. Interperforator flow is bidirectional, with directionality of flow dependent on perforator perfusion pressures. With adequate perfusion pressure, a single perforator can vascularize multiple perforasomes via interperforator flow.

2. Design of the flap and orientation of the skin paddle should be in the same direction as the linking vessels, which are axial in the extremities and perpendicular to the midline in the trunk. Linking vessels allow for interperforator communication between perforators from the

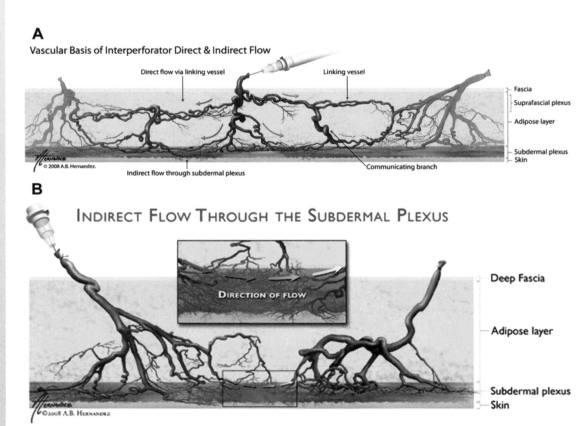

**Fig. 1.** (*A, B*) Linking vessels, direct and indirect. (*Courtesy of* Alexandra B. Hernandez, M.A. of Gory Details Illustration; with permission.)

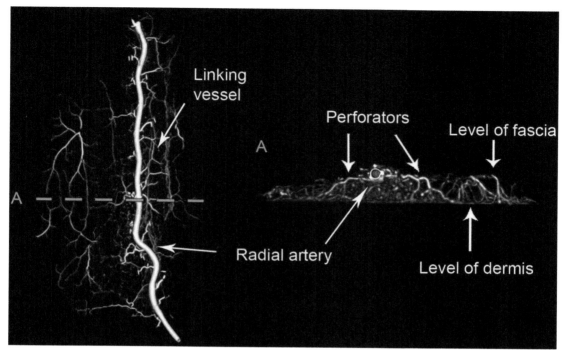

**Fig. 2.** Linking vessels parallel to long axis of limb and parallel to source artery.

same underlying source arteries and with perforators of adjacent source arteries (**Fig. 2**).

3. Perforators from the same source artery are preferentially filled by interperforator flow. In addition, if a source artery has minimal perforating vessels along its vascular path, there is a decrease in the axial pattern of its vascular distribution because there are fewer interperforator linking vessels (**Fig. 3**).

4. Directionality of a perforator can be determined based on its proximity to an articulation. Perforators found adjacent to an articulation have preferential directionality away from the articulation, whereas perforators between 2 articulations or at the midpoint of the trunk have multidirectional flow (**Fig. 4**).

These principles explain how large volumes of soft tissue can be harvested, because hyperperfusion of a single perforator can capture multiple adjacent perforasomes, with preferential flow in the direction of the linking vessels, reflecting the path of the underlying source artery.[41]

## PERFORATOR HOT SPOT VERSUS COLD SPOT

There are nearly 400 perforators in the body, on each of which a pedicle-based flap can be raised, allowing multiple alternative reconstructive options.[13,40,42,43] Perforator flaps have been described for reconstruction of the breast, head and neck, and extremities. The perforators are not distributed evenly, because the body has areas of higher perforator density, called hot spots, and areas of lower perforator density, called cold spots (**Fig. 5**). Hot spots are consistently found in the same areas of the body. In the extremities, they are found typically adjacent to articulations and midway between 2 articulations, whereas in the trunk they are found parallel to the anterior and posterior midline, and midaxillary regions.[44–47] Knowledge of hot-spot territories allows optimal surgical planning of the flap, and permits quicker surgical dissection in cold spots.

## PERFUSION PRINCIPLES: PERFORATOR LOCATION AND ANGLE OF PERFUSION

The volume of soft tissue that can safely be harvested in a pedicle perforator flap (PPF) depends on the ability of the dominant perforator to adequately perfuse the entire flap. Principles that aid in optimizing the vascularity of a flap include the relative position of the dominant perforator within the flap, and the angle of perfusion. Designing flaps with the primary perforating vessel positioned centrally allows for greater interperforator flow by preserving the linking vessels (direct and indirect) and the communicating vessels, resulting in a greater number of adjacent

Perfusion in Multiple Perforasomes via Linking Vessels

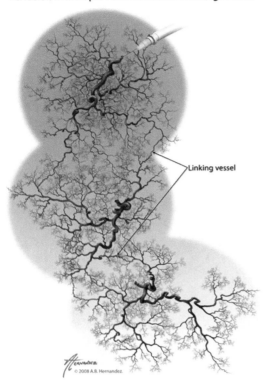

**Fig. 3.** Preferential filling of interperforator flow within same source artery. (*Courtesy of* Alexandra B. Hernandez, M.A. of Gory Details Illustration; with permission.)

perforasomes that are vascularized. Eccentric positioning of a perforator decreases the volume of tissue that can safely be harvested.[48] However, if great care is taken to ensure that the linking

vessels are parallel to the long axis of the designed flap, complications of flap loss can be avoided or minimized (**Fig. 6**).

The angle of perfusion of a perforator is defined as the angle of vascular perfusion flowing away from the perforator and confined by the mechanical borders of the flap. The angle is measured at the proximal aspect of the flap. In a cadaveric study of anterolateral thigh flaps, area of perfusion and percentage of flap perfusion were evaluated based on differing angles of perfusion, by using computed tomography (CT) angiography. Decreasing the angle of perfusion resulted in a significant decrease in the volume and percentage of flap perfusion. An acute angle of perfusion (60°) is thought to be disruptive of interperforator flow by failing to incorporate linking vessels between adjacent perforators, and thus decreasing flap perfusion.[48] The flap vascularization by the dominant perforator can be optimized by positioning the perforator in the central portion of the flap and by avoiding an acute angle of perfusion at the proximal aspect of the flap. These modifications allow for increased interperforator flow by incorporating critical linking vessels, resulting in a robustly perfused flap.

## BENEFITS OF PERFORATOR FLAPS

PPF allow complex locoregional reconstruction while avoiding microsurgical free-flap reconstruction and monitoring.[40] The main advantages of perforator flaps include sparing of underlying muscle, decreased donor site morbidity, decreased operative times, and improved aesthetic outcome by supplying like with like for optimal texture, thickness, and color match (**Fig. 7**). The KPIF is a

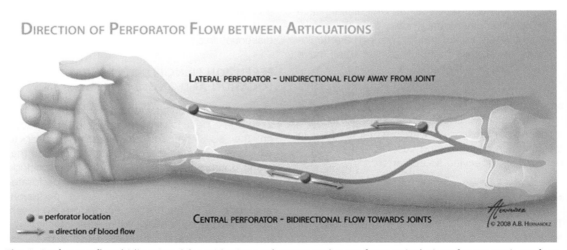

**Fig. 4.** Perforator flow bidirectional for midpoint perforators and away from articulations for eccentric perforators. (*Courtesy of* Alexandra B. Hernandez, M.A. of Gory Details Illustration; with permission.)

**A**

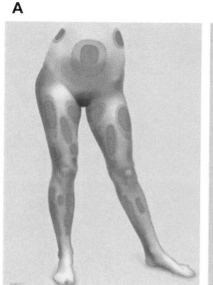
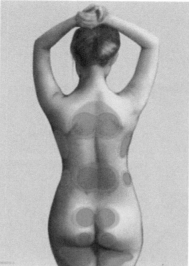
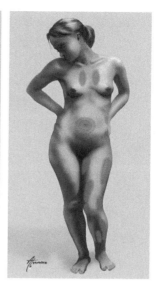

**B**

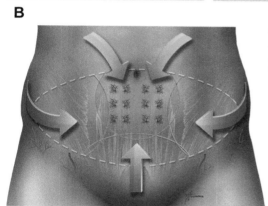

**Fig. 5.** (*A*) Hot spot and cold spots of perforator distribution throughout the body. (*B*) Perforator hot spot concentrated around the umbilicus in the abdomen. (*Courtesy of Alexandra B. Hernandez, M.A. of Gory Details Illustration; with permission.*)

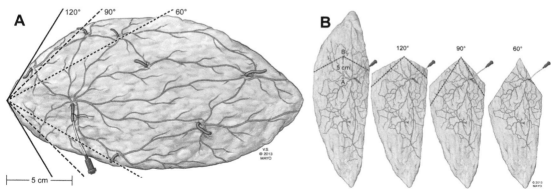

**Fig. 6.** (*A, B*) Angle of perfusion of PPF. The more eccentric the perforator is located within the flap, the wider the angle of perfusion needs to be in order to incorporate as many linking vessels as possible and maximize perfusion. (Copyright © Mayo Foundation for Medical Education and Research. All rights reserved.)

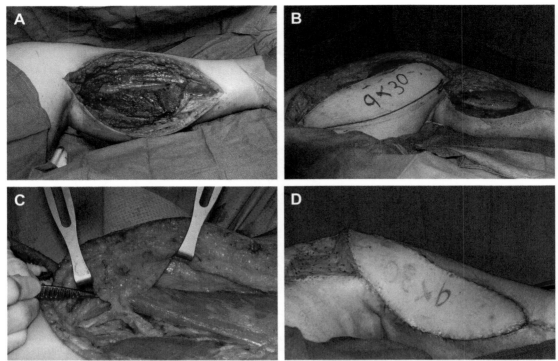

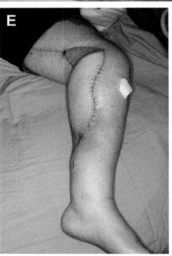

**Fig. 7.** (*A–D*) PPF based on a perforator from the superficial femoral artery. Flap was used for coverage of a soft tissue defect following postsarcoma resection in the medial-proximal left leg. (*E*) Final result with stable coverage four weeks after surgery.

single flap based on multiple perforators that has shown excellent reconstructive outcomes for large defects while avoiding free-flap reconstruction and allowing shorter operative times, fairly pain-free postoperative course, and shorter duration of hospitalization, and is ideal for patients with multiple comorbidities who are unable to undergo prolonged complex reconstructive procedures (**Fig. 8**).

## PATIENT SELECTION AND PREOPERATIVE PLANNING

Each patient presents a unique challenge to the reconstructive surgeon because each patient introduces individual-specific comorbidities, including prior trauma, reconstructive surgery, prior irradiation, and smoking, all of which affect the vascularity and mobility of the adjacent tissue. When evaluating a patient for reconstruction with a

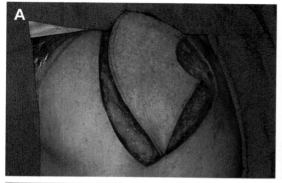
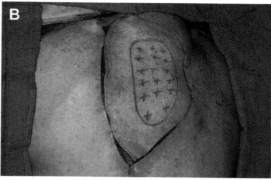
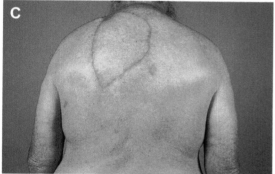

**Fig. 8.** (*A–C*) Keystone flap for coverage of central upper back defect following melanoma excision. Note the multiple perforators preserved within the central portion of the flap. The flap area peripheral to these perforators was undermined for additional advancement with minimal tension.

KPIF or PPF, it is critical to evaluate the defect and the quality of the adjacent tissue, particularly noting the soft tissue laxity. Preoperative imaging is not routinely indicated for identification of perforators, because sound knowledge of perforator location based on the hot-spot principle, in conjunction with Doppler evaluation of the adjacent tissue, is sufficient (**Fig. 9**). Radiographic studies that are preoperatively obtained by the oncologic team for evaluation of tumor invasiveness, including CT or MRI, can help identify large perforators in the vicinity of the malignancy. In circumstances requiring the evaluation of traumatic wounds involving extremities, imaging can be obtained of the vascular anatomy to assess vascular injury with angiography or CT angiography.[40,42]

## PEDICLE PERFORATOR FLAPS

PPF have introduced a paradigm shift in the planning of reconstructive surgery, particularly introducing a significant element of freedom in flap design, resulting in multiple options for wound closure.[49] Using the hot-spot principle, and familiarity with the location of dominant perforators, PPF can be harvested on any substantially sized perforator with the aid of a Doppler.[40,42] Depending on the location of the pedicle in the designed flap and the length of pedicle dissected, flaps can achieve

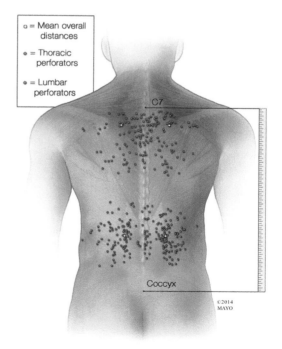

**Fig. 9.** Perforator density distribution in the back with a hot-spot concentration within 10 cm from the midline. (Copyright © Mayo Foundation for Medical Education and Research. All rights reserved.)

significant rotational freedom. The propeller flap can achieve complete 180° rotation with appropriate surgical planning and execution.[40] PPF can be used for reconstruction of defects located on the trunk, head and neck, and extremities.[40] Examples of commonly used perforators for PPF include perforators from the superficial femoral artery, deep inferior epigastric artery, profunda artery, descending branch of lateral circumflex femoral artery, and lateral superior genicular artery.

## FREESTYLE PERFORATOR FLAP

However, it is important to understand that PPF are not limited to known dominant perforators, and there is no need to rely on conventional flap design. This liberty has resulted in the freestyle perforator concept of designing a flap on any dominant perforator adjacent to the defect for ad hoc reconstruction (**Fig. 10**). The ability to raise a freestyle flap on a single dominant pedicle has been further revolutionized by Wei and Mardini,[50] by raising freestyle free perforator flaps.

## PEDICLE PERFORATOR FLAP DESIGN

PPF are conventionally designed with an elliptical skin paddle, but can be altered to meet the reconstructive requirements (eg, triangular pedicle perforator flap for V-Y advancement; **Fig. 11**). Flaps are harvested larger than the anticipated defect to account for limited tissue laxity, allow

for flap inset under minimal tension, and to accommodate postoperative swelling.[42] Perforators are identified in the tissue adjacent to the defect with a Doppler.[40] All Doppler-able perforators are marked on the skin, and a line is drawn over the path of the dominant axial vessels connecting the perforators, with specific marking of the most dominant perforator.[42] Dominant perforator identification is not necessary when the skin island is advanced as a multiperforator flap.

A skin paddle is then designed incorporating the most dominant perforator, with the long axis of the flap oriented parallel to the directionality of vascular flow, which is oriented axially along the extremities and perpendicular to midline in the trunk.[39] Doing so facilitates the inclusion of linking vessels and increases the likelihood of primary closure of the donor site.[40] The surgeon should plan backup options for reconstruction before wholly committing to a designed PPF. An initial exploratory incision is made on one side of the planned flap, with care taken to avoid the violation of potential secondary reconstructive options.[40,42] The dominant perforator is surgically isolated and evaluated with the Doppler, and confirmed visually to be of adequate caliber (>0.5 mm). The pedicle can be further dissected to gain additional length for flap advancement.

If the perforator is of adequate quality, the flap is incised circumferentially along the planned skin paddle margin and advanced into the defect. Flap perfusion is reevaluated clinically and with the

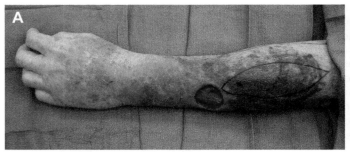
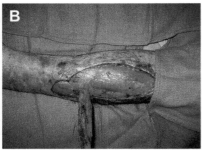
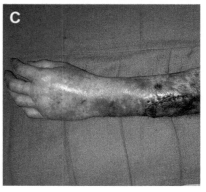

**Fig. 10.** (*A–C*) Freestyle PPF for coverage of a dorsal forearm soft tissue defect. A suitable freestyle perforator with a strong arterial and venous Doppler signal was identified and selected close to the defect.

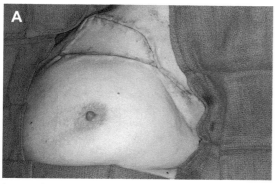
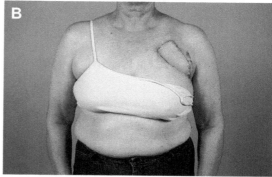

**Fig. 11.** (*A, B*) Freestyle V-Y triangular perforator advancement flap for melanoma reconstruction in the left upper chest.

Doppler to verify minimal changes in flow after advancement. The flap is inset under minimal tension, and the donor site is routinely closed primarily, although in rare circumstances a skin graft might be required for coverage (**Fig. 12**).

## PROPELLER FLAP

The propeller flap is a single perforator flap that requires specific mention because of its significant rotational capability, attributable to the location of the dominant perforator within the skin paddle.

The elliptical flap is based on a perforator located eccentrically closer to the defect, allowing a significant angle of rotation.[42] The perfusion of the flap is enhanced by the inclusion of axial linking vessels within the flap, and by the direction of flow of the perforator. Similar principles of flap elevation, pedicle evaluation, and intraoperative monitoring are followed as previously discussed for PPF. The pedicle can be dissected to the source vessel to increase flap mobility and rotational capability, and to decrease the likelihood of vessel twisting or kinking. The flap is dissected either in the

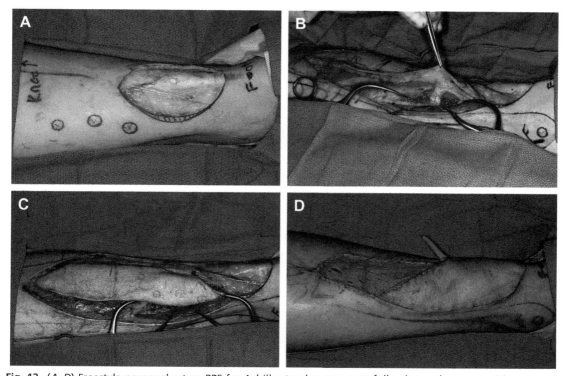

**Fig. 12.** (*A–D*) Freestyle peroneal artery PPF for Achilles tendon coverage following melanoma excision.

subfascial or suprafascial plane, and inset into the defect by rotating the flap in the direction of least vessel twist or kink (**Fig. 13**).[40,42]

## KEYSTONE PERFORATOR ISLAND FLAP: INTRODUCTION

The KPIF is a single multiperforator advancement flap based on random fasciocutaneous or musculocutaneous perforators that allows coverage of soft tissue defects by transfer of adjacent tissue with adequate soft tissue laxity.[51] This flap can be the primary reconstructive option or be planned as an adjunct for supplemental soft tissue coverage. Knowledge of hot spots of perforasomes allows KPIF skin islands to be based on regularly identified musculocutaneous and fasciocutaneous perforators, which are never surgically identified, resulting in decreased operative times (**Fig. 14**).[51,52] The inclusion of multiple perforators allows increased vascularity and resilience of the flap (**Fig. 15**).

The KPIF is named after the keystone of an arch in Roman architecture, and is described as a curvilinear trapezoidal design flap.[35,53] Behan[35] described the use of the flap for large elliptical defects, with the transfer of adjacent tissue for better color and contour match. The flap is designed as 2 opposing V-Y flaps that are oriented parallel to the long axis of the defect. The defect usually has a 3:1 long axis to short axis ratio. The ablative surgeon should plan the excisional defect to be elliptical, with the long axis parallel to the line of cutaneous nerves, veins, and/or known perforators to allow for possible preservation of cutaneous sensation.[35,39] The long axis of the flap should follow

maximal axiality of flow from dominant perforators, allowing for capture of multiple perforators, which are oriented axially in the extremities, and perpendicular to the midline in the trunk.[39]

Advancement of the KPIF into the defect along the short axis creates redundancy and subsequent laxity of the soft tissue in the long axis of the flap, which results in an increase in the length of the flap along its short axis, which is the area of greatest tension during closure.[35,52,54] The V-Y advancement closure at each end of the flap in the long axis further decreases the size of the donor site defect, and as a result decreases the tension of wound closure.[35] Harvesting the KPIF with significant soft tissue laxity allows for wound closure without excessive tension by distributing the laxity to the entire flap, and typically avoids the need for adjunct procedures for donor site closure.[35,52,54]

## KEYSTONE PERFORATOR ISLAND FLAP: MODIFICATIONS

Originally, the short axis of the KPIF was designed to have a 1:1 ratio with the defect short axis, and the limbs of the flap were angled at 90° to the long axis of the defect.[35,42,53] However, modifications in the design and harvest of the flap grants greater liberty to the reconstructive surgeon to maximize tissue use and to decrease risk of complications. Modifications include:

1. Increase the ratio of flap size to defect size
2. Deepithelialization for dead-space obliteration
3. Circumferential incision of deep fascia
4. Distally based or proximally based keystone rotation flap[35]

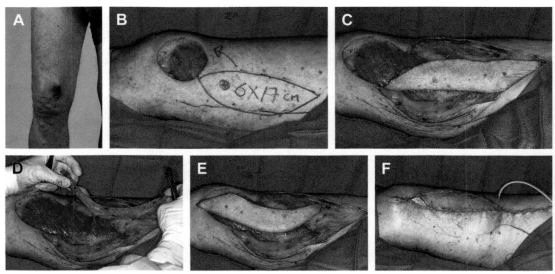

**Fig. 13.** (*A–F*) Freestyle perforator flap based on a distal dominant perforator from the superficial femoral artery.

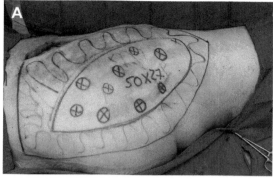

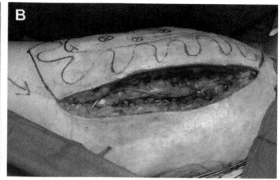

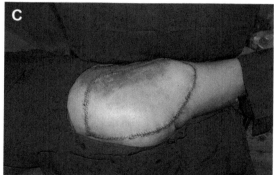

Fig. 14. (A–C) Keystone flap for trochanteric wound coverage following infected hardware removal. Note the preservation of perforators (hot spot) within the central portion of the flap. Peripheral undermining was performed for maximal flap advancement.

5. Bilateral opposing keystone flap
6. Asymmetric limb angulation for avoidance of critical structures

The flap size can be made larger depending on the adjacent tissue laxity, with flap to defect short axis ratios routinely 3:1 or 4:1 and in rare circumstances up to 5:1.[39] The increase in flap size decreases the tension of wound closure, and allows the integration of additional perforators by which well-vascularized tissue can be advanced into the defect (Fig. 16). The flap should be planned with the hot spot located in the central portion of the KPIF for optimal flap perfusion. Larger flaps are designed if the quality of adjacent tissue is compromised by surgical undermining, radiation therapy, adjacent surgical procedures, or an inflammatory process.[39,42] For reconstruction of defects in the inguinal region, when a notably large KPIF has been harvested, excess soft tissue can be deepithelialized and used for obliteration of empty space (Fig. 17). This maneuver can be

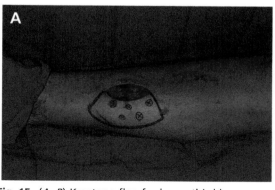

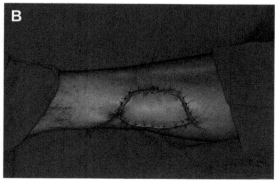

Fig. 15. (A, B) Keystone flap for lower third leg coverage following skin cancer resection. Note long axis of the keystone flap is designed parallel to the long axis of the limb, and concentrated over a maximal number of perforators to enhance vascularity. The keystone flap should be designed to be wide enough to incorporate as many suitable perforators as possible.

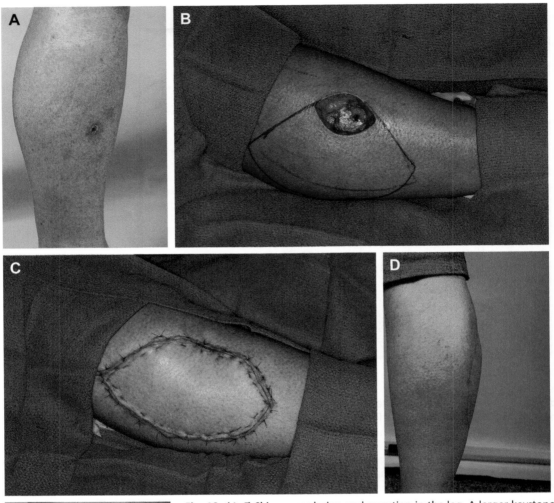

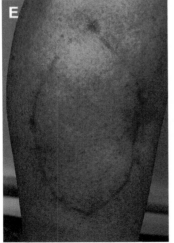

**Fig. 16.** (*A–E*) Skin cancer lesion and resection in the leg. A larger keystone flap relative to the defect size ratio (4:1) was designed because of a lack of soft tissue laxity. Circumferential skin and fascia incisions were performed, as well as peripheral flap undermining, in order to allow proper advancement and tension-free closure.

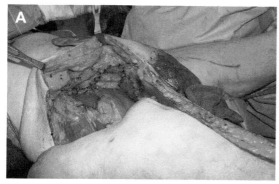

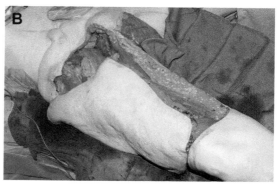

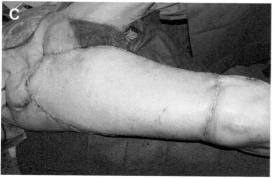

Fig. 17. (A–C) Large anterior thigh keystone flap used for coverage of groin soft tissue defect following sarcoma resection. Note that part of the proximal edge of the keystone flap was de-epithelialized for empty space obliteration of the groin and lower abdomen.

performed in combination with local muscle transposition, especially when there is concern for vessel exposure (**Fig. 18**).[39]

Mobility of the KPIF is significantly increased by incising the deep fascia. Originally, this was limited to the fascia along the greater (also known as the outer) curvature of the flap; however, the authors routinely incise the deep fascia in the progressive manner until appropriate mobility and laxity has been obtained.[39] Our experience has shown that greater flap mobility can be achieved, with almost complete circumferential incision of the deep fascia with sparing of the proximal and distal attachments or complete circumferential incision without risking flap viability.[39,55] When KPIF flaps are designed over muscle bellies and undergo complete circumferential incision, significant flap mobility is gained. Furthermore, approximately 50% of the flap can be dissected proximally or distally in the subfascial plane, by which the KPIF can obtain significant rotation to allow for closure of defects across joints or for compound fractures with exposed bone.[35]

Occasionally, a defect is too large for a single KPIF, necessitating the use of an adjunct procedure or reconstruction with bilateral opposing keystone flaps for additional soft tissue coverage (see **Fig. 18**). The KPIF allows the recruitment of native tissue with similar color, texture, and thickness, and less contour deformity, compared with a free flap, PPF, or propeller flap. A second KPIF should always be designed on the contralateral side of the defect as a backup flap, to be raised and advanced when indicated.[39] Conventional KPIF designs describe the limbs to be at 90° or perpendicular to the long axis of the defect, which introduces unnecessary surgical constraints and can result in iatrogenic injury.[35] KPIF can be designed with asymmetric limbs to avoid critical structures, including joint creases and lymphatic basins, reducing the risk for joint contracture and lymphedema.[39] Furthermore, limbs should be designed to align with the natural aesthetic lines along the midaxial lines to minimize deformity and to create more aesthetically natural contour.

## KEYSTONE PERFORATOR ISLAND FLAP: PLANNING AND PROCEDURE

Reconstruction with a KPIF requires an elliptical defect, ideally located near a known hot spot. The long axis of the elliptical defect is oriented parallel to the line of cutaneous nerves, veins, and known perforators, which is longitudinal in the extremities and perpendicular to the midline on the trunk.[35] The primary KPIF is planned on the side of the defect with greater soft tissue laxity, with a second KPIF planned on the contralateral side as a backup option. Perforator localization with the use of Doppler in the adjacent tissue helps with

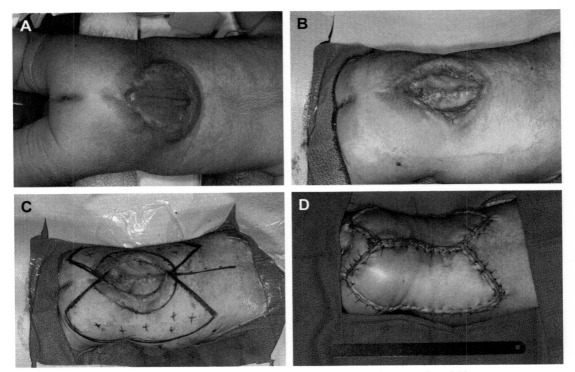

**Fig. 18.** (A–D) Bilateral keystone flaps for coverage of a myelomeningocele in a 4-day-old boy.

identification of perforator capture and ensures the optimal central positioning of the perforator in the flap. The KPIF is oriented with the long axis following the axiality of flow from perforators, which follows the path of the underlying source artery, thus ensuring the capture of linking vessels.[39] The short axis of the KPIF should be the same size or larger than the defect. The short axis of the KPIF does not include any areas of tissue undermining adjacent to the defect along the lesser curvature of the flap, because this area is void of viable perforating vessels. Smaller flaps are avoided when extensive undermining has taken place.[39,55] The limbs of the flap can be designed independent of each other (asymmetric) to avoid crossing joint creases, lymphatic basins, or other local critical structures.

After satisfactory design of the KPIF, the flap can be advanced in multiple variations until adequate mobility and laxity are achieved,[42] including:

1. Complete circumferential skin incision.
2. Complete circumferential skin incision with progressive fascial release along the greater curvature.
3. Complete circumferential skin and fascial release, which also allows for significant flap rotation.[56]
4. Incision of the skin and fascia limited to the limbs of the KPIF.

5. Limited exposure or minimally invasive (endoscopic) fascial release of the greater curvature, with skin and fascial release of the KPIF limbs.
6. Limited skin incision along the greater curvature, with incision of the flap limbs and complete circumferential fascial release.

Greater flap mobility can also be obtained by undermining the adjacent tissue, or by subfascial undermining of the flap. However, it is of paramount significance to only perform subfascial dissection in known cold spots to avoid injury to perforating vessels and potentially risk flap survival. If additional soft tissue coverage is needed, bilateral opposing keystone flaps can be raised. Furthermore, other flaps, such as PPF, V-Y advancement flaps, or rotation flaps, can be used in conjunction with KPIF for wound closure (**Fig. 19**). Defects in the inguinal region can be reconstructed with a large KPIF, with portions of the flap deepithelialized for dead-space obliteration.[39]

## KEYSTONE PERFORATOR ISLAND FLAP: CLOSURE

The surgical site is closed in multiple layers, typically beginning by reapproximating the defect at the midline with the lesser curvature of the KPIF.[50] The closing tension might be too great in some

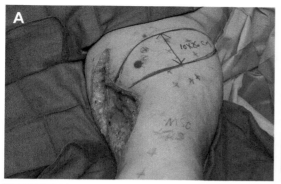

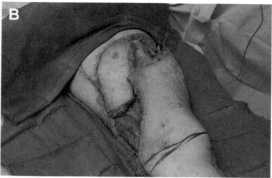

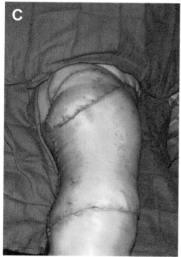

**Fig. 19.** (*A–C*) Left thigh sarcoma resection defect covered with a combination of a freestyle PPF and anterior thigh keystone flap. A keystone flap was used to supplement the pedicle perforator flap.

instances, warranting the closure of the edges with progressive tissue advancement to the midline. Advancement of the larger KPIF tissue into the smaller defect creates flap laxity along the long axis, which results in an increase of the short axis of the KPIF. The flap shortens along the long axis and widens along the short axis with progressive closure, adopting a rounder shape. The limbs of the KPIF are then closed in a V-Y fashion, and the greater curvature of the flap is finally reapproximated. Progressive tension suture and 3-point suture techniques can be used for redistribution of tension and for dead-space obliteration.[39] Routine surgical drain placement is not necessary, unless indicated for the primary defect, or if extensive soft tissue undermining has taken place.[39,51] Avoid drain placement adjacent to flap hot spots to prevent unintentional distortion of the underlying perforators.

## KEYSTONE PERFORATOR ISLAND FLAP AND PEDICLE PERFORATOR FLAP: COMPLICATIONS

The most common complications are typically minor, involving wound separation and delayed wound healing, which are treated conservatively with local wound care.[37,39,51,57] Risk of wound complications is increased by an active smoking history and preoperative irradiation.[51] Major complications with flap compromise resulting in partial or total flap loss are rare (less than 10%).[35,51] Modifications to the KPIF are safe, with no events of partial or total flap loss noted in a recent retrospective study of 42 consecutive KPIF-based reconstructions.[39]

## KEYSTONE PERFORATOR ISLAND FLAP: ADVANTAGES

KPIF have many advantages compared with microsurgical free flap–based reconstruction, including:

1. Shorter operative times than free flap or single perforator flaps, with quick flap elevation and inset (2–3 hours).[51,58,59]
2. Avoid technical demands of perforator dissection.[39]
3. High reproducibility, technically easy flap harvest, and reliable vascularity.[39,51]

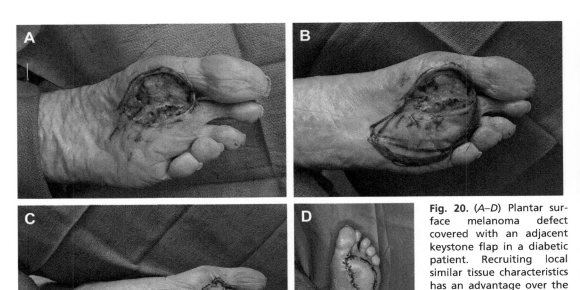

Fig. 20. (A–D) Plantar surface melanoma defect covered with an adjacent keystone flap in a diabetic patient. Recruiting local similar tissue characteristics has an advantage over the plantar surface.

4. Single-region donor site, allowing superior aesthetic match by advancing adjacent tissue with similar color and mechanical qualities such as texture, thickness, color match (**Fig. 20**).[39,51]
5. Transfer of sensate tissue for reconstruction.[35,39]
6. Ideal for patients with significant medical co-morbidities who are unable to undergo prolonged operative procedures.
7. Avoid need for postoperative flap monitoring.[39]
8. Decreased postoperative pain, postoperative edema, earlier patient ambulation, and shorter duration of hospitalization.[35]

## KEYSTONE PERFORATOR ISLAND FLAP: DISADVANTAGES AND CONTRAINDICATIONS

Limitations of the KPIF primarily depend on the availability of perforators and the laxity of the adjacent soft tissue. Reconstruction of scalp defects with a KPIF is contraindicated because of the lack of perforators.[51] Relative contraindications include wounds that have been irradiated, undergone significant undermining, or are currently in an inflammatory state, because these conditions compromise the vascularity and laxity of the flap.[51] Contour deformities usually improve through a combination of tissue creep and stress relaxation, and are typically less severe compared with reconstruction with perforator or propeller flaps.[37,39,44]

Larger flaps have longer incisions, which can result in more noticeable scarring, so it is essential to plan flaps along aesthetic lines.[39,42]

## SUMMARY

The increase in wealth of vascular anatomy knowledge, including the perforasome theory and identification of perforator hot spots, has led to major advances and freedom in reconstructive surgery. Tissue selection for locoregional reconstruction should be based on known hot spots and dominant perforators, and flaps should be designed to maximize interperforator flow through linking vessels. The PPF and KPIF have allowed the transfer large volumes of soft tissue for reconstruction and have minimized donor site morbidity, avoiding technically challenging microsurgical free-flap reconstruction and achieving superior aesthetic outcomes, and has resulted in minimal postoperative monitoring, decreased patient reported pain, and shorter periods of hospitalization. These advantages allow patients with significant medical comorbidities to undergo essential, complex surgical reconstruction and avoid the risks inherent with long periods of general anesthesia. Future understanding of vascular anatomy will allow additional modifications, leading to increasing surgical liberty in the planning and execution of reconstructive flaps, with the eventual goal of optimizing patient care and surgical outcomes.

## REFERENCES

1. Koshima I, Soeda S. Inferior epigastric artery skin flaps without rectus abdominis muscle. Br J Plast Surg 1989;42:645–8.
2. Kroll SS, Rosenfield L. Perforator-based flaps for low posterior midline defects. Plast Reconstr Surg 1988; 81:561–6.
3. Milton SH. Experimental studies on island flaps: 1. The surviving length. Plast Reconstr Surg 1971;48: 574–8.
4. Hyakusoku H, Yamamoto T, Fumiiri M. The propeller flap method. Br J Plast Surg 1991;44:53–4.
5. Hallock GG. The propeller flap version of the adductor muscle perforator flap for coverage of ischial or trochanteric pressure sores. Ann Plast Surg 2006;56:540–2.
6. Teo TC. The propeller flap concept. Clin Plast Surg 2010;37:615–26.
7. Schaverien MV, Hamilton SA, Fairburn N, et al. Lower limb reconstruction using the islanded posterior tibial artery perforator flap. Plast Reconstr Surg 2010;125:1735–43.
8. Lu TC, Lin CH, Lin CH, et al. Versatility of the pedicled peroneal artery perforator flaps for soft-tissue coverage of the lower leg and foot defects. J Plast Reconstr Aesthet Surg 2011;64:386–93.
9. Hallock GG. A paradigm shift in flap selection protocols for zones of the lower extremity using perforator flaps. J Reconstr Microsurg 2013;29:233–40.
10. Gir P, Cheng A, Oni G, et al. Pedicled perforator (propeller) flaps in lower extremity defects: a systematic review. J Reconstr Microsurg 2012;28: 595–601.
11. Nelson JA, Fischer JP, Brazio PS, et al. A review of propeller flaps for distal lower extremity soft tissue reconstruction: is flap loss too high? Microsurgery 2013;33:578–86.
12. Lazzeri D, Huemer GM, Nicoli F, et al. Indications, outcomes, and complications of pedicled propeller perforator flaps for upper body defects: a systematic review. Arch Plast Surg 2013;40: 44–50.
13. Taylor GI, Palmer JH. The vascular territories (angiosomes) of the body: experimental study and clinical applications. Br J Plast Surg 1987;40:113–41.
14. Atik B, Tan O, Mutaf M, et al. Skin perforators of back region: anatomical study and clinical applications. Ann Plast Surg 2008;60:70–5.
15. Hallock GG. Anatomic basis of the gastrocnemius perforator based flap. Ann Plast Surg 2001;47: 517–22.
16. Hamdi M, Spano A, Van Landuyt K, et al. The lateral intercostal artery perforators: anatomical study and clinical application in breast surgery. Plast Reconstr Surg 2008;121:389–96.
17. Hamdi M, Van Landuyt K, de Frene B, et al. The versatility of the inter-costal artery perforator (ICAP) flaps. J Plast Reconstr Aesthet Surg 2006;59:644–52.
18. Heitmann C, Guerra A, Metzinger SW, et al. The thoracodorsal artery perforator flap: anatomic basis and clinical application. Ann Plast Surg 2003;51:23–9.
19. Koshima I, Moriguchi T, Soeda S, et al. The gluteal perforator-based flap for repair of sacral pressure sores. Plast Reconstr Surg 1993;91:678–83.
20. Kato H, Hasegawa M, Takada T, et al. The lumbar artery perforator based island flap: anatomical study and case reports. Br J Plast Surg 1999;52:541–6.
21. Minabe T, Harii K. Dorsal intercostal artery perforator flap: anatomical study and clinical applications. Plast Reconstr Surg 2007;120:681–9.
22. Moscatiello F, Masia J, Carrera A, et al. The "propeller" distal anteromedial thigh perforator flap: anatomic study and clinical applications. J Plast Reconstr Aesthet Surg 2007;60:1323–30.
23. Mun GH, Lee SJ, Jeon BJ. Perforator topography of the thoracodorsal artery perforator flap. Plast Reconstr Surg 2008;121:497–504.
24. Ogawa R, Hyakusoku H, Murakami M, et al. An anatomical and clinical study of the dorsal intercostal cutaneous perforators, and application to free microvascular augmented subdermal vascular network (ma-SVN) flaps. Br J Plast Surg 2002;55: 396–401.
25. Rad AN, Singh NK, Rosson GD. Peroneal artery perforator-based propeller flap reconstruction of the lateral distal lower extremity after tumor extirpation: case report and literature review. Microsurgery 2008;28:663–70.
26. Thione A, Valdatta L, Buoro M, et al. The medial sural artery perforators: anatomic basis for a surgical plan. Ann Plast Surg 2004;53:250–5.
27. Saint-Cyr M, Schaverien M, Arbique G, et al. Three- and four-dimensional computed tomographic angiography and venography for the investigation of the vascular anatomy and perfusion of perforator flaps. Plast Reconstr Surg 2008;121:772–80.
28. Saint-Cyr M, Schaverien M, Rohrich RJ. Preexpanded second intercostal space internal mammary artery pedicle perforator flap: case report and anatomical study. Plast Reconstr Surg 2009;123: 1659–64.
29. Saint-Cyr M, Wong C, Schaverien M, et al. Perforasome theory vascular anatomy and clinical implications. Plast Reconstr Surg 2009;124:1529.
30. Schaverien M, Saint-Cyr M, Arbique G, et al. Arterial and venous anatomies of the deep inferior epigastric perforator and superficial inferior epigastric artery flaps. Plast Reconstr Surg 2008;121:1909–19.
31. Schaverien M, Saint-Cyr M, Arbique G, et al. Three- and four-dimensional arterial and venous anatomies

of the thoracodorsal artery perforator flap. Plast Reconstr Surg 2008;121:1578–87.

32. Schaverien M, Saint-Cyr M, Arbique G, et al. Three- and four-dimensional computed tomographic angiography and venography of the anterolateral thigh perforator flap. Plast Reconstr Surg 2008;121: 1685–96.

33. Wong C, Saint-Cyr M, Arbique G, et al. Three- and four-dimensional computed tomography angiographic studies of commonly used abdominal flaps in breast reconstruction. Plast Reconstr Surg 2009; 124:18–27.

34. Wong C, Saint-Cyr M, Rasko Y, et al. Three- and four-dimensional arterial and venous perforasomes of the internal mammary artery perforator flap. Plast Reconstr Surg 2009;124:1759–69.

35. Behan FC. The keystone design perforator island flap in reconstructive surgery. ANZ J Surg 2003;73: 112–20.

36. Behan FC, Sizeland A, Porcedu S, et al. Keystone island flap: an alternative reconstructive option to free flaps in irradiated tissue. ANZ J Surg 2006;76: 407–13.

37. Moncrieff MD, Bowen F, Thompson JF, et al. Keystone flap reconstruction of primary melanoma excision defects of the leg: the end of the skin graft? Ann Surg Oncol 2008;15:2867–73.

38. Peters LJ. Keystone island flaps: a radiation oncologist's perspective. ANZ J Surg 2006;76:1127.

39. Mohan AT, Rammos CK, Akhavan AA, et al. Evolving concepts of keystone perforator island flaps (KPIF): principles of perforator anatomy, design modifications, and extended clinical applications. Plast Reconstr Surg 2016;137:1909–20.

40. Lecours C, Saint-Cyr M, Wong C, et al. Freestyle pedicle perforator flaps: clinical results and vascular anatomy. Plast Reconstr Surg 2010;126:1589–603.

41. Rubino C, Coscia V, Cavazzuti AM, et al. Haemodynamic enhancement in perforator flaps: the inversion phenomenon and its clinical significance: a study of the relation of blood velocity and flow between pedicle and perforator vessels in perforator flaps. J Plast Reconstr Aesthet Surg 2006;59:636–43.

42. Mohan AT, Sur YJ, Zhu L, et al. The concept of propeller, perforator, keystone, and other local flaps and their role in the evolution of reconstruction. Plast Reconstr Surg 2016;138:710e–29e.

43. Saint-Cyr M, Schaverien MV, Rohrich RJ. Perforator flaps: history, controversies, physiology, anatomy, and use in reconstruction. Plast Reconstr Surg 2009; 4:132e–45e.

44. Saint-Cyr M, Schaverien M, Wong C, et al. The extended anterolateral thigh flap: anatomical basis and clinical experience. Plast Reconstr Surg 2009; 123:1245–55.

45. Wong C, Saint-Cyr M, Mojallal A, et al. Perforasomes of the DIEP flap: vascular anatomy of the lateral versus medial row perforators and clinical implications. Plast Reconstr Surg 2010;125:772–82.

46. Aho JM, Laungani AT, Herbig KS, et al. Lumbar and thoracic perforators: vascular anatomy and clinical implications. Plast Reconstr Surg 2014; 134:635e–45e.

47. Bailey SH, Saint-Cyr M, Wong C, et al. The single dominant medial row perforator DIEP flap in breast reconstruction: three-dimensional perforasome and clinical results. Plast Reconstr Surg 2010;126:739–51.

48. Laungani AT, Christner J, Primus JA, et al. Study of the impact of the location of a perforator in the perfusion of a perforator flap: the concept of "Angle of Perfusion". J Reconstr Microsurg 2017;33:49–58.

49. Mardini S, Al-Mufarrej FM, Jeng SF, et al. Free-style free flaps. In: Blondeel PN, Morris SF, Hallock GG, et al, editors. Perforator flaps: anatomy, technique, & clinical applications, vol. 2, 2nd edition. St Louis (MO): Quality Medical; 2013. p. 1245–60.

50. Wei FC, Mardini S. Free-style free flaps. Plast Reconstr Surg 2004;114:910–6.

51. Khouri JS, Egeland BM, Daily SD, et al. The keystone island flap: use in large defects of the trunk and extremities in soft-tissue reconstruction. Plast Reconstr Surg 2011;127:1212–21.

52. Pelissier P, Santoul M, Pinsolle V, et al. The keystone design perforator island flap: part I. Anatomic study. J Plast Reconstr Aesthet Surg 2007;60:883–7.

53. Behan F, Findlay M, Lo CH. The keystone perforator island flap concept. Sydney (Australia): Churchill Livingstone; 2012.

54. Shayan R, Behan FC. Re: the "keystone concept": time for some science. ANZ J Surg 2013;83: 499–500.

55. Behan FC, Paddle A, Rozen WM, et al. Quadriceps keystone island flap for radical inguinal lymphadenectomy: a reliable locoregional island flap for large groin defects. ANZ J Surg 2013;83:942–7.

56. Monarca C, Rizzo MI, Sanese G. Keystone flap: freestyle technique to enhance the mobility of the flap [corrected]. ANZ J Surg 2012;82:950–1.

57. Rao AL, Janna RK. Keystone flap: versatile flap for reconstruction of limb defects. J Clin Diagn Res 2015;9:PC05–7.

58. Rubino C, Figus A, Mazzocchi M, et al. The propeller flap for chronic osteomyelitis of the lower extremities: a case report. J Plast Reconstr Aesthet Surg 2009;62:e401–4.

59. Pignatti M, Pasqualini M, Governa M, et al. Propeller flaps for leg reconstruction. J Plast Reconstr Aesthet Surg 2008;61:777–83.

# Unique Techniques or Approaches in Microvascular and Microlymphatic Surgery

Jin Bo Tang, MD[a,*], Luis Landín, MD, PhD[b],
Pedro C. Cavadas, MD, PhD[c], Alessandro Thione, MD, PhD[c],
Jing Chen, MD[d], Gemma Pons, MD, PhD[e],
Jaume Masià, MD, PhD[e]

## KEYWORDS

- Microsurgical flaps • Arm transplant • Toe-to-hand transfer • Microlymphatic surgery
- Breast reconstruction

## KEY POINTS

- Strategies for treating donor-site–depleted patients who require transfer of soft tissue or bone.
- Fillet flaps from a severely traumatized lower extremity can be implanted to the forearm for temporary storage and transferred back to cover the amputated stump of the lower extremity.
- Updates and summaries of arm transplant and postsurgical treatment.
- The cosmetics of toe-to-hand transfer can be improved through insertion of free tissue transfers to the volar aspect of the transferred toe.
- Diagnostic images and surgical treatment of breast lymphedema.

Video content accompanies this article at http://www.plasticsurgery.theclinics.com.

## INTRODUCTION

Half a century after the advent of microsurgery, limited opportunities for straightforward innovations remain. However, many challenging clinical problems persist. Some of those difficult problems have been overcome with novel techniques and approaches. The lead editor (JBT) of this issue invited a panel of senior surgeons known for innovation to discuss their unique techniques and approaches to topics not covered by independent articles in this issue. The editor is pleased to present the wisdom, technique, and experience of these well-reputed surgeons.

## FLAP PREFABRICATION FOR DONOR-SITE–DEPLETED PATIENTS

Jin Bo Tang: for years you and your colleagues have faced some of the most difficult situations in reconstructive microsurgery and treated those patients with innovative approaches. Can you

The authors have nothing to disclose.
[a] Department of Hand Surgery, The Hand Surgery Research Center, Affiliated Hospital of Nantong University, 20 West Temple Road, Nantong 226001, Jiangsu, China; [b] Plastic & Reconstructive Surgery, Hospital Universitario La Paz, Paseo de la Castellana, 261, Madrid 28046, Spain; [c] Reconstructive Surgery Unit, Clinica Cavadas, Paseo Facultades 1, bajo 8, Valencia 46021, Spain; [d] Department of Hand Surgery, Affiliated Hospital of Nantong University, 20 West Temple Road, Nantong 226001, Jiangsu, China; [e] Department of Plastic Surgery, Hospital de la Santa Creu I Sant Pau, Universitat Autònoma de Barcelona, Sant Quintí 89, Barcelona 08026, Spain
* Corresponding author.
E-mail address: jinbotang@yahoo.com

Clin Plastic Surg 44 (2017) 403–414
http://dx.doi.org/10.1016/j.cps.2016.11.007
0094-1298/17/© 2017 Elsevier Inc. All rights reserved.

summarize your current approaches for donor-site–depleted patients who have already undergone multiple microsurgical transfers, for whom lack of good donor tissues presents a problem?

## Pedro Cavadas and Alessandro Thione

Complex reconstruction usually entails the use of specialized tissues. Such patients often have already been operated on, and optimal donor sites may be depleted. Flap prefabrication may allow the use of the required specialized tissues when the native donor areas are not available. Flap prefabrication comprises vascular induction with a vascular carrier, flap preassembly (mainly skeletal), and pregrafting (or prelamination). First described in the early 1990s, flap prefabrication has never become popular, in part because of its technical difficulty.[1] Pregrafting has been well described and is not discussed here.

### Vascular induction

Vascular induction is a modality of prefabrication that exploits natural wound healing and spontaneous vascular reconnection around vascularized tissue. The vascular carrier is usually thin microvascular subcutaneous tissue with a long pedicle, implanted under the surface to be transferred.[2] Radial forearm or dorsalis pedis flaps are the most useful carriers; anterolateral thigh (ALT) flaps do not have a pedicle long enough for most indications. The pedicle should be planned to allow pedicled transfer of the prefabricated flap if possible. In facial reconstruction this is usually the case. The pink supraclavicular skin, the submental beard, or the hairy scalp can be transferred as a prefabricated flap for facial resurfacing in unfavorable cases. The external nose can be reconstructed with a prefabricated supraclavicular flap in the absence of frontal donor areas, using a radial forearm flap as a carrier (**Fig. 1**). The entire nose can be

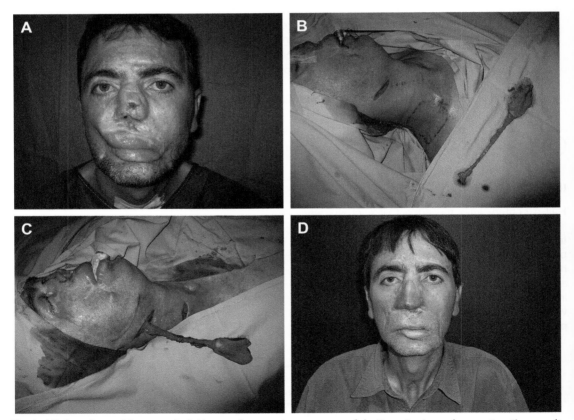

**Fig. 1.** (*A*) A patient with severe facial burn, after previous unsuccessful attempts at nasal reconstruction resulting in infected and exposed alloplastic material and depletion of both frontal forehead flaps. (*B*) The supraclavicular pink skin was used for flap prefabrication. A subcutaneous radial forearm flap was placed subdermally and anastomosed to the facial vessels. (*C*) Two months later the prefabricated flap was elevated and transferred as a pedicle flap for nasal external coverage. The remnants of the local flaps were recycled for internal lining. (*D*) End result after nasal reconstruction. The perioral area was reconstructed with submental flaps.

prefabricated in the supraclavicular area using a dorsalis pedis flap for internal lining and vascular induction of the overlying pink skin, along with cartilage pregrafting in patients with multiple unsuccessful attempts with depletion of optimal donor areas (**Fig. 2**).

### Skeletal preassembly

The number of possible donor areas for long cortical bone flaps is limited. In cases requiring reconstruction of long segments of bone, without available fibular donor areas and with poor indication of bone transport techniques, preassembly of smaller segments of bone to form a longer segment is an option. The construction is completed remotely, piggy-backing the vascular pedicles and with simplified plate-and-screw fixation. Once healed, the whole block can be free-transferred to the bone defect, allowing more formal internal fixation. The iliac crest free flap and the scapular angular bone flap can be piggy-backed and connected to the descending branch of the lateral circumflex femoral vessels distal to the cutaneous perforator. Minimal plate fixation reduces interference with blood flow. For example, a 20-cm long construct can be used for reconstruction of a massive femoral defect in an irradiated limb, combined with trifocal lengthening of the tibia (**Fig. 3**).

Prefabrication is a staged procedure that requires dissection and transfer of scarred tissues and vessels. It is complex, difficult to plan, and usually of long duration, calling for significant patient compliance. In return, it allows the transfer of nonanatomic tissue combinations or, in complex cases, may bypass the depletion of optimal native donor areas of specialized tissue.

## ECTOPIC STORAGE OF FILLET FLAPS FROM THE LOWER EXTREMITY

Jin Bo Tang: ectopic implantation of an amputated hand for temporary storage at other anatomical sites has been reported over several decades and is currently used by some surgeons. Although ectopic implantation of a flap is uncommon, I know you have unique experience with this procedure. Our readers would appreciate hearing your thoughts and experience. To me, a better term is ectopic storage of a fillet flap, and this is neither implantation nor replantation; it is a temporary storage of a fillet flap. Please comment on a possible better terminology for this unique method.

### Luis Landín

Reconstruction of the mangled leg typically results in 2-year outcomes equivalent to those of amputation.[3,4] The energy expenditure of walking is exponentially related to the length of the lower extremity.[5] Therefore, we perform revascularization or replantation of the lower extremity in

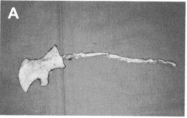
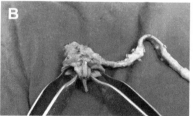
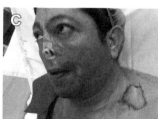
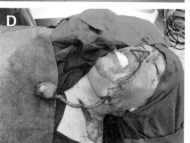
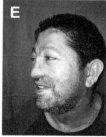

**Fig. 2.** (*A*) Dorsalis pedis flap with long anterior tibial pedicle for complex nasal reconstruction in a patient with multiple previous attempts at reconstruction. Both frontal flaps had been used and lost because of recurrent infection. To minimize risk of infection, a remote complete prefabrication was performed. (*B*) The dorsalis pedis flap was used for internal lining and as a vascular carrier of the supraclavicular skin. Frugal skeletal construction was performed to maximize the contact surface between the vascular carrier and the overlying supraclavicular skin. (*C*) At 2 months the nose was ready for transfer. The skin was incised peripherally and sutured again to improve vascular supply from the underlying carrier. (*D*) The composite prefabricated flap, including the internal lining (dorsalis pedis), cartilage skeleton, and overlying supraclavicular skin, was transferred as a pedicle to the nasal defect. Because the skeleton was not manipulated at this stage, the risk of infection was minimal. (*E*) End result. There is a relative lack of fine details. The result is a compromise between enough skeletal support and unimpeded contact between the dorsalis pedis and the supraclavicular skin.

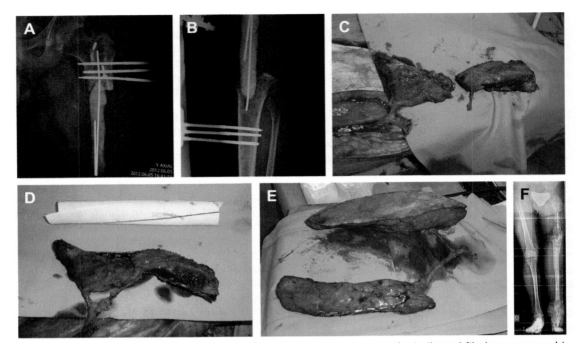

**Fig. 3.** (*A, B*) Massive defect of the left femur after radionecrosis and sepsis. The ipsilateral fibula was not usable and the contralateral one had been previously used. Bone transport was not feasible in irradiated fields. (*C*) The remaining iliac crest was elevated as a 10-cm vascularized bone. The only remaining thoracodorsal artery was used to elevate a 10-cm scapular angular bone. This flap was connected to the descending branch of the right circumflex femoral vessels, after the take-off of the cutaneous ALT perforator. (*D*) The iliac crest was anastomosed to the thoracodorsal vessels of the previous flap and it was plated to the scapula with a locking 3.5-mm reconstruction plate, creating a 20-cm bone flap. (*E*) Two months later, the preassembled flap was elevated including the ALT skin paddle on the circumflex femoral vessels and transferred to the left side. The pedicle was anastomosed to the pedicle of a previous latissimus dorsi flap end to side. Bone was fixed with a long locking compression plate. Because of hardware infection, the plate was removed at 1 month and replaced by an Ilizarov construct. The tibia was lengthened by bifocal callotaxis to compensate the short femur. (*F*) Final result with stable skeletal healing.

patients with trauma less than the age of 60 years and retain almost the full length of the lower extremity (Video 1).

Crush injury associated with traumatic amputation of the lower limb is usually extensive and does not permit replantation. However, from the amputated part, fillet flaps can be harvested for coverage of the amputated stump or other tissue defects (**Fig. 4**). Ectopic implantation of the fillet flaps allows for serial surgical debridement and adjuvant surgical procedures on the remaining stump and permits a period of several days to determine delimitation and necrosis of borderline tissues (**Fig. 5**).

Ectopic implantation requires radical debridement of the fillet flap. In the heavily crushed foot when the sole remains uninjured, we favor filleting a sole flap (**Fig. 6**). Our favorite recipient vessels for ectopic implantation of a sole flap are the radial artery and its accompanying veins (**Fig. 7**), because they provide a long pedicle when the

ectopically implanted sole flap is transferred back to the lower extremity. However, occupational therapy is demanding, because a few days after ectopic implantation both the fillet part and the stump become edematous and the vessels and nerves granulate, hampering vascular anastomoses. If the ectopically implanted part is elevated based on a long pedicle, the clinicians can search for recipient vessels proximal to the injury zone at the stump, maximizing the chances for success. When the implanted flap is transferred back to the lower extremity, the flap remains edematous for long periods. Although it may take months for the sole of the foot to adapt to the curvature of the leg stump, coverage is excellent and permits prosthesis adaptation with few aesthetic sequelae in the forearm (**Fig. 8**, Video 2).

Ectopic storage should be considered for inclusion in reconstructive surgery terminology. It clarifies the point that the procedure is intended to salvage the amputated part in an otherwise

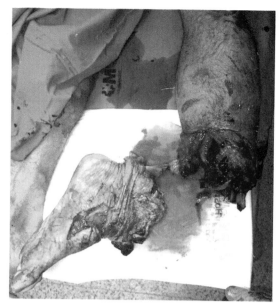

**Fig. 4.** Crushed stump at the level of middle third of the tibia. The distal third of the tibia was lost. The foot was deemed to be not replantable. However, the sole of the foot was uninjured.

mangled stump the viability of which is questionable. Thus, vascularized storage is the goal, whereas the specific anatomic region is less important. In addition, it connotes the temporary nature of the procedure.

## ARM TRANSPLANTATION

Jin Bo Tang: arm transplants have been rare, but I know you and your colleagues performed bilateral arm transplant.[6,7] Please describe your experience, and please provide a concise review of

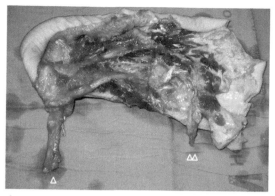

**Fig. 6.** Sole fillet flap from the amputated foot. The posterior (*1 triangle*) and anterior (*2 triangles*) tibial vessels and the plantar nerves were preserved, in continuity with the plantar fat pad.

arm transplant cases reported to date, and compare the unique postoperative care of an arm transplant with that of a hand transplant.

### Luis Landín

Arm donation poses notable risks that must be avoided. Massive bleeding in the donor is a potential complication that may compromise donor hemodynamic stability and hamper multiorgan donation. Thus upper-limb donation must be performed under the same setup used for donation of thoracoabdominal organs.

In the recipient, the vascularization of the distal third of the muscles and periosteum should be preserved to prevent allograft-bone nonunion. Bone union has often been reported despite maintenance of immunosuppression with

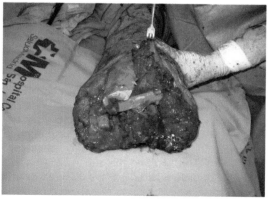

**Fig. 5.** The stump was clean after being debrided twice and underwent an Ertl procedure.

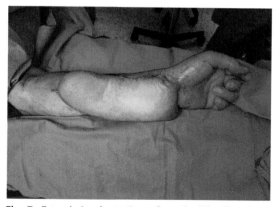

**Fig. 7.** Ectopic implantation of a sole fillet flap from the foot in the forearm of the patient. The anterior tibial artery was anastomosed to the radial artery and 2 accompanying veins were anastomosed. The posterior tibial vein was anastomosed to the innominate vein.

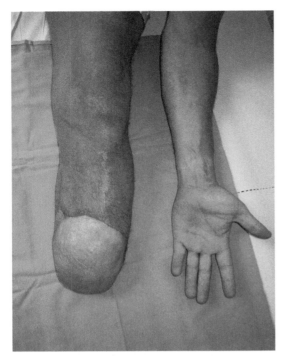

**Fig. 8.** The fillet flap was transferred back to cover the amputated stump of the leg, and the forearm is also shown after taking away the fillet flap.

healing-impairing regimes like sirolimus.[8] However-er, we and others have observed delayed bone union in arm transplants.[9] In addition, biceps and triceps necrosis is another possible complication after aggressive distal humerus dissection, as was our experience in Madrid. The wounds required serial debridement before healing, and full-dose immunosuppressive therapy had to be delayed, which triggered a Banff grade III (out of IV) rejection in the early postoperative period. In the late period, a bipolar latissimus dorsi transfer permitted elbow flexion.

The required levels of immunosuppression are commonly high among arm transplant recipients. It has been our and others' experience that rejection episodes did not respond to therapy adjustment but instead required lymphocyte depletion, via administering either alemtuzumab or thymo-globuline.[10] To date no study has determined whether larger amounts of allograft require higher doses of immunosuppression, but it seems plausible and has been a clinical observation in arm, leg, and combined transplants. However, high doses of immunosuppression pose a notable risk of neoplasm, as was the case with a bilateral leg recipient.[11]

To date 2 patients have received arm transplants in Poland, another patient in Germany,

and 2 other patients in Spain. Although it may be considered macrovascular surgery, it has yet to be defined as a straightforward surgical or medical procedure. For the Polish patients, limited success was reported without secondary surgeries.[9] Little information has been released on the transplant patient in Germany. By contrast, the patient operated on by Drs Cavadas and Tang in 2008 in Valencia, Spain, has shown excellent results and is able to drive. That patient underwent extensive secondary procedures, and we use the same surgical approach. As we have also observed, medical complications do develop in these patients, because they are prone to diabetes and hypertension. The second arm transplant in Spain was performed by Dr Tang in Madrid in 2014. In the second case, because of our patient's impending kidney failure, we switched the immunosuppressive regime from the calcineurin inhibitor tacrolimus to a combination of the CTLA-4 (cytotoxic T-lymphocyte antigen 4) costimulation-blocker belatacept and sirolimus. This combination triggered a heavy rejection episode, but creatinine clearance was not further impaired (unpublished data). In the setting of acute rejection, lymphocytes cross the dermoepidermal junction to reach the epidermis, causing dermatitis in the skin of the allograft. Lymphocytes are also detected close to the vessels in the muscles in deep biopsies.[6]

## THUMB AND FINGER RECONSTRUCTION: AESTHETIC REFINEMENTS

Jin Bo Tang: microsurgical toe-to-hand transfer is a mature and classic technique.[12,13] What remains to be improved is the cosmetic appearance of the toes that have been moved to the hand. What methods do you recommend to improve toe cosmetics of the toe in the hand?

### Jing Chen

Cosmetics of transferred second toes has been a concern to many surgeons, especially the narrow neck of the toes. Methods of aesthetic refinements in second-toe–thumb transfer are summarized in **Fig. 9**. Various flaps can be inserted into the narrow neck of the transferred second toe. To eliminate the bulbous pulp and the narrow neck of the second toe, Zhang and colleagues[14] used a pedicle flap from the fibular side of the great toe to insert into the ventral surface of the second toe before the second toe was freely transferred (see **Fig. 9**). The flap and the second toe have a common pedicle based on the plantar artery, veins, and nerves, which was dissected proximally to the site between the first dorsal and plantar metatarsal arteries. Then the flap was rotated

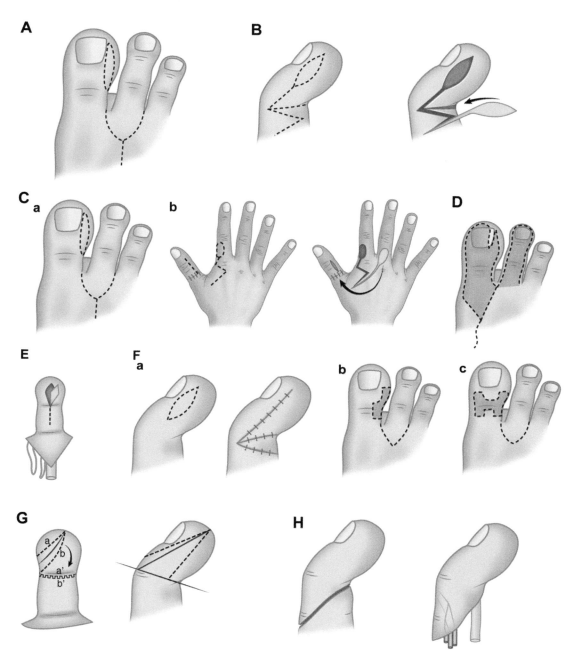

**Fig. 9.** The methods to refine cosmetics of the transferred toes. (A) A pedicled flap from fibular side of the great toe inserted into the second toe. (B) A pedicled flap from fibular or tibial side of the second toe inserted into the narrow neck of the second toe. (C) A flap from the fibular side of the great toe pedicled with the fibular proper plantar digital artery (a) combined or not combined with a dorsal index finger flap (b), was inlaid with the second toe at the same time. (D) The second-toe transfer for thumb reconstruction interchanging the entire skin-nail flap from the great toe with another from the second toe. (E). The diamond-shaped pulp flap of the second toe was rotated 180° and inserted into the narrow neck of the second toe. (F) A pedicled flap from the fibular side of the second toe (a) or/and a pedicled flap from fibular (b) or/and tibial side (c) of the great toe were inserted into the narrow neck and plantar side of the second toe. (G) A triangular flap was converted from the pulp to the neck of the second toe. (H) A tongue-shaped flap (5–8 mm long, 3–5 mm wide) was added to the vascular pedicle of the second toe.

180°, and inserted into the incision to increase the circumference of the second toe. Li and colleagues[15] designed a pedicle flap from the fibular or tibial side of the second toe. The width of that flap was the difference between the circumference of the toe tip and the circumference of the narrow neck of the second toe (see **Fig. 9**). The flap was rotated 90° at a pivot 1.5 mm distal to the proximal interphalangeal joint of the second toe and was inserted into an incision made at the narrow neck of the toe (see **Fig. 9**). A pedicled flap from the fibular aspect of the great toe can be made and combined with the dorsal island flap of the index finger, then inserted into the second toe at the same time (see **Fig. 9**).[16] If the diameter of the second toe needs to be increased further, the dorsal island flap from an index finger can be harvested to insert into an additional incision in the second toe (see **Fig. 9**).[17] Liu and colleagues[18] rotated a diamond-shaped pulp flap from the second toe 180° and inserted it into the narrow neck of the free second toe (see **Fig. 9**). Wang and colleagues[19] used 3 kinds of pedicled flaps for this purpose: the fibular side of the second toe, and either an H-shaped or a T-shaped flap from the fibular side of the great toe (see **Fig. 9**). These flaps were brought to the ventral side of the second toe (alone or together) to relieve the constriction below the toe pulp.

Zhao and colleagues[20] described a modified second-toe transfer (**Fig. 10**). First, a neurovascular island flap called a keyhole flap is raised on the lateral aspect of the great toe. The flap is 30 mm long and 20 mm wide at its widest point. The pedicle of the flap is dissected proximally to establish continuity with the first dorsal metatarsal artery. An I-shaped incision is made on the distal part of the pulp of the second toe. The flap is brought into the volar incision through a subcutaneous tunnel and sutured. Second, a transverse incision is made 2 mm proximal to the distal border of the eponychium; the length of the incision is the width of the nail. The skin strip and eponychium are excised, and the 2 edges are sutured together. Third, 2 oval skin excisions are made on each side of the tip of the pulp and the skin ellipses are excised, along with a wedge of subcutaneous tissue extending down to the bone. Then the wound is sutured to reduce the bulbous appearance.

The twisted-toe technique is another way to achieve more acceptable appearance and functional outcome compared with the great toe or trimmed great toe transfer. The twisted-toe flap has already been well described in the literature.[21,22]

Motion at toe joints is not ample for thumb or finger movement, especially when the transfer includes the metatarsophalangeal joint. This phenomenon relates to the nature of small joints (their difficulty in restoring motion, as seen in finger joint repair, flap coverage, or replantation[23–32]) and differences in anatomy of the toe and finger or thumb joints.

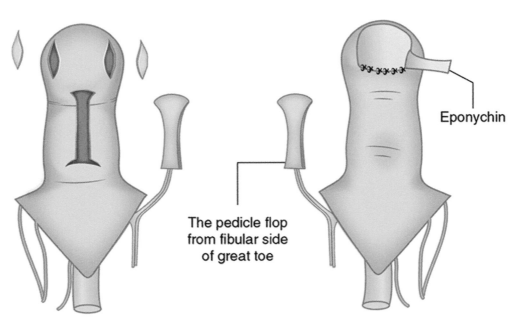

The pedicle flop from fibular side of great toe

Eponychin

**Fig. 10.** (A) A flap from the adjacent side of the great toe was harvested and inserted into the volar aspect of the second toe, with skin excisions on each side of the toe tip. (B) Excising the eponychium to lengthen the nail.

# THE RATIONAL APPROACH FOR BREAST CANCER–RELATED LYMPHEDEMA

Jin Bo Tang: can you explain and introduce your current algorithm for treatment of breast cancer–related lymphedema?

### Gemma Pons and Jaume Masià

Lymphedema is one of the most serious complications of breast cancer therapy, and its treatment is a challenging problem for plastic surgeons. Although more conservative surgery has been introduced, it continues to be a prevalent iatrogenic problem that strongly affects quality of life. Despite the persistent lack of consensus about surgical treatment of lymphedema, we have developed an algorithm, BCN (Barcelona) lymphedema algorithm for surgical treatment (BLAST), based on a detailed preoperative assessment (**Fig. 11**). After reviewing anamnestic data and performing a clinical examination, we can determine the lymphedema stage according to the International Society of Lymphedema.[33] Diagnostic imaging techniques are used to analyze each case, to understand the pathophysiology of the lymphedema and to select the right surgical indication for each patient. Accordingly, our assessment protocol includes indocyanine green (ICG) lymphography,[34] lymphoscintigraphy, magnetic resonance (MR) lymphography, and computed tomography (CT) angiography.

We consider ICG lymphography the essential preoperative test in our assessment protocol, because it permits differentiation between a functional and nonfunctional lymphatic system. After injecting the ICG into the interdigital spaces, the functional lymphatic channels are visualized in

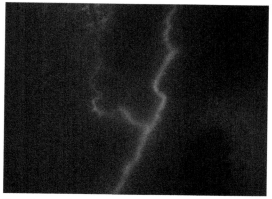

**Fig. 12.** ICG lymphography image showing fluorescent linear lymphatic channels.

real time as fluorescent channels on a display (**Fig. 12**). Information obtained during the preoperative assessment is of paramount importance, because only patients with a functional lymphatic system can be offered reconstructive surgical techniques (ie, lymphaticovenular anastomosis and lymph node transfer). Patients without functional lymphatic channels are candidates for reductive techniques.

The lymphaticovenular anastomosis technique[35] (**Fig. 13**) consists of locating lymphatic vessels and anastomosing to subdermal veins through a 2-cm to 3-cm incision in the affected upper limb. Information obtained by ICG lymphography and MR lymphography are key to locating functional lymphatic channels and making surgery feasible.

Lymph node transfer[36] (**Fig. 14**) is based on replacing previously resected axillary lymph nodes with a free flap that is rich in lymphatic tissue (ie, containing 3–5 lymph nodes). Our preferred donor

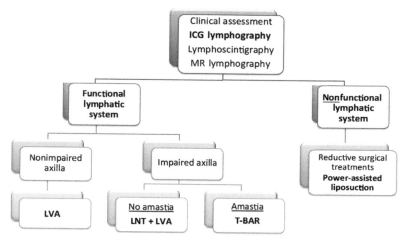

**Fig. 11.** BLAST (Barcelona lymphodema algorithm for surgical treatment). LNT, lymph node transfer; LVA, Lymphaticovenous anastomosis; T-BAR, total breast anatomy restoration.

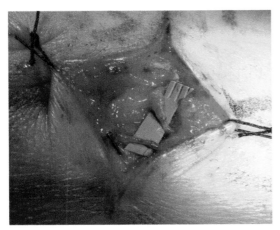

**Fig. 13.** Two lymphatic vessels anastomosed termino-terminal with subdermal venules.

site is the superficial inferior epigastric area, which is nourished by superficial circumflex iliac vessels. We currently study the donor site preoperatively with CT angiography. Intrapreoperatively, we perform reverse mapping of the donor limb to minimize potential donor-site morbidity. When we choose to approach lymphedema and autologous breast reconstruction simultaneously with an abdominal perforator flap, we raise a compound abdominal flap (a deep inferior epigastric artery perforator or superficial inferior epigastric artery) including lymph nodes with double vascularization. In addition, in some cases we perform lymphaticovenous anastomosis in the upper limb. This complex approach is known as total breast anatomy restoration.[37]

Reductive surgical treatment is offered when preoperative assessment indicates a nonfunctional lymphatic system and nonpitting lymphedema. The most effective reductive technique we use is liposuction, as described by Brorson and colleagues.[38]

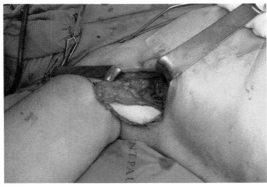

**Fig. 14.** Vascularized lymph node flap transferred to the axillary area.

We consider preoperative assessment essential to selecting patients who will benefit maximally from lymphedema surgery and to determine whether reconstructive or reductive surgery is indicated. Although we are still searching for a definitive lymphedema treatment, the algorithm we present has considerably improved our long-term results. Further progress in diagnostic imaging will allow us to improve our understanding of the physiopathology of lymphedema and to undertake larger comparative studies with the goal of identifying a definitive surgical treatment of lymphedema.

## SUMMARY

Several methods can be used for identifying tissues for transfer in donor-site–depleted patients. A fillet flap can be temporarily stored in other parts of the body and transferred back to the site of tissue defect, including covering the amputated stump of the lower extremity. Human arm transplant is rare and has some unique concerns for the surgery and postsurgical treatment. Cosmetics of the narrow neck of transferred second toes can be improved with insertion of a flap. Lymphedema of the breast after cancer treatment can be diagnosed with several currently available imaging techniques and treated surgically with lymphaticovenous anastomosis.

## SUPPLEMENTARY DATA

Supplementary data related to this article can be found at http://dx.doi.org/10.1016/j.cps.2016.11.007.

## REFERENCES

1. Khouri RK, Upton J, Shaw WW. Principles of flap prefabrication. Clin Plast Surg 1992;19:763–71.
2. Pribaz JJ, Maitz PK, Fine NA. Flap prefabrication using the "vascular crane" principle: an experimental study and clinical application. Br J Plast Surg 1994;47:250–6.
3. Cavadas PC, Landin L, Ibanez J, et al. Infrapopliteal lower extremity replantation. Plast Reconstr Surg 2009;124:532–9.
4. Bosse MJ, MacKenzie EJ, Kellam JF, et al. An analysis of outcomes of reconstruction or amputation after leg-threatening injuries. N Engl J Med 2002;347: 1924–31.
5. Gonzalez EG, Corcoran PJ, Reyes RL. Energy expenditure in below-knee amputees: correlation with stump length. Arch Phys Med Rehabil 1974;55:111–9.
6. Landin L, Cavadas PC, Garcia-Cosmes P, et al. Perioperative ischemic injury and fibrotic degeneration

of muscle in a forearm allograft: functional follow-up at 32 months post transplantation. Ann Plast Surg 2011; 66:202–9.

7. Cavadas PC, Landin L, Ibanez J. Bilateral hand transplantation: result at 20 months. J Hand Surg Eur Vol 2009;34:434–43.

8. Cavadas PC, Hernan I, Landin L, et al. Bone healing after secondary surgery on hand allografts under sirolimus-based maintenance immunosuppression. Ann Plast Surg 2011;66:667–9.

9. Jablecki J, Kaczmarzyk L, Domanasiewicz A, et al. Result of arm-level upper-limb transplantation in two recipients at 19- and 30-month follow-up. Ann Transplant 2012;17:126–32.

10. Cavadas PC, Ibanez J, Thione A, et al. Bilateral trans-humeral arm transplantation: result at 2 years. Am J Transplant 2011;11:1085–90.

11. Cavadas PC, Thione A, Blanes M, et al. Primary central nervous System posttransplant lymphoproliferative disease in a bilateral transfemoral lower extremity transplantation recipient. Am J Transplant 2015;15:2758–61.

12. Nikkah D, Martin N, Pickford M. Paediatric toe-to-hand transfer: an assessment of outcomes from a single unit. J Hand Surg Eur Vol 2016;41: 281–94.

13. Sabapathy SR, Elliot D, Venkatramani H. Pushing the boundaries of salvage in mutilating upper limb injuries: techniques in difficult situations. Hand Clin 2016;32:585–97.

14. Zhang JL, Ren ZY, Wang CQ. Digital reconstruction by transferring the free second toe inlaid with the composite pedicle flap from fibular side of the great toe. Chin J Microsurg 2001;24:252–3.

15. Li Z, Lao KC, Zhang CJ, et al. The finger reconstruction by transferring the free second toe inlaid with the lateral flap from the second toe. Chin J Hand Surg 2006;24:380.

16. Zhang JL, Xie ZR, Xiao JB, et al. A new surgical treatment for digital reconstruction by the second toe transfer. Chin J Microsurg 2007;10:331–3.

17. Zhang JL, Xie ZR, Xiao JB, et al. A new surgery treatment for thumb reconstruction by one-stage plasty free second toe transfer. Chin J Microsurg 2008;31:335–7.

18. Liu GJ, Guo DL, Li JQ, et al. The finger reconstruction by transferring the free second toe inlaid with the diamond shaped flap from the pulp of the second toe. Chin J Repair Reconstr Surg 2007;21: 1389–91.

19. Wang BS, Zhen XJ, Wang XH, et al. Reconstruction of finger with reshaped second toe. Chin J Microsurg 2008;31:411–3.

20. Zhao J, Tien HY, Abdullah S, et al. Aesthetic refinements in second toe-to-thumb transfer surgery. Plast Reconstr Surg 2010;126:2052–9.

21. Iglesias M, Butron P, Serrano A. Thumb reconstruction with extended twisted toe flap. J Hand Surg Am 1995;20:731–6.

22. Kempny T, Paroulek J, Marik V, et al. Further developments in the twisted-toe technique for isolated thumb reconstruction: our method of choice. Plast Reconstr Surg 2013;131:871e–9e.

23. Breahna A, Siddiqui A, Fitzgerald O'Connor E, et al. Replantation of digits: a review of predictive factors for survival. J Hand Surg Eur Vol 2016;41: 753–7.

24. Ma Z, Guo F, Qi J, et al. Effects of non-surgical factors on digital replantation survival rate: a meta-analysis. J Hand Surg Eur Vol 2016;41: 157–63.

25. Cheah AE, Yao J. Hand fractures: indications, the tried and true and new innovations. J Hand Surg Am 2016;41:712–22.

26. Erken HY, Akmaz I, Takka S, et al. Reconstruction of the transverse and dorsal-oblique amputations of the distal thumb with volar cross-finger flap using the index finger. J Hand Surg Eur Vol 2015;40: 392–400.

27. Liodaki E, Xing SG, Mailaender P, et al. Management of difficult intra-articular fractures or fracture dislocations of the proximal interphalangeal joint. J Hand Surg Eur Vol 2015;40:16–23.

28. Zhang G, Ju J, Li L, et al. Combined two foot flaps with iliac bone graft for reconstruction of the thumb. J Hand Surg Eur Vol 2016;41:745–52.

29. Wang H, Chen C, Li J, et al. Modified first dorsal metacarpal artery island flap for sensory reconstruction of thumb pulp defects. J Hand Surg Eur Vol 2016;41:177–84.

30. Chen QZ, Sun YC, Chen J, et al. Comparative study of functional and aesthetically outcomes of reverse digital artery and reverse dorsal homodigital island flaps for fingertip repair. J Hand Surg Eur Vol 2015;40:935–43.

31. Lee SH, Jang JH, Kim JI, et al. Modified anterograde pedicle advancement flap in fingertip injury. J Hand Surg Eur Vol 2015;40:944–51.

32. Usami S, Kawahara S, Yamaguchi Y, et al. Homodigital artery flap reconstruction for fingertip amputation: a comparative study of the oblique triangular neurovascular advancement flap and the reverse digital artery island flap. J Hand Surg Eur Vol 2015;40:291–7.

33. International Society of Lymphology. The diagnosis and treatment of peripheral lymphedema: 2013 consensus document of the international society of lymphology. Lymphology 2013;46:1–11.

34. Yamamoto T, Narushima M, Yoshimatsu H, et al. Dynamic indocyanine green (ICG) lymphography for breast cancer-related arm lymphedema. Ann Plast Surg 2014;73:706–9.

35. Koshima I, Inagawa K, Urushibara K, et al. Supermi-
    crosurgical lymphaticovenular anastomosis for the
    treatment of lymphedema in the upper extremities.
    J Reconstr Microsurg 2000;16:437–42.
36. Becker C. Autologous lymph node transfers.
    J Reconstr Microsurg 2016;32:28–33.
37. Masia J, Pons G, Nardulli ML. Combined surgical
    treatment in breast cancer-related lymphedema.
    J Reconstr Microsurg 2016;32:16–27.
38. Brorson H. Liposuction in lymphedema treatment.
    J Reconstr Microsurg 2016;32:56–65.

# New Frontiers in Robotic-Assisted Microsurgical Reconstruction

Amir E. Ibrahim, MD[a], Karim A. Sarhane, MD, MSc[b],
Jesse C. Selber, MD, MPH[c],*

## KEYWORDS

- Robotic surgery • Minimally invasive surgery • Reconstructive microsurgery • Da Vinci system
- Lymphedema surgery • Microvascular surgery

## KEY POINTS

- Designed 30 years ago for a neurosurgery biopsy, robotic surgery has revolutionized the field of minimally invasive surgery.
- It has recently been introduced into reconstructive surgery with burgeoning applications in microsurgery.
- Robotic surgery combines properties of conventional microsurgery, endoscopic surgery, and tele-surgery, making it an ideal platform for challenging microsurgery cases.
- We present the clinical applications of robotic microsurgery, highlighting its distinct advantages over conventional microsurgery.
- We outline the main limitations preventing its widespread use, and the salient research and educational projects aiming at overcoming these limitations.

The use of robotics in surgery has been on an exponential increase over the last 10 years. With its enhanced precision, greater degrees of freedom, superior 3-dimensional vision, improved resolution, and tremor elimination, robotic surgery has opened a new era of minimally invasive procedures. Its use has spread across various surgical specialties, including plastic and reconstructive surgery, with demonstrable efficacy and patient safety. One of the most encouraging application of robots in reconstructive surgery is microsurgery. Microsurgery is a unique field that requires the highest levels of precision for optimal outcomes and success rates. In no surgical field is this level of precision more crucial than in microsurgery. The advent of robotic surgery and its unique features (including complete tremor elimination and up to 5:1 motion scaling) has offered microsurgeons "suprahuman" levels of precision. In addition, with its high-definition 3-dimensional optics and up to 10× magnification, robotics provide a potentially ideal setup for performing the delicate manipulations required in microsurgery. Its minimally invasive possibilities also allow microsurgeons to operate in confined spaces, obviating the need for open, more morbid approaches, which in turn can enhance functional outcomes. Finally, owing advanced computerized imaging systems, robotic surgery is able to incorporate additional

The authors have nothing to disclose.
[a] Division of Plastic Surgery, Department of Surgery, American University of Beirut Medical Center, P.O. Box 11-0236, Riad El-Solh/Beirut 1107 2020, Lebanon; [b] Department of Surgery, University of Toledo Medical Center, 3000 Arlington Avenue, MS 1095, Toledo, OH 43614, USA; [c] Department of Plastic Surgery, University of Texas MD Anderson Cancer Center, Unit 1488, 1400 Pressler Street, Houston, TX 77030, USA
* Corresponding author.
E-mail address: jcselber@mdanderson.org

Clin Plastic Surg 44 (2017) 415–423
http://dx.doi.org/10.1016/j.cps.2016.12.003

visual guidance (fluorescence and near infrared imaging), which benefits cases that use navigation of various types.

In view of all these strategic advantages over conventional microsurgical, 3 main applications of robotic microsurgery have been established: (1) robotic microvascular surgery used principally in transoral reconstruction, (2) robotic microneural surgery used mainly in shoulder and brachial plexus surgery, (3) robotic lymphaticovenous bypass used for lymphedema surgery. In this paper, we provide a critical appraisal of these 3 applications based on the literature and on our own experience in the field. We also present new clinical applications of robotic microsurgery in urology, neurosurgery, ophthalmology, and otology, underscoring the versatility of this novel microsurgical technology. Finally, we outline our curricular strategy for an effective and tailored robotic microsurgical training that might propagate the use of this new technology and further expand the boundaries of microsurgery.

## ROBOTIC MICROVASCULAR SURGERY

In 2010, the senior author reported his first series of transoral robotic reconstruction of oropharyngeal defects showing favorable results with good functional outcomes.[1] The first robotic microvascular anastomosis was performed in this series, and exemplified the distinct advantages of the robot for microsurgery.[2] These included 100% tremor elimination, motion scaling (up to 5:1), and the possibility to work with full precision in confined spaces. The facial artery (a common recipient artery in head and neck reconstruction) is difficult to access, because it is sheltered by the mandibular ramus, coursing obliquely beneath the digastric and stylohyoid muscles. When a tracheostomy and ventilator tubing are also present, the space available to perform the anastomosis may be further restricted. The robot's enhanced precision and superior visualization, as well as long slender arms allow such anastomosis in confined spaces to be performed more easily, and can sometimes limit additional access incisions (**Fig. 1**). Song and colleagues[3] also made use of these key features of robotic surgery to perform a microvascular anastomosis of a radial forearm flap (recipient vessel: facial artery) to reconstruct an oropharyngeal defect after resecting a tonsillar tumor (T3 N0 M0, stage III). In this case, the neck dissection was performed through a retroauricular incision, which made conventional microsurgery very difficult to perform through that narrow space.

## ROBOTIC MICRONEURAL SURGERY

Despite great advances in techniques, satisfactory functional recovery after peripheral nerve repair is seldom achieved. Part of the problem resides in the microimperfections of such a delicate repair. An imprecise nerve coaption impedes neuroregeneration. It is technically challenging to perfectly match the internal nerve fascicles (an essential requirement emphasized by Millesi[4–6]) using standard microsurgical techniques. Furthermore, it is equally important to ensure gentle handling of the injured stumps during the repair of the various layers of the nerve. The benefits of robotic surgery over conventional microsurgery (disappearance of physiologic tremor, 3-dimensional vision, high definition/magnification, superior ergonomics, and amplification of surgeons' dexterity) have generated interest in microneural surgery. This application in robotic microsurgery was pioneered by Livernaux[7] who demonstrated the feasibility of robotic microneural repair on fresh nerves using either an anatomic (epiperineural repair) or a neurotrophic technique (nerve regrowth guide). These promising results allowed the same group to perform robotic intraneural microdissection of peripheral nerve tumors, allowing them to identify of the fascicles with greater accuracy and safety.[8]

Livernaux's group also tested the robotic platform in brachial plexus reconstruction.[9] The brachial plexus is a complex anatomic environment composed of an intricate, weblike array of nerves and multiple intertwined connections, all of which pose challenges for dissection, exposure, and coaptation. Traditionally, access to the brachial plexus necessitated a long incision with a considerable amount of dissection; this has often resulted in substantial scarring and adhesions, which compromised the quality of repair and decrease functional outcomes. For these reasons, closed injuries are frequently not explored acutely and rather managed with observation. This strategy however leads to a delay of 3 to 6 months before exploration and nerve repair, which might not only result in denervation muscle atrophy, but might also decrease the intrinsic ability of the nerve to regenerate.[10] Although endoscopic approaches might alleviate the morbidity of early exploration by reducing the incision size, the technique does not allow meticulous nerve dissection and finely tuned microneural repair. Because of the ability to perform minimally invasive repair, robotic microsurgery might facilitate early exploration (**Fig. 2**).

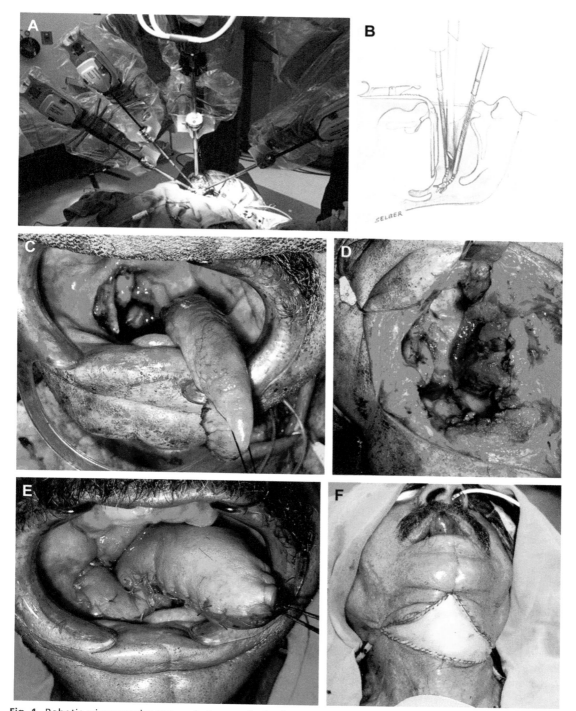

**Fig. 1.** Robotic microvascular surgery in transoral robotic reconstructive surgery. Transoral robotic reconstruction requires a mouth retractor to set the interdental opening. The robotic endoscope and 2 robotic instrument arms are introduced through the mouth and converge on the target oropharyngeal anatomy. External view (*A*) and depiction of internal view (*B*) is shown. (*C–F*) Case presentation. A 75-year-old man presented with a history of right neck metastatic squamous cell carcinoma. He was found to have a large recurrence. He underwent a pull-through resection, leaving a defect that extended from the tip of the tongue to the epiglottis (*C*, view through the mouth; *D*, the lateral pharyngotomy). The anterior inset was performed through the mouth by hand, because was the most distal portion of the pharyngeal inset through the pharyngotomy. The remaining inset, unreachable through the mouth or neck, was completed robotically (*E*). A second skin paddle was used to resurface the neck (*F*).

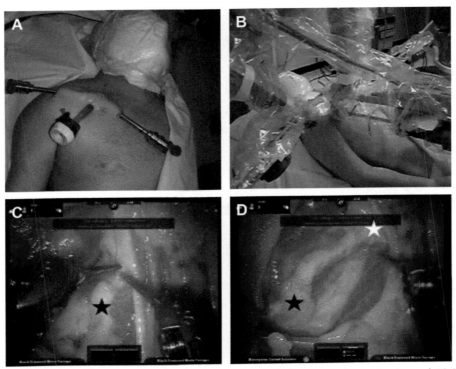

**Fig. 2.** Robotic microneural surgery. Anatomic repair of a rat sciatic nerve using epiperineural 10-0 stich (*A*). Result of the repair (*B*). Preparation of a robot-assisted endoscopic repair of the right supraclavicular brachial plexus. Three trocars in place (*C*). Robot in place ready to operate; note that the stand of the robot is at the head of the opposite side (*D*). (The *black star* shows the transplant model. The *white star* shows the C5 portion upstream of the graft.)

Facca and colleagues[11] presented their experimental and clinical experience in robotic-assisted surgery of the shoulder girdle and brachial plexus. In their cadaveric studies, they were able to dissect the supraclavicular brachial plexus and adjacent anatomic structures (jugular vein, omohyoid muscle, phrenic nerve, scalene muscles, and nerve roots from C4 to C7). A complete dissection and full exposure of the supraclavicular portion of the brachial plexus was achieved successfully. They were also able to graft a nerve segment into an artificially created gap by performing separate epineural and perineural repairs with 10-0 nylon. Moreover, the robot demonstrated feasibility in performing nerve transfers[12,13] and more recently in neurolysis (intercostal and phrenic nerve harvest) for potential brachial plexus reconstruction.[14,15]

## ROBOTIC LYMPHEDEMA SURGERY

The unique features of robotic surgery (ultraprecision and 100% tremor filtration) are currently being expanded to the field of supermicrosurgery, specifically to lymphedema surgery. This is a niche microsurgical discipline that requires extraordinary levels of precision and tissue handling. Lymphaticovenular bypasses are typically performed end-to-end using 11-0 or 12-0 nylon sutures on a 50-μm needle.[16] These are extremely technically challenging procedures, and may exceed in certain cases the limits of human precision. The suprahuman precision afforded by the robot, as well as it is superior picture clarity and advanced imaging system, can be of great benefit in this setting.

The senior author has performed several lymphovenous bypass surgeries using the Da Vinci robot and found it to be promising for this application. In addition to tremor elimination, the robotic visual system allowed rapid transitioning between near-infrared laser vision and normal bright field vision, which provided a dynamic method for mapping the lymphatic vascular network and visualizing indocyanine green diffusion patterns. This allowed a better identification of lymphatic insufficiency and pressure gradients, which is key for lymphedema surgery. Set up for robotic lymphatic microsurgery is relatively straightforward. The robotic arms are placed at about 45° above the target anatomy and in direct proximity to the external incision (**Fig. 3**).

## ROBOTIC MICROSURGERY INVADING OTHER SPECIALTIES

New directions for robotic microsurgical applications are being explored in the fields of urology, neurosurgery ophthalmology, and otology (**Fig. 4**).

### *Urology*

In urology, microsurgical applications include robotic assisted vasoepididymostomy (for vasectomy reversal), subinguinal varicocelectomy, denervation of the spermatic cord (for chronic orchalgia), vasovasostomy (for bilateral vasal obstruction), and testicular artery reanastomosis (in case iatrogenic injuries occur).[17–19] Parekattil and Moran[19] presented their experience with these techniques and concluded that the use of robotic assistance in microsurgical vasovasostomy may have benefit over conventional techniques in decreasing operative duration and significantly improving early semen analysis measures. As for robotic-assisted microsurgical subinguinal varicocelectomy, this technique seems to be feasible, and there are potential advantages in decreasing operative duration and improving surgeon efficiency.[20]

### *Neurosurgery*

Although the use of endoscope-assisted microsurgery in brain surgery was not widely adopted by neurosurgeons (owing to technical constraints), the advent of robotic microsurgery with its augmented reality, stereoendoscopy, and jointed-wrist instruments may create a shift in neurosurgery toward minimally invasive neurosurgical

techniques.[21] The University of Calgary, Canada has recently built a new robotic platform (NeuroArm) for microneurosurgery.[22] Similar to the Da Vinci system, NeuroArm is based on a "master–slave" control in which commanded hand-controller movements are replicated by the robot arms.[23,24] The manipulator consists of 2 arms, each with has 8 degrees of freedom, with end effectors that mimic a surgeon's hand and interface with microinstruments. The console provides visual, auditory, and tactile feedback, creating an immersive environment for the neurosurgeon. Furthermore, the robot is MRI compatible, allowing real-time imaging during procedures to account for brain shift. The NeuroArm was designed to perform standard techniques (biopsy, microdissection, thermocoagulation, fine suturing), allowing procedures such as lesionectomy and aneurysm clipping to be performed. Early reports from the NeuroArm case series have been promising,[22] and further clinical studies are required to determine the feasibility of integrating robotics into the workflow of microneurosurgery.

### *Ophthalmology*

Many robotic systems have been developed and investigated to explore the potential of expanding the capabilities of retinal microsurgery. These include untethered microrobots (enabling sutureless and precise ophthalmic procedures, like targeted drug delivery and epiretinal membrane peeling),[25] and handheld robotic devices for microsurgery: "Micron," a filter shown in an ex vivo experiment to reduce unintentional motion yet preserving intuitive eye-hand coordination[26]; and "SMART," a microforceps shown in a biologic tissue model to significantly improve targeted grasping and peeling.[27] Also, experiments were performed using a "master–slave" teleoperated microsurgical system for vitreoretinal surgery. This system was

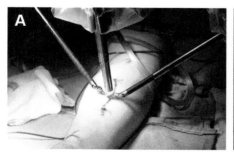
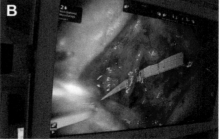

**Fig. 3.** Robotic lymphovenous bypass. The robotic camera is positioned in the middle, and the 2 arms are on either side of the forearm (*A*). A third arm with a "fine tissue forceps" attachment serves as a stationary assistant, and the surgeon is able to toggle back and forth between arms 1 and 3, depending on which arm is being used to position the vessel, and which is being used to suture. Black Diamond Micro Needle drivers (Intuitive Surgical) replace the larger jawed needle drivers used during the inset, and a 9-0 nylon suture is used for the anastomosis. Lymphovenous bypass completed (*B*).

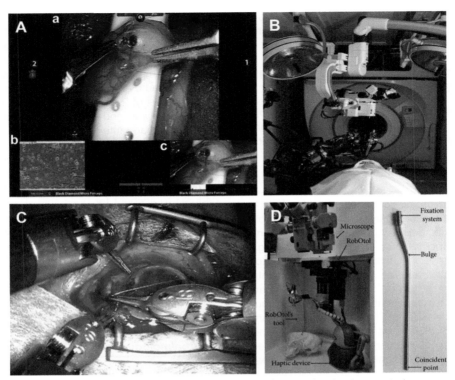

**Fig. 4.** Robotic microsurgery invading other fields. *Urology*: Robotic-assisted microsurgical vasectomy reversal. (a) Main view from the camera system of the da Vinci robotic platform, (b) real-time image from the left side with the andrology optical microscope (original magnification, ×100), and (c) view from the right side with the VITOM camera view for enhanced magnification. (*A*) *Neurosurgery*: NeuroArm (University of Calgary, Alberta, Canada) is a MRI-computable master/slave system capable of several surgical tasks (*B*). *Ophthalmology*: Robotically assisted pterygium surgery. Suture of the conjunctival graft: The graft is sutured to the edges of the excision area with 6 interrupted 8-0 polyglactin sutures and 2 Black Diamond Microforceps (*C*). *Otology*: RobOtol, a teleoperated system for middle ear microsurgery. The surgeon uses a microscope and commands the robot with the haptic device, a Phantom Omni (Sensable, Wilmington, MA); to avoid visual obstruction by the robot, a bulge is designed on the tool (*D*).

conceived to provide micrometer accurate manipulation within the eye,[28,29] and demonstrated on a pig's eye experiment superior operability in microcannulation of retinal vessels as compared with the traditional manual procedure.[30] More recently, the DaVinci Si HD robotic surgical system (Intuitive Surgical; Sunnyvale, CA) was tested on freshly enucleated pig eyes for pterygium surgery[31] then clinically on a 73-year-old patient (using Kenyon technique, excision coupled with a conjunctival autograft),[32] and proved to be feasible for ocular surface microsurgery, including dissection, excision, graft preparation, and graft suture using 8-0 polyglactine sutures.

## Otology

Middle ear surgery involves handling the smallest and the most fragile bones of the human body and hence requires microsurgical gestures with submillimetric levels of precision. Outcomes of these delicate operations may be improved with robotic assistance.[33] Recently, a teleoperated system, RobOtol, was developed to enhance gesture accuracy and handiness in microsurgical procedures of the middle ear.[34] The system was tested virtually in 2 challenging procedures (stapedotomy and stapedioplasty). The authors noted that robotic microsurgery prevented involuntary movements on the ossicular chain (which may result in severe damage, including rupture of the incus-malleus joint or incus luxation), while safely placing a prosthesis piston on the long process of the incus.

## Limitations of Robotic Microsurgery

The current limitations of the robotic platform for microsurgery are suboptimal optics of the endoscope (as compared with the operating microscope), absence of standard microsurgical instruments, and lack of haptic feedback. These differences can be overcome with better quality, fixed distance lenses fitted to the stereoscopic optical system of the robot. Also, more delicate microsurgical robotic instruments are required, which would bear greater resemblance to traditional microsurgical instruments and accommodate basic forms of haptic feedback. Only 1 study has assessed haptics objectively and concluded it was not crucial to completing an accurately tied knot with a microsurgical suture.[35] Subjects tied knots and tightened them with eyes open and closed with robotic assistance. No difference in suture breakage and poor tightening was observed.[35] The senior author's experience is that microsurgery is 90% visual, and most of what we imagine we are feeling, we are actually seeing, and our brain is supplying the illusion of sensation. The small amount of haptic feedback that is real, however, is a very important component and, at this time, constitutes a barrier to robotics playing a more active role in microsurgery.

### Robotic Microsurgical Training

Considering the technical complexity of robotic microsurgery and the consequences of failure, systematic teaching modules and comprehensive learning assessment tools are needed to ensure appropriate training and safe use. Unlike many other robotic versions of open procedures, robotic microsurgery combines the same principles as conventional microsurgery (for which a number of training modules already exist[36,37]) with an additional skill set unique to the surgical robot.

To measure this mixture of skills and better evaluate trainees, the senior author created the Structured Assessment of Robotic Microsurgery Skills.[38] This evaluation system combines the Structured Assessment of Microsurgical Skills scoring system with other validated skill domains pertaining specifically to robotic surgery.[39] Microsurgical skills are assessed by 3 parameters (1, dexterity; 2, visuospatial ability; and 3, operative flow), and the robotic skills by 5 additional ones (1, camera movement; 2, depth perception; 3, wrist articulation; 4, atraumatic tissue handling; and 5, atraumatic needle handling). Each parameter is scored from 1 to 5, with 1 being the worst and 5 the best. The overall performance and overall skill level are also assessed independently.[40]

The senior author applied this new robotic microsurgical evaluation tool on surgeons with varying levels of expertise (clinical fellows, research fellows, and experienced microsurgeons), and was able to plot the maturation process of these skills.[38] This new assessment system was validated with excellent consistency and high levels of interrater reliability. The authors noticed improvement in all robotic microsurgical skills and overall performance across our heterogeneous group of learners. There was an initial steep increase in technical skills acquisition, then followed by gradual improvement, and a steady decrease in operative times.

In a prior study of conventional microsurgical assessment data using the Structured Assessment of Microsurgical Skills,[41] moderately experienced subjects improved their skills through the middle and upper range of scores.[41–43] By contrast, in the robotic microsurgery study, subjects with no prior experience in robotic microsurgery moved through all but the highest level of Structured Assessment of Robotic Microsurgical Skills scores to achieve proficiency.[42–45] Furthermore, all groups demonstrated an ability to gain proficiency in robotic microsurgical anastomosis with minimal robot-specific training, indicating that the technical aspects of robotic microsurgery can be gained by learners with no prior microsurgery or robotic experience.[46] Prior experience with conventional microsurgery did, however, improve the acquisition of robotic technical proficiency in certain areas (but was not necessary).

## SUMMARY

Robotic microsurgery is a growing discipline in robotic surgery whose future and impact on multiple disciplines is anticipated to be groundbreaking. It has already found numerous clinical applications in various microsurgical areas, and is allowing procedures never possible before to be performed with ease and certainty. It is currently experiencing rapid innovation with new robotic instrumentation that might enable tactile feedback, real-time Doppler monitoring, hydrojet and fiberoptic $CO_2$ laser dissection, and enhanced visual acuity and optics.[19] Equally important, it is also trending toward customized education and curricular design with individual assessment, targeted feedback, and competency-based learning. All these efforts will further increase its popularity, facilitate its widespread use, and allow more complex microsurgical procedures to be performed pushing further the frontiers of microsurgery.

## REFERENCES

1. Selber JC. Transoral robotic reconstruction of oropharyngeal defects: a case series. Plast Reconstr Surg 2010;126:1978–87.

2. Longfield EA, Holsinger FC, Selber JC. Reconstruction after robotic head and neck surgery: when and why. J Reconstr Microsurg 2012;28:445–50.

3. Song HG, Yun IS, Lee WJ, et al. Robot-assisted free flap in head and neck reconstruction. Arch Plast Surg 2013;40:353–8.

4. Millesi H. Factors affecting the outcome of peripheral nerve surgery. Microsurgery 2006;26:295–302.

5. Millesi H. The nerve gap. Theory and clinical practice. Hand Clin 1986;2:651–63.

6. Millesi H. The current state of peripheral nerve surgery in the upper limb. Ann Chir Main 1984;3:18–34.

7. Nectoux E, Taleb C, Liverneaux P. Nerve repair in telemicrosurgery: an experimental study. J Reconstr Microsurg 2009;25:261–5.

8. Tigan L, Miyamoto H, Hendriks S, et al. Interest of telemicrosurgery in peripheral nerve tumors: about a series of seven cases. Chir Main 2014;33:13–6.

9. Garcia JC, Lebailly F, Mantovani G, et al. Telerobotic manipulation of the brachial plexus. J Reconstr Microsurg 2012;28:491–4.

10. Scheib J, Höke A. Advances in peripheral nerve regeneration. Nat Rev Neurol 2013;9:668–76.

11. Facca S, Hendriks S, Mantovani G, et al. Robot-assisted surgery of the shoulder girdle and brachial plexus. Semin Plast Surg 2014;28:39–44.

12. Naito K, Facca S, Lequint T, et al. The Oberlin procedure for restoration of elbow flexion with the da Vinci robot: four cases. Plast Reconstr Surg 2012;129:707–11.

13. Porto de Melo PM, Garcia JC, Montero EF, et al. Feasibility of an endoscopic approach to the axillary nerve and the nerve to the long head of the triceps brachii with the help of the Da Vinci Robot. Chir Main 2013;32:206–9.

14. Miyamoto H, Serradori T, Mikami Y, et al. Robotic intercostal nerve harvest: a feasibility study in a pig model. J Neurosurg 2016;124:264–8.

15. Porto de Melo P, Miyamoto H, Serradori T, et al. Robotic phrenic nerve harvest: a feasibility study in a pig model. Chir Main 2014;33:356–60.

16. Chang DW. Lymphaticovenular bypass for lymphedema management in breast cancer patients: a prospective study. Plast Reconstr Surg 2010;126:752–8.

17. Kuang W, Shin PR, Matin S, et al. Initial evaluation of robotic technology for microsurgical vasovasostomy. J Urol 2004;171:300–3.

18. Tojuola B, Kartal I, Brahmbhatt J, et al. Targeted robotic assisted microsurgical denervation of the spermatic cord for the treatment of chronic scrotal content pain: single center, large series review. J Urol 2015;193:e836.

19. Parekattil SJ, Moran ME. Robotic instrumentation: evolution and microsurgical applications. Indian J Urol 2010;26:395–403.

20. Gudeloglu A, Brahmbhatt JV, Parekattil SJ. Robot-assisted microsurgery in male infertility and andrology. Urol Clin North Am 2014;41:559–66.

21. Marcus HJ, Seneci CA, Payne CJ, et al. Robotics in keyhole transcranial endoscope-assisted microsurgery: a critical review of existing systems and proposed specifications for new robotic platforms. Neurosurgery 2014;10:84–95.

22. Pandya S, Motkoski JW, Serrano-Almeida C, et al. Advancing neurosurgery with image-guided robotics. J Neurosurg 2009;111:1141–9.

23. Louw DF, Fielding T, McBeth PB, et al. Surgical robotics: a review and neurosurgical prototype development. Neurosurgery 2004;54:525–36.

24. McBeth PB, Louw DF, Rizun PR, et al. Robotics in neurosurgery. Am J Surg 2004;188:68S–75S.

25. Ullrich F, Bergeles C, Pokki J, et al. Mobility experiments with microrobots for minimally invasive intraocular surgery. Invest Ophthalmol Vis Sci 2013;54:2853–63.

26. Maclachlan RA, Becker BC, Tabarés JC, et al. Micron: an actively stabilized handheld tool for microsurgery. IEEE Trans Robot 2012;28:195–212.

27. Song C, Park DY, Gehlbach PL, et al. Fiber-optic OCT sensor guided "SMART" micro-forceps for microsurgery. Biomed Opt Express 2013;4:1045–50.

28. Wei W, Goldman R, Simaan N, et al. Design and theoretical evaluation of micro-surgical manipulators for orbital manipulation and intraocular dexterity. In: Proceedings 2007 IEEE international conference on robotics and automation. IEEE; Angelicum University, Roma, Italy, 2007. p. 3389–95.

29. Yu H, Shen JH, Joos KM, et al. Design, calibration and preliminary testing of a robotic telemanipulator for OCT guided retinal surgery. In: 2013 IEEE International Conference on Robotics and Automation. IEEE; Angelicum University, Roma, Italy, 2013. p. 225–31.

30. Ida Y, Sugita N, Ueta T, et al. Microsurgical robotic system for vitreoretinal surgery. Int J Comput Assist Radiol Surg 2012;7:27–34.

31. Bourcier T, Nardin M, Sauer A, et al. Robot-assisted pterygium surgery: feasibility study in a nonliving porcine model. Transl Vis Sci Technol 2015;4:9.

32. Bourcier T, Chammas J, Becmeur P-H, et al. Robotically assisted pterygium surgery: first human case. Cornea 2015;34:1329–30.

33. Miroir M, Nguyen Y, Szewczyk J, et al. Design, kinematic optimization, and evaluation of a teleoperated system for middle ear microsurgery. ScientificWorldJournal 2012;2012:907372.

34. Kazmitcheff G, Nguyen Y, Miroir M, et al. Middle-ear microsurgery simulation to improve new robotic procedures. Biomed Res Int 2014;2014:891742.

35. Panchulidze I, Berner S, Mantovani G, et al. Is haptic feedback necessary to microsurgical suturing?

Comparative study of 9/0 and 10/0 knot tying operated by 24 surgeons. Hand Surg 2011;16:1–3.

36. Hino A. Training in microvascular surgery using a chicken wing artery. Neurosurgery 2003;52:1495–7.

37. Seyhan T, Ozerdem OR. Microsurgery training on discarded abdominoplasty material. Plast Reconstr Surg 2006;117:2536–7.

38. Alrasheed T, Liu J, Hanasono MM, et al. Robotic microsurgery: validating an assessment tool and plotting the learning curve. Plast Reconstr Surg 2014;134:794–803.

39. Dulan G, Rege RV, Hogg DC, et al. Developing a comprehensive, proficiency-based training program for robotic surgery. Surgery 2012;152:477–88.

40. Selber JC, Alrasheed T. Robotic microsurgical training and evaluation. Semin Plast Surg 2014; 28:5–10.

41. Selber JC, Chang EI, Liu J, et al. Tracking the learning curve in microsurgical skill acquisition. Plast Reconstr Surg 2012;130:550e–7e.

42. Chan WY, Matteucci P, Southern SJ. Validation of microsurgical models in microsurgery training and competence: a review. Microsurgery 2007;27: 494–9.

43. Chan W, Niranjan N, Ramakrishnan V. Structured assessment of microsurgery skills in the clinical setting. J Plast Reconstr Aesthet Surg 2010;63: 1329–34.

44. Balasundaram I, Aggarwal R, Darzi LA. Development of a training curriculum for microsurgery. Br J Oral Maxillofac Surg 2010;48:598–606.

45. Temple CL, Ross DC. A new, validated instrument to evaluate competency in microsurgery: the University of Western Ontario Microsurgical Skills Acquisition/Assessment instrument [outcomes article]. Plast Reconstr Surg 2011;127: 215–22.

46. Karamanoukian RL, Bui T, McConnell MP, et al. Transfer of training in robotic-assisted microvascular surgery. Ann Plast Surg 2006;57:662–5.

# The Advent of Vascularized Composite Allotransplantation

Curtis L. Cetrulo Jr, MD[a,b,]*, Zhi Yang Ng, MD[a,b],
Jonathan M. Winograd, MD[a], Kyle R. Eberlin, MD[a]

## KEYWORDS

- Allotransplantation • Composite tissue grafting • Tissue transfer

## KEY POINTS

- The ultimate utility of VCA is the provision of functional restoration and improvement in quality of life.
- To this end, developments in peripheral nerve regeneration may allow for greater functional return after upper extremity loss at more proximal levels (ie, upper arm, above elbow).
- Additional advances in the treatment of autoimmune dermatologic disease may provide new insights into mechanisms to achieve tolerance of skin in VCA.
- The future of VCA is bright and most likely involves advances in basic science and clinical protocols to achieve the ultimate goal of immunologic tolerance.

Modern microsurgical techniques have made possible a broad spectrum of novel means for the reconstruction of complex bone and soft tissue defects. These techniques, in combination with developments in transplant immunology, have led to successful hand and facial allotransplantation and achievement of the highest rung in the reconstructive ladder – truly replacing like with like.

The utilization of contemporary microsurgical technique in the context of vascularized composite allotransplantation (VCA) (1) permits successful technical execution and feasibility of VCA, (2) facilitates the study of immunologic tolerance in VCA preclinical models, and (3) optimizes functional VCA outcomes.

## TECHNICAL FEASIBILITY

To date, the world experience in VCA includes more than 100 upper extremity, 30 craniofacial,

and various other types of composite soft tissue transplants, including the abdominal wall, lower extremity, and genitourinary region across different patient age groups. At the Massachusetts General Hospital (MGH), the authors have performed a left upper extremity VCA in a left-hand dominant patient who was 9 years' status–post 50% burns of his total body surface area with prior extensive débridement and skin grafting and a metacarpal amputation of his left hand without excellent function. His burns resulted in the absence of cutaneous veins in the forearm, which presented a challenge for venous outflow of the allograft. This technical challenge was successfully overcome with a volar forearm fasciocutaneous extension technique (**Fig. 1**) incorporating proximal vascular anastomoses and distal neurorrhaphies for the synergistic effect of improved perfusion and minimizing the length of neural regeneration to expedite functional recovery.[1] At

The authors have nothing to disclose.
a Division of Plastic and Reconstructive Surgery, Massachusetts General Hospital, 15 Parkman Street, Wang ACC #435, Boston, MA 02114, USA; b Vascularized Composite Allotransplantation Laboratory, Center for Transplantation Sciences, Massachusetts General Hospital, Charlestown Navy Yard, Building 149, 13th Street, Suite 9019, Boston, MA 02129, USA
* Corresponding author.
E-mail address: CCETRULO@mgh.harvard.edu

Clin Plastic Surg 44 (2017) 425–429
http://dx.doi.org/10.1016/j.cps.2016.12.007

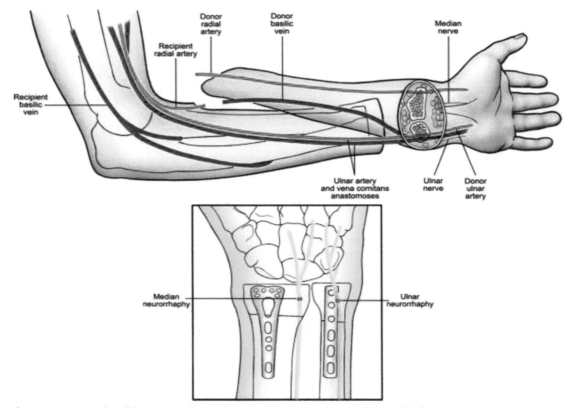

**Fig. 1.** Operative plan: (1) osteosynthesis at 3 cm proximal to radiocarpal joint; (2) ulnar artery and vena comitans anastomoses in distal forearm proximal to wrist crease; radial artery, vena comitans, and basilic vein anastomoses in proximal forearm immediately distal to antecubital fossa; (3) digital flexors adjusted to achieve natural cascade and single-weave, Brown side-to-side tenorrhaphy for all tendons; and (4) median and ulnar neurorrhaphies at wrist flexion crease. (*Reproduced from* Eberlin KR, Leonard DA, Austen WG Jr, et al. The volar forearm fasciocutaneous extension: a strategy to maximize vascular outflow in post-burn injury hand transplantation. Plast Reconstr Surg 2014;134:733; with permission.)

3 years' post-VCA, the patient has regained good strength and sensibility in the left hand, with an intrinsic power of 4/5 and a Disabilities of Arm, Shoulder and Hand score of 27.

Despite the ever-increasing numbers and types of VCAs, patients who have received such allografts are necessarily maintained on various combinations of lifelong immunosuppressive regimens that are modeled after those used in solid organ transplantation. The potential sequelae of such chronic immunosuppression are well known, and patients who are recipients of VCA have developed myriad complications, including chronic allograft loss, metabolic disorders, renovascular dysfunction, opportunistic infections, and neoplasms.[2]

## IMMUNOLOGIC TOLERANCE APPROACHES
### Mixed Chimerism

Building on the clinical success of the authors' transplant center colleagues in achieving immunosuppression-free renal transplantation based on the establishment of mixed chimerism,[3] the authors' current laboratory efforts in VCA are directed at the adoption of this approach for the induction of immunologic tolerance. This protocol involves nonmyeloablative conditioning and hematopoietic stem cell transplantation (HSCT) of the VCA recipient so that coexistence of the immune cells of both donor and recipient can be achieved in the absence of destructive immunologic responses (**Fig. 2**).

### Importance of Stable Mixed Chimerism

The authors have recently demonstrated, for the first time, that all components of a fasciocutaneous VCA, including the epidermis, can be accepted indefinitely in a unique MGH miniature swine model. Using the authors' previously described protocol, haplomatched animals (SLA^AC donors and SLA^AD recipients) are

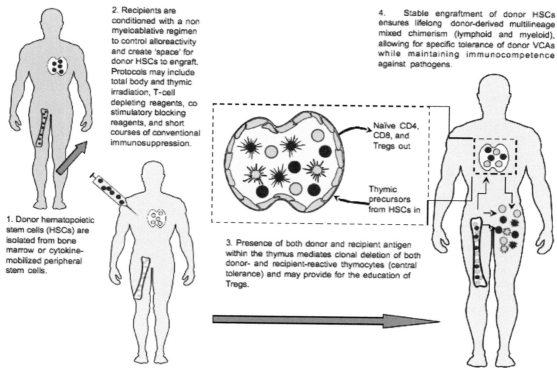

**Fig. 2.** Mixed chimerism: donor hematopoietic stem cells (blue) are transplanted into the VCA recipient (pink) and migrate to the thymus where both donor and recipient alloreactive cells undergo deletion, thereby permitting organ or VCA allograft acceptance.

conditioned with 100 cGy of total body irradiation and CD3 immunotoxin for T cell depletion followed by HSCT with cytokine-mobilized peripheral blood mononuclear cells to establish stable mixed chimerism. VCA performed 100 days later led to indefinite survival, which provides proof of concept of the importance of stable mixed chimerism in VCA; when VCA was performed concomitant to HSCT, indefinite survival was again achieved, which laid the grounds for the development of a clinically relevant protocol.[4]

Harvesting bone marrow (BM) from the donor in a day 0 combined HSCT and VCA approach would, therefore, represent the most clinically viable approach to achieve mixed chimerism. Furthermore, the extent of HLA matching of donors and recipients in clinical VCA is unpredictable; hence, it is imperative that any protocol for tolerance induction is robust enough to overcome full HLA mismatches. The authors' studies have shown, however, that when donor BM was used as the cell source for HSCT, using the same protocol described previously, in fully mismatched swine, only transient mixed chimerism was generated and neither VCA tolerance nor improved survival was attained once immunosuppression was withdrawn.[5] Overall, these findings suggest that

stable mixed chimerism and, in turn, increased conditioning and resulting toxicity would be required in clinical VCA.

## Delaying Mixed Chimerism

Preliminary studies of a day 0 donor BM transplantation (DBMT) and VCA protocol with additional recipient conditioning in the form of thymic irradiation have resulted in various complications, including neck abscesses, embolic phenomena, and, most importantly, failure of BM engraftment in haplomatched swine. The challenges of a day 0 concurrent DBMT and VCA approach have led to the adoption of delaying tolerance induction, whereby the allograft is transplanted under the cover of standard immunosuppression and donor BM stored at the time of transplant.

Nonhuman primate (NHP) studies by the authors' solid organ transplantation colleagues in kidney and lung transplantation have shown that a delay period of 4 months allowed for resolution of the perioperative inflammatory milieu and enabled engraftment for stable mixed chimerism after DBMT in haplomatched animals. The authors have adopted this delayed tolerance induction protocol (**Fig. 3**) in NHP studies of VCA.

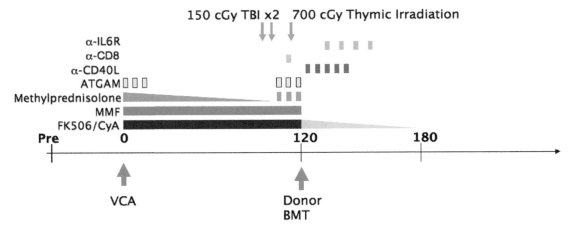

**Fig. 3.** Delayed tolerance induction protocol: VCA is performed on day 0 after induction therapy with antithymocyte globulin (ATGAM) and maintained thereafter on standard triple immunosuppression for 4 months. Prior to BM transplantation (BMT), the recipient is initiated on conditioning with total body and thymic irradiation, ATGAM; post-BMT, anti-CD40L and anti-IL-6 are infused for costimulatory blockade and to up-regulate regulatory T cells (Tregs) to promote tolerance. The recipient is then maintained on calcineurin inhibitor monotherapy for another 30 days before tapering to complete withdrawal over the next 30 days. CyA, cyclosporine-A; FK506, tacrolimus; MMF, mycophenolate mofetil; TBI, total body irradiation.

## Immunogenetics and Skin Immunobiology

In addition to developing tolerance protocols, the MGH miniature swine model used in the authors' VCA studies allows investigating the role of major histocompatibility complex (MHC) matching. As described previously, after the establishment of mixed chimerism with the authors' protocol,[4] haplomatched animals accepted VCA indefinitely and a similar result has been observed in MHC class II–mismatched animals. In MHC class I–mismatched animals, however, the epidermis of the VCA is rejected after cessation of immunosuppression despite persisting mixed chimerism and donor-specific unresponsiveness based on in vitro immunologic assays.[6] This led to the hypothesis that there was a local mechanism operational at the level of the skin behind complete VCA acceptance.

Flow cytometric analysis of serial VCA and host skin biopsies from the authors' swine studies have provided further insight for these observations. In haplomatched and MHC class II–mismatched chimeras, donor and host contributions to the cutaneous immune cell populations (including Foxp3[+] regulatory T cells and Langerhans cells) equilibrate and result in VCA acceptance; in MHC class I–mismatched chimeras, progressive infiltration of recipient-type CD8[+] T cells with loss of donor-derived T cells and Langerhans cells is observed in VCA skin on withdrawal of immunosuppression, consistent with acute rejection both clinically and on histology. Similarly, the authors have observed an almost complete turnover of

skin-resident immune cells to recipient-type in NHP VCA studies during the delay period when on standard immunosuppression prior to DBMT. Remarkably, protocol biopsies of the authors' clinical hand transplant patient have also detected recipient-type T cells despite the absence of acute rejection episodes to date.

Overall, further investigation into the skin immune system is required for both understanding of rejection or acceptance of VCA and protective immunity in immunologically active tissues posttransplant. In turn, immunomodulatory targets directed at specific components of the skin may lead to further novel therapeutic options.

## FUTURE OF VASCULARIZED COMPOSITE ALLOTRANSPLANTATION

Much of the current literature on VCA pertains to skin-bearing composite allografts, such as that of the upper extremities, face, and abdominal wall. Recent extension of VCA to non–skin-bearing entities, such as the uterus and larynx, may represent a new domain of VCA in the form of muscular and cartilaginous allotransplantation. Although uterine transplantation has demonstrated its efficacy in allowing women to become pregnant and carry to term, removal of the transplanted womb after it has served its purpose (ie, delivery of a child) represents a totally different paradigm to current VCA because immunosuppression would only be required for the duration when the uterine allograft is in situ. The risk-benefit ratio of such temporary VCAs may, therefore, be more acceptable to both physicians and patients. The incidence and risks of acute and chronic rejection in such buried, non–skin-bearing forms of VCA are also poorly understood at present.

The ultimate utility of VCA is the provision of complete functional restoration. To this end, developments in peripheral nerve regeneration and the neurotrophic effect of calcineurin inhibitors may allow for greater functional return even after more proximal amputation levels, such as the elbow and upper arm. Additional advances in the treatment of autoimmune dermatologic disease may provide new insights into mechanisms of achieving skin tolerance in VCA. The future of VCA is bright and will most likely involve advances in basic science and clinical protocols to achieve the ultimate goal of immunologic tolerance.

## REFERENCES

1. Eberlin KR, Leonard DA, Austen WG Jr, et al. The volar forearm fasciocutaneous extension: a strategy to maximize vascular outflow in post-burn injury hand transplantation. Plast Reconstr Surg 2014;134: 731–5.

2. Petruzzo P, Dubernard JM. The international registry on hand and composite tissue allotransplantation. Clin Transplant 2011;247–53.

3. Kawai T, Cosimi AB, Spitzer TR, et al. HLA-mismatched renal transplantation without maintenance immunosuppression. N Engl J Med 2008; 358:353–61.

4. Leonard DA, Kurtz JM, Mallard C, et al. Vascularized composite allograft tolerance across MHC barriers in a large animal model. Am J Transplant 2014;14: 343–55.

5. Leto Barone AA, Kurtz JM. Effects of Transient donor chimerism on rejection of mhc-mismatched vascularized composite allografts in swine. Vascularized Composite Allotransplantation 2015;2:1–8.

6. Shanmugarajah K, Powell H, Leoanrd DA, et al. The effect of MHC antigen matching between donors and recipients on skin tolerance of vascularized composite allografts. Am J Transplant 2016. http://dx.doi.org/10.1111/ajt.14189.

# Index

*Note:* Page numbers of article titles are in **boldface** type.

Printed and bound by CPI Group (UK) Ltd, Croydon, CR0 4YY

08/05/2025

01864699-0013